Modern Management of High Grade Glioma, Part I

Guest Editors

ISAAC YANG, MD
SEUNGGU J. HAN, MD

NEUROSURGERY
CLINICS OF NORTH AMERICA

www.neurosurgery.theclinics.com

Consulting Editors
ANDREW T. PARSA, MD, PhD
PAUL C. McCORMICK, MD, MPH

April 2012 • Volume 23 • Number 2

SAUNDERS an imprint of ELSEVIER, Inc.

W.B. SAUNDERS COMPANY
A Division of Elsevier Inc.

1600 John F. Kennedy Blvd. • Suite 1800 • Philadelphia, PA 19103-2899

http://www.theclinics.com

NEUROSURGERY CLINICS OF NORTH AMERICA Volume 23, Number 2
April 2012 ISSN 1042-3680, ISBN-13: 978-1-4557-3897-7

Editor: Jessica McCool

Neurosurgery Clinics of North America (ISSN 1042-3680) is published quarterly by Elsevier Inc., 360 Park Avenue South, New York, NY 10010-1710. Months of issue are January, April, July, and October. Business and Editorial Offices: 1600 John F. Kennedy Blvd., Suite 1800, Philadelphia, PA 19103-2899. Customer Service Office: 11830 Westline Industrial Drive, St. Louis, MO 63146. Periodicals postage paid at New York, NY, and additional mailing offices. Subscription prices are $346.00 per year (US individuals), $531.00 per year (US institutions), $378.00 per year (Canadian individuals), $649.00 per year (Canadian institutions), $483.00 per year (international individuals), $649.00 per year (international institutions), $170.00 per year (US students), and $233.00 per year (international students). International air speed delivery is included in all *Clinics* subscription prices. All prices are subject to change without notice. **POSTMASTER:** Send address changes to *Neurosurgery Clinics of North America*, Elsevier Periodicals Customer Service, 11830 Westline Industrial Drive, St. Louis, MO 63146. **Customer Service: 1-800-654-2452 (US and Canada). From outside the US and Canada, call: 1-314-453-7041. Fax: 1-314-453-5170. E-mail: JournalsCustomerService-usa@elsevier.com (for print support) and journalsonlinesupport-usa@elsevier.com (for online support).**

Reprints. For copies of 100 or more, of articles in this publication, please contact the Commercial Reprints Department, Elsevier Inc., 360 Park Avenue South, New York, NY 10010-1710. Tel. (212) 633-3812; Fax: (212) 462-1935; E-mail: reprints@elsevier.com.

Neurosurgery Clinics of North America is covered in *MEDLINE/PubMed (Index Medicus), EMBASE/Excerpta Medica, and Current Contents/Clinical Medicine (CC/CM).*

Cover image from the American Association for Cancer Research: Vredenburgh JJ, Desjardins A, Herndon JE, et al. Bevacizumab plus irinotecan in recurrent glioblastoma multiforme. J Clin Oncol 2007;25(30):4722–9; with permission for print use only.

Printed and bound by CPI Group (UK) Ltd, Croydon, CR0 4YY

Transferred to Digital Print 2012

Contributors

CONSULTING EDITORS

ANDREW T. PARSA, MD, PhD
Associate Professor, Principal Investigator,
Brain Tumor Research Center, Reza and
Georgianna Khatib Endowed Chair in Skull
Base Tumor Surgery, Department of
Neurological Surgery, University of California,
San Francisco, San Francisco, California

PAUL C. McCORMICK, MD, MPH, FACS
Herbert & Linda Gallen Professor of
Neurological Surgery, Department of
Neurological Surgery, Columbia University
Medical Center, New York, New York

GUEST EDITORS

ISAAC YANG, MD
Assistant Professor, University of California,
Los Angeles, David Geffen School of Medicine
at UCLA, UCLA Department of Neurosurgery;
UCLA Jonsson Comprehensive Cancer
Center, UCLA Brain Tumor Program,
Los Angeles, California

SEUNGGU J. HAN, MD
Department of Neurological Surgery, University
of California, San Francisco, San Francisco,
California

AUTHORS

MANISH K. AGHI, MD, PhD
Department of Neurological Surgery,
University of California, San Francisco,
San Francisco, California

KRISTEN A. BATICH, BA
Department of Pathology, Duke University
Medical Center, Durham, North Carolina

MITCHEL S. BERGER, MD
Professor and Chairman, UCSF Brain Tumor
Research Center; Department of Neurological
Surgery, University of California,
San Francisco, San Francisco, California

JOHN A. BOOCKVAR, MD
Associate Professor; Co-Director, Department
of Neurological Surgery, Weill Cornell Brain
Tumor Center, Weill Cornell Medical College,
New York–Presbyterian Hospital, New York,
New York

JAN-KARL BURKHARDT, MD
Department of Neurological Surgery, New
York–Presbyterian Hospital, Weill Cornell
Medical College, New York, New York

JOAQUIN Q. CAMARA-QUINTANA, BS
Department of Neurosurgery, Stanford
University, Stanford, California

JOSE A. CARRILLO, MD
Assistant Professor of Neurology,
Department of Neurology, University
of California, Irvine, Orange, California

EDWARD F. CHANG, MD
Assistant Professor, UCSF Epilepsy Center;
Department of Neurological Surgery,
University of California, San Francisco,
San Francisco, California

BRYAN D. CHOI, AB
Division of Neurosurgery, Department
of Surgery; Department of Pathology,
Duke University Medical Center, Durham,
North Carolina

FRANCES CHOW, BA
UCLA Department of Neurosurgery;
David Geffen School of Medicine,
University of California, Los Angeles,
Los Angeles, California

NICOLE CREMER, BS
UCLA Department of Neurosurgery;
David Geffen School of Medicine,
University of California, Los Angeles,
Los Angeles, California

ANTONIO A.F. DE SALLES, MD, PhD
Department of Neurosurgery and Radiation
Oncology, David Geffen School of Medicine,
University of California, Los Angeles,
Los Angeles, California

PAULA EBOLI, MD
Department of Neurological Surgery,
Cedars-Sinai Medical Center, Los Angeles,
California

DARIO J. ENGLOT, MD, PhD
Resident, UCSF Epilepsy Center; Department
of Neurological Surgery, University of
California, San Francisco, San Francisco,
California

MICHELLE L. FEINBERG, MD
Department of Neurological Surgery, George
Washington University Medical Center,
Washington, DC

ALLAN H. FRIEDMAN, MD
Division of Neurosurgery, Department of
Surgery, Duke University Medical Center,
Durham, North Carolina

PAUL A. GARCIA, MD
Professor, UCSF Epilepsy Center; Department
of Neurology, University of California,
San Francisco, San Francisco, California

ALESSANDRA A. GORGULHO, MD, MSc
Department of Neurosurgery, David Geffen
School of Medicine, University of California,
Los Angeles, Los Angeles, California

SEUNGGU J. HAN, MD
Department of Neurological Surgery, University
of California, San Francisco, San Francisco,
California

JETHRO HU, MD
Department of Neurological Surgery,
Cedars-Sinai Medical Center, Los Angeles,
California

ARMAN JAHANGIRI, BS
Department of Neurological Surgery,
University of California, San Francisco,
San Francisco, California

CHAE-YONG KIM, MD, PhD
Department of Neurosurgery, Seoul National
University Bundang Hospital, Bundang-gu,
Seongnam-si, Gyeonggi-do, Korea;
Department of Neurosurgery, Seoul National
University College of Medicine, Seoul, Korea

YOUNG-HOON KIM, MD
Department of Neurosurgery, Seoul National
University Bundang Hospital, Bundang-gu,
Seongnam-si, Gyeonggi-do, Korea;
Department of Neurosurgery, Seoul National
University College of Medicine, Seoul, Korea

WON KIM, MD
UCLA Department of Neurosurgery;
David Geffen School of Medicine,
University of California, Los Angeles,
Los Angeles, California

GORDON LI, MD
Department of Neurosurgery, Stanford
University, Stanford, California

JOSHUA LUCAS, MD
Department of Neurosurgery, University
of Southern California, Los Angeles,
California

ANKIT I. MEHTA, MD
Division of Neurosurgery, Department
of Surgery, Duke University Medical Center,
Durham, North Carolina

CLAUDIA A. MUNOZ, MD, MPH
Assistant Professor of Neurosurgery,
Department of Neurology, University
of California, Irvine, Orange, California

DANIEL T. NAGASAWA, MD
UCLA Department of Neurosurgery;
David Geffen School of Medicine,
University of California, Los Angeles,
Los Angeles, California

SEEMA NAGPAL, MD
Clinical Assistant Professor of Neurology,
Neurosciences, and Neurosurgery, Division
of Neuro-oncology, Department of Neurology,
Stanford Advanced Medicine Center,
Stanford, California

RYAN T. NITTA, PhD
Department of Neurosurgery, Stanford
University, Stanford, California

CHIRAG G. PATIL, MD, MS
Assistant Professor, Department of
Neurosurgery, Director, Center for
Neurosurgical Outcomes Research,
Cedars-Sinai Medical Center, Los Angeles,
California

HOWARD A. RIINA, MD
Department of Neurological Surgery,
New York–Presbyterian Hospital,
Weill Cornell Medical College, New York,
New York

ASHIMA SAINI, MD
Assistant Professor, Department of Radiation
Oncology, George Washington University
Medical Center, Washington, DC

JOHN H. SAMPSON, MD, PhD, MHSc
Division of Neurosurgery, Department of
Surgery; Department of Pathology,
Duke University Medical Center,
Durham, North Carolina

MICHAEL T. SELCH, MD
Department of Radiation Oncology,
David Geffen School of Medicine,
University of California, Los Angeles,
Los Angeles, California

JONATHAN H. SHERMAN, MD
Assistant Professor of Neurosurgery,
Director of Surgical Neuro-oncology,
Director of Stereotactic Radiosurgery,
Department of Neurological Surgery,
George Washington University Medical Center,
Washington, DC

BENJAMIN J. SHIN, BS
Department of Neurological Surgery,
New York–Presbyterian Hospital,
Weill Cornell Medical College, New York,
New York

MICHAEL E. SUGHRUE, MD
Department of Neurological Surgery,
Comprehensive Brain Tumor Center,
University of Oklahoma, Oklahoma City,
Oklahoma

JENNIFER A. SWEET, MD
Department of Neurological Surgery, George
Washington University Medical Center,
Washington, DC

**BENEDICT BENG TECK TAW, MBBS,
FRCSEd(SN), FCSHK**
Division of Neurosurgery, Department
of Surgery, University of Hong Kong,
Hong Kong, SAR, China

JOSHUA J. WIND, MD
Resident, Department of Neurological Surgery,
George Washington University Medical Center,
Washington, DC

ISAAC YANG, MD
Assistant Professor, University of California,
Los Angeles, David Geffen School of Medicine
at UCLA, UCLA Department of Neurosurgery;
UCLA Jonsson Comprehensive Cancer
Center, UCLA Brain Tumor Program,
Los Angeles, California

ANDREW YEW, MD
UCLA Department of Neurosurgery;
David Geffen School of Medicine,
University of California, Los Angeles,
Los Angeles, California

RICHARD YOUNG, MD
Resident, Department of Neurological Surgery,
George Washington University Medical Center,
Washington, DC

GABRIEL ZADA, MD
Department of Neurosurgery,
University of Southern California,
Los Angeles, California

Contents

The insula is a functionally and anatomically complex cortical structure that can be affected by both low-grade and high-grade gliomas. This complexity often prevents many neurosurgeons from attempting to surgically manage insular gliomas. This article reviews the anatomic and functional uniqueness of the insula and the surgical outcomes and lessons learned from previously reported surgical series. Successful management of insular gliomas, defined as maximal resection of the tumor without postoperative neurologic morbidity, can be achieved through a sophisticated understanding of the neurovascular structure of the insular region and an intraoperative functional mapping using cortico-subcortical electrical stimulation.

Many neurosurgeons take a nihilistic approach to surgical treatment of gliomas, stating the inability to achieve a cure. Where this idea comes from is somewhat nebulous to most neurosurgeons. A review of the scientific studies supporting the commonly held beliefs about gliomas shows that these ideas regarding the surgical treatment of gliomas are based on overgeneralizations of data from older studies. One should avoid the temptation to apply them to the greater concept of what gliomas are, how they behave, and what should be done, but rather we should continue to scientifically evaluate the role of surgical resection in glioma treatment.

Surgery remains one of the oldest and still most important forms of treatment for patients with glioma. The advantages of surgical resection for glioma must be balanced with the potential of operative morbidity to surrounding eloquent brain. To that end, advances in functional brain mapping allow for safer operations with more aggressive surgical resections. A brief history of motor mapping as well as its present day use in aiding resection of eloquent gliomas is discussed.

High-grade gliomas (HGGs), including anaplastic astrocytoma and glioblastoma multiforme, are the most common primary brain tumors, and are often associated with seizures. Seizure control is a critical but often underappreciated goal in the treatment of patients harboring these malignant lesions. Patients with HGG who also have medically intractable seizures should be considered for a palliative resection guided by electrocorticography and functional mapping. Antiepileptic drugs remain the mainstay of seizure treatment in HGG, and antiepileptic medication should be started after a tumor-related seizure, but should not be used prophylactically in the absence of seizure activity.

The purpose of this article is to update the neurosurgical field on current molecular markers important to glioblastoma biology, treatment, and prognosis. The highlighted biologic markers in this article include epidermal growth factor receptor (EGFR), EGFR variant III (EGFRvIII), phosphatase and tensin homolog deleted on chromosome 10 (PTEN), and O6-methylguanine-DNA methyltransferase (MGMT).

The purpose of this article is to update the neurosurgical community on the role of adjuvant radiation therapy in the management of patients with high-grade glioma. This information guides clinicians in the multidisciplinary management of these patients via a review of the literature describing current treatment paradigms as well as new avenues of investigation.

Radiotherapy has become a part of the standard treatment of high-grade gliomas. Studies have shown that high-dose radiation results in more effective tumor control but at the cost of radionecrosis and other radiation-related side effects. Despite advancing techniques in stereotaxy and precise radiotherapy delivery techniques, studies published for stereotactic radiosurgical treatment of high-grade gliomas have not been unanimous, with large trials showing no survival benefit compared with conventional conformal radiotherapy. New imaging modalities have been studied with the hope to improve accuracy in the planning of radiosurgical treatments. However, further large scale studies are needed to confirm these results.

The development of radiologic criteria for the assessment of response to treatment in high-grade gliomas (HGGs) has evolved considerably over the past few decades since the original response criteria based on computed tomography imaging. Accuracy and objectivity in the assessment of response to treatment of HGGs is necessary for altering treatment regimens, establishing accurate provider communication, and improving the quality of clinical trials. Future studies assessing emerging advanced neuroimaging techniques will facilitate the development of even more accurate evidence-based radiologic response criteria.

The standard of care for newly diagnosed malignant glioblastoma entails postoperative radiotherapy and adjuvant chemotherapy with temozolomide. There has been an increase in the incidence of enhancing and progressive lesions seen on magnetic resonance imaging (MRI) following treatment. Conventional MRI with gadolinium contrast is unable to distinguish between the effects of treatment and actual tumor recurrence. New modalities have provided additional information for distinguishing treatment effects from tumor progression but are not 100% sensitive or specific in diagnosing progression. Novel radiographic or nonradiographic biomarkers with sensitivity and specificity verified in large randomized clinical trials are needed to detect progression.

The 1,3-bis(2-chloroethyl)-1-nitrosourea (BCNU; carmustine) polymer wafer (Gliadel) was developed for use in malignant glioma to deliver higher doses of chemotherapy directly to tumor tissue while bypassing systemic side effects. Phase III clinical trials for patients with newly diagnosed malignant gliomas demonstrated a small, but statistically significant, improvement in survival. However, the rate of complications, including an increase in cerebrospinal fluid leaks and intracranial hypertension, has limited their use. This article reviews the current data for use of BCNU wafers in malignant gliomas.

Irinotecan, cisplatin, and nitrosoureas have a long history of use in brain tumors, with demonstrated efficacy in the adjuvant treatment of malignant gliomas. In the era of temozolomide with concurrent radiotherapy given as the standard of care, their use has shifted to treatment at progression or recurrence. Now with the widespread use of bevacizumab in the recurrent setting, irinotecan and other chemotherapies are seeing increased use in combination with bevacizumab and alone in the recurrent setting. The activity of these chemotherapeutic agents in brain tumors will likely ensure a place in the armamentarium of neuro-oncologists for many years.

This article provides historical and recent perspectives related to the use of temozolomide for the treatment of glioblastoma multiforme. Temozolomide has quickly become part of the standard of care for the modern treatment of stage IV glioblastoma multiforme since its approval in 2005. Yet despite its improvements from previous therapies, median survival remains approximately 15 months, with a 2-year survival rate of 8% to 26%. The mechanism of action of this chemotherapeutic agent, conferred advantages and limitations, treatment resistance and rescue, and potential targets of future research are discussed.

Glioblastoma multiforme constitutes the most common primary brain tumor and carries a grim prognosis for patients treated with conventional therapy including surgery, radiation therapy, and chemotherapy. There has been a recent revival of selective intra-arterial delivery of targeted agents for the treatment of glioblastoma multiforme. Because these agents are less toxic and their delivery leads to a higher tumor–drug concentration, this combination may provide a better outcome in patients with high-grade glioma. This article discusses early experiences in patients who received superselective intra-arterial cerebral infusion of bevacizumab, cetuximab, and temozolamide after blood–brain barrier disruption with mannitol.

Glioblastoma multiforme is a malignant primary brain tumor for which no cure has been developed. However, with aggressive surgical resection, radiation, and the advent of temozolomide, the overall survival of patients with glioblastomas has improved significantly. Despite this multimodal treatment, glioblastoma invariably recurs. Although treatment options for glioblastoma recurrence are limited, one promising therapy is bevacizumab (Avastin). The role of Avastin in the management of recurrent glioblastomas is reviewed.

The diffuse nature of gliomas has long confounded attempts at achieving a definitive cure. The advent of computed tomography and magnetic resonance imaging made it increasingly apparent that gliomas could have a multifocal or multicentric appearance. Treating these tumors is the summit of an already daunting challenge, because the obstacles that must be surmounted to treat gliomas in general, namely, their heterogeneity, diffuse nature, and ability to insidiously invade normal brain, are more conspicuous in this subset of tumors.

Neurosurgery Clinics of North America

VISIT THE CLINICS ONLINE!

Access your subscription at:
www.theclinics.com

Preface

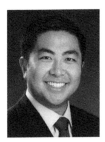 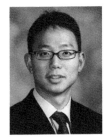

Isaac Yang, MD   Seunggu J. Han, MD
Guest Editors

Malignant glioblastoma is the most common and lethal primary brain tumor, and arguably the most challenging disease entity encountered in the fields of neuro-oncology and neurosurgery. Currently, average survival of a patient with malignant glioma remains approximately just over one year. Malignant glioma is a grave diagnosis for patients, their families, their treating clinicians. The devastating nature of its diagnosis has come to public attention after Senator Kennedy's recent struggle with the disease.

Over the past two decades, treatment for malignant gliomas has evolved into that of a multidisciplinary approach, which includes maximal surgical resection when feasible, followed by radiation and chemotherapy. Each of these arms represent the result of many clinical trials and studies. Multiple trials are currently ongoing to determine if any variations in technique or agent in these modalities will further improve outcomes. At recurrence, few standard therapies are available, and many investigators are continuing to study the application of a number of novel modalities and agents in this setting.

This first part of a two-part issue of *Neurosurgery Clinics of North America* aims to provide for clinicians, researchers, and investigators, an organized and expansive survey with critical scientific analysis of the currently available therapies for patients with malignant gliomas, as well as the clinical evidence behind each of these modalities from a world-class assembly of leading investigators and expert clinicians. It will also focus on special considerations when the tumor is in challenging locations requiring language or motor mapping, when they are multifocal, or when they occur in the pediatric population. Novel modalities currently under active study will also be reviewed, including alternative radiation modalities such as radiosurgery, adjuvants to radiotherapy such as radiosensitizers, delivery of chemotherapeutic agents intra-arterially

or directly into the surgical bed, immunotherapy, nanotechnology, and other targeted molecular therapy agents. These contributions from some of the world's foremost and leading brain tumor investigators represent some of the premiere efforts in increasing our knowledge and information on modern therapy for glioblastoma.

We hope this critical analysis and thorough survey will provide clinicians and research scientists with a comprehensive and systematic overview of modern brain tumor therapy and further stimulate future studies and investigations against glioblastoma. It is our aim that this text may be utilized effectively as a resource to neurosurgeons, neuroscientists, neuro-oncologists, experimental researchers, clinical practitioners, and all others alike who aim to further their knowledge and explore in-depth critical investigations in brain tumor therapy. Our most sincere hope is that these endeavors will continue to improve and make advances in our glioma therapies that will translate into making the lives of our brain tumor patients better.

Isaac Yang, MD
UCLA Department of Neurosurgery
University of California, Los Angeles
David Geffen School of Medicine at UCLA
695 Charles East Young Drive South
UCLA Gonda 3357
Los Angeles, CA 90095–1761, USA

Seunggu J. Han, MD
Department of Neurological Surgery
University of California, San Francisco
505 Parnassus Avenue, M779
San Francisco, CA 94117, USA

E-mail addresses:
IYang@mednet.ucla.edu (I. Yang)
HanSJ@neurosurg.ucsf.edu (S.J. Han)

Neurosurg Clin N Am 23 (2012) xiii
doi:10.1016/j.nec.2012.02.003

neurosurgery.theclinics.com

Note to Readers: Authors John D. Rolston, MD, PhD, Sharanya Arcot Desai, BE, MSc, Nealen G. Laxpati, BS, and Robert E. Gross, MD, PhD would like to acknowledge the support of Steve M. Potter, PhD during the preparation of their article, "Electrical Stimulation for Epilepsy: Experimental Approaches," which appeared in the October 2011 issue of *Neurosurgery Clinics of North America*, Epilepsy Surgery: The Emerging Field of Neuromodulation.

John D. Rolston, MD, PhD

doi:10.1016/j.nec.2012.02.004

neurosurgery.theclinics.com

Current Surgical Management of Insular Gliomas

Young-Hoon Kim, MD[a,b], Chae-Yong Kim, MD, PhD[a,b],*

KEYWORDS

- Insula • Gliomas • Maximal resection
- Neurologic morbidity • Intraoperative functional mapping

In 1809, Johann Christian Reil (1759–1813), the German anatomist, physiologist, and psychiatrist, first described the island (or insula) of Reil.[1,2] This anatomically and functionally complex structure is located in the depth of the sylvian fissure, overlies the basal ganglia block, and is hidden by the opercula of the frontal, parietal, and temporal lobes. It is thought to play roles in autonomic sensation, gustatory function, olfaction, memory, drive, auditory–vestibular function, and the motor integration and motor planning of speech in the dominant hemisphere.[3–5] The insula is also associated with cardioregulatory and vasomotor functions, pain perception, and bio-behavioral dysfunction characteristics of schizophrenia.[6] Moreover, the insula is adjacent to essential peri-sylvian language areas (ie, Broca areas and Wernicke areas and their association fibers, the primary auditory area, and both the primary motor and sensory areas).

Therefore, intrinsic tumors located in the insular and peri-insular areas present with a variety of ill-defined symptoms and neurologic signs dominated by a single entity, such as motor dysphasia with or without lower facial paresis.[1,7,8] The anatomic complexity of the insula and its functionally critical nature have caused radical insula operations to be taboo among neurosurgeons for a long time, and they have often recommended a conservative strategy for the treatment of intrinsic insular tumors.[9] However, since the seminal 1992 study by Yasargil and colleagues,[2] which demonstrated that it was possible to extirpate intrinsic insular tumors with less risk than initially thought, some experienced neurosurgeons have reported favorable outcomes of insular tumor surgery based on a detailed understanding of the pertinent anatomy and the application of modern microneurosurgical techniques.[5,10–15]

Nonetheless, achieving both maximal resection and a favorable functional outcome in intrinsic insular tumor surgery has been challenging for most neurosurgeons. This article reviews the anatomic and surgical characteristics of insular gliomas (which are the most frequent intrinsic tumor in the insula) and evaluates the reported oncological and functional outcomes after insular glioma surgery.

ANATOMY OF INSULAR GLIOMA AND SURGICAL APPROACHES

A detailed understanding of the complex anatomy of the insula and its surrounding structures is required for the removal of insular gliomas with minimal morbidity. The insula, a well-defined cerebral cortical surface, is a pyramidal structure whose 3 sides meet at a peak called the insular apex, the most lateral projection of the insula. The central sulcus separates the larger anterior portion from the smaller posterior portion. The anterior portion is composed of 3 short gyri (ie, the anterior, middle, and posterior short insular gyri) as well as the transverse gyrus and the accessory gyrus. The posterior portion is composed of the anterior and posterior long insular gyri. The limen insulae, a white matter

a Department of Neurosurgery, Seoul National University Bundang Hospital, 166 Gumi-ro, Bundang-gu, Seongnam-si, Gyeonggi-do 463-707, Korea
b Department of Neurosurgery, Seoul National University College of Medicine, 101 Daehangno, Jongno-gu, Seoul 110-744, Korea
* Corresponding author. Department of Neurosurgery, Seoul National University Bundang Hospital, 166 Gumi-ro, Bundang-gu, Seongnam-si, Gyeonggi-do 463-707, Korea.
E-mail address: chaeyong@snu.ac.kr

Neurosurg Clin N Am 23 (2012) 199–206
doi:10.1016/j.nec.2012.01.010
1042-3680/12/$ – see front matter © 2012 Elsevier Inc. All rights reserved.

structure in the anterobasal portion of the insula, parallels the course of the lateral olfactory stria, extending from the anterior perforated substance medially to the insular pole along what is known as the sylvian stem.[4,16]

In the central portion of the insula, the extreme capsule, claustrum, external capsule, putamen, and globus pallidus lie in a lateral-to-medial direction. The perimeter of the insula is provided by the anterior, superior, and inferior peri-insular sulci, which separate the insula from the fronto–orbital, fronto–parietal, and temporal opercula, respectively. These are critical internal landmarks that define the internal extent of the insula for the neurosurgeon.[1,4,11] Superior to the central portion of the insula, at the level of the superior peri-insular sulcus, is the corticospinal tract in the corona radiata; the uncinate fasciculus is located anteroinferiorly, and the arcuate fasciculus is located posteriorly along the same sulcus. The anterior and posterior limits of the insula are defined as the meeting point of the anterior with the superior peri-insular sulcus and that of the superior with the inferior peri-insular sulcus, respectively.

The course and supply of the middle cerebral artery (MCA) and its perforating vessels are most important for insular glioma surgery. The blood supply of insular gliomas is largely derived from the M2 segment of the MCA through its short- and medium-sized perforating vessels. Devascularization of an insular glioma can be achieved by advertent coagulation and cutting each of the M2 perforators after subpial dissection. Long perforating vessels of the M2 overlying the posterior portion of the insula supply the corona radiate, particularly the corticospinal and thalamocortical fibers, and they therefore must be preserved during surgery.[11,17,18] The M1 segment of the MCA lies at the anteroinferior portion of the insula, extending laterally from the carotid bifurcation under the anterior perforated substance, and it supplies the basal ganglia and internal capsule via lateral lenticulostriate perforating vessels. The mean distance from the insular apex to the most lateral lenticulostriate artery is less than 1.5 cm, and the neurosurgeon must preserve the first lenticulostriate artery encountered, which is usually located in the medial side of the tumor, without creating a dense hemiplegia.[11,18,19]

Yasargil and colleagues[2] reported an extensive surgical series of limbic and paralimbic intrinsic tumors (including insular gliomas), and they demonstrated for the first time that microsurgery is possible for tumors occupying that region without critical neurologic deterioration. They proposed a classification scheme for tumors in paralimbic regions. In this scheme, type 3a tumors (purely insular tumors), type 3b tumors (those infiltrating the peri-sylvian opercula), and type 5 tumors (those extending to other paralimbic areas) were included in the broad category of insular gliomas.

Tables 1 and **2** present the summarized data of the patients with insular gliomas in the previously reported surgical series. The traditional approach for insular gliomas had been the trans-sylvian approach because of the seminal work of Yasargil and colleagues.[2] The advantages of the trans-sylvian approach include a direct corridor to the insular region, the possibility of a wide surgical view by widely opening the sylvian fissure, and the great familiarity of this approach to neurosurgeons. However, the risk of vascular damage, in particular to the perforating vessels, by means of the trans-sylvian approach to the insular region, is never negligible. Therefore, in recently reported papers,[5,13,14] a transcortical approach (ie, a transopercular approach) has been used as an alternative or adjunctive method to the traditional trans-sylvian approach. A transcortical approach by means of subpial dissection prevents injuries to and iatrogenic spasms of the MCA and its branches. In addition, intraoperative monitoring, such as of somatosensory-evoked potentials and motor-evoked potentials, is necessary to preserve the integrity of the peri-insular regions. Likewise, awake craniotomy enables the neurosurgeon to monitor the language function of the patient, which is especially important for tumors in the dominant hemisphere.[20]

CLINICAL CHARACTERISTICS AND DIAGNOSIS OF INSULAR GLIOMAS

Insular gliomas are the most frequent intrinsic tumor in the insular region, and they accounted for up to 25% of all low-grade gliomas (LGGs) and 10% of all high-grade gliomas (HGGs) in a recent epidemiologic study.[21] Sanai and colleagues[5] reported characteristics that distinguish insular gliomas from other gliomas beyond the critical neurologic nature and anatomic complexity of the insula. There is a clear tendency toward low-grade histology that is unique to the insula and distinct from other regions, and this propensity may be caused by a particular microenvironment within the insula or by the nature of the originating glioma cells that propagate these tumors. Additionally, patients with insular gliomas generally show a prolonged and slowly progressing clinical course. However, an unpredictable natural course is characteristic of insular gliomas of both low- and high-grade histology. The representative surgical series reported that LGGs accounted for 36% to 74% of insular tumors, and the median age of the patients ranged from 36 to 41 years (see **Table 1**).

Table 1
Demographical and clinical data of the patients with insular gliomas in previous representative reports

Author, Year	Total Number	Age (Range)	Sex	Description of Seizure	Presenting Symptoms and Signs	Histology	F/U Duration (Range)
Yasargil et al,[2] 1992	80	Peak age 41–50 y	NA	SPS (5%) CPS (28%) 2nd GTCS (13%) GTCS (10%) Absence (15%) Others (4%)	Seizure (78%) Sensorimotor hemideficit (26%) Speech impairment (26%) Neuropsychological defect (35%) Visual acuity decrease (10%) Visual field defect (10%)	LGG (44%) HGG (56%)	NA
Vanaclocha et al,[15] 1997	23	Median 40 y (12–64 y)	Male (65%) Female (35%)	NA	NA	LGG (70%) HGG (30%)	Median 2.5 y (1–6.5 y)
Lang et al,[18] 2001	22	Median 36 y (2–78 y)	Male (32%) Female (68%)	Total (64%)	Seizure (64%) Weakness/hemiparesis (32%) Dysphasia/dysnomia (18%)	LGG (50%) HGG (50%)	Median 1.2 y (0.2–4 y)
Moshel et al,[12] 2008	38	Mean 38 y (15–59 y)	Male (61%) Female (39%)	SPS (8%) CPS (34%) GTCS (29%)	Seizure (71%) Hemiparesis (8%) Hemianesthesia (8%) Dysphasia (16%) Headache (29%) Memory deficits (8%) Visual problems (3%)	LGG (74%) HGG (26%)	NA
Duffau,[13] 2009	51	Mean 36 y (19–57 y)	Male (59%) Female (41%)	SPS (69%) GTCS (29%) Intractable (35%)	Seizure (98%) Intracerebral hemorrhage (2%) Hemiparesis (2%)	LGG (100%) HGG (0%)	Median 4 y (0.3–10.1 y)
Simon et al,[14] 2010	94	Median 41 y (9–77)	Male (61%) Female (39%)	Total (82%) Intractable (13%)	Seizure (82%) Hemiparesis or dysphasia (24%)	LGG (36%) HGG (64%)	Median 3.1 y (0–17.1 y)
Sanai et al,[5] 2010	104	Median 40 y (18–75)	Male (40%) Female (60%)	Total (72%)	Seizure (72%) Sensory impairments (13%) Headache (7%) Languade deficits (5%) Incidental (4%)	LGG (60%) HGG (40%)	Median 4.2 y (1.4–10.2 y)

Abbreviations: CPS, complex partial seizure; F/U, follow-up; GTCS, generalized tonic–clonic seizure; HGG, high-grade glioma; LGG, low-grade glioma; NA, not available; SPS, simple partial seizure.

Table 2
Surgical and functional outcome of the patients with insular gliomas in previous representative reports

Author, Year	Total Number	Approach	Extent of Resection	Immediate N/D	Permanent N/D	Survival Data	F/U Duration (Range)
Yasargil et al,[2] 1992	80	Trans-sylvian	NA	NA	Total (11%)	NA	NA
Vanaclocha, et al,[15] 1997	23	Trans-sylvian	GTR (87%) STR (13%)	Total (26%) Hemiparesis (22%) Dysphasia (4%)	Total (0%)	Alive at last F/U (87%)	Median 2.5 y (1–6.5 y)
Lang et al,[18] 2001	22	Trans-sylvian (36%) + ATL (36%) + transopercular (28%)	>90% (45%) 75%–90% (27%) <75% (28%)	Total (36%) Weakness (18%) Speech impairment (27%)	Total (9%) Weakness (9%)	Alive at last F/U (68%)	Median 1.2 y (0.2–4 y)
Moshel et al,[12] 2008	38	Trans-sylvian	GTR (55%) NTR (18%) STR (26%)	Total (16%) Hemiparesis (16%) Dysphasia (3%)	Total (13%) Hemiparesis (13%) Dysphasia (5%)	NA	NA
Duffau,[13] 2009	51	Transopercular (94%) Transsylvian (6%)	GTR (16%) STR (61%) PR (24%)	Total (59%) Hemiparesis (37%) Dysphasia (20%) Athymhormic syndrome (14%) FCMS (8%)	Total (4%) Hemiparesis (4%)	Alive at last F/U (82%)	Median 4 y (0.3–10.1 y)
Simon et al,[14] 2010	94	Trans-sylvian (25%) Transopercular (50%) Combined (25%)	>90% (42%) 70%–90% (51%) <70% (7%)	NA	Total (20%) Hemiparesis (13%) Dysphasia (5%)	a	Median 3.1 y (0–17.1 y)
Sanai et al,[5] 2010	104	Transcortical	>90% (23%) 80%–90% (39%) 60%–80% (28%) <60% (11%)	Total (14%) Motor deficits (9%) Speech deficits (5%)	Total (6%) Motor deficits (5%) Speech deficits (1%)	Alive at last F/U (91%)	Median 4.2 y (1.4–10.2 y)

Abbreviations: ATL, anterior temporal lobectomy; FCMS, Foix-Chavany-Marie syndrome; F/U, follow-up; GTR, gross total removal; NA, not available; N/D, neurologic deficits; NTR, near total removal; PR, partial removal; STR, subtotal removal.
a The 5-year overall survival (OS) and progression-free survival (PFS) rates in WHO grade 2 gliomas were 68% and 58%, respectively. The median OS and PFS in anaplastic astrocytomas were 61 months and 51 months, respectively. The 5-year OS and PFS rates in anaplastic oligodendrogliomas were 83% and 80%, respectively.

Medically intractable epilepsy is the most common presenting symptom of patients with insular gliomas, especially those with LGGs. According to previous reports,[2,5,12–14,18] 64% to 98% of patients with insular tumors suffer from intractable epilepsy, among whom simple and complex partial seizures accounted for 33% to 69% of cases and generalized seizures 23% to 29% of cases (see **Table 1**). The semiology of insular epilepsy reflects the diverse characteristics of the region's functional anatomy.[22] It may present as temporal lobe epilepsy[8,22–24] or frontal lobe epilepsy,[22,25] manifesting as a simple partial seizure with respiratory, viscero-sensitive, or oroalimentary features.[7,26] Spreading to the suprasylvian opercular cortex in the frontal or parietal lobe may induce facial sensory disturbances or tonic–clonic laryngeal constriction, gustatory illusions and hypersalivation with postictal facial paresis.[8,27] Spreading to the infra-sylvian operculum in the temporal lobe may produce auditory hallucinations or sensory dysphasia.[1,28]

Regarding HGGs in the insular region, the presenting symptoms (such as headache, sensorimotor impairment, or language disturbance) are associated with mass effects and peri-tumoral vasogenic edema. Cognitive dysfunction is often induced by regional edema, electrophysiological abnormalities, and adverse effects of antiepileptic drugs.[29,30] Various clinical symptoms and neurologic signs, including memory impairment, attention deficits, and visual disturbances may manifest due to the functional complexity of the insula (see **Table 1**).

Magnetic resonance imaging (MRI) is the gold standard diagnostic tool for insular gliomas. The exact location and boundary of the tumor and the relationship between the tumor and adjacent vessels must be preoperatively defined by MRI scans with cerebral angiography. Their proximity to functionally critical cerebral cortex, white matter tracts, and basal ganglia make the recently developed functional evaluation methods crucial to insular glioma surgery. Functional MRI,[31] magnetoencephalography,[32] and positron emission topography[33] provide useful information regarding functional–anatomic correlations, and diffusion tensor imaging with tractography reveals specific white matter tracts.[34]

SURGICAL RESULTS AND ONCOLOGICAL OUTCOME

In microsurgery for insular gliomas, both maximal resection for oncological control and a functional outcome without a catastrophic neurologic impairment are essential aspects. Since the seminal work of Yasargil and colleagues,[2] several groups have achieved favorable resection outcomes (see **Table 2**). Gross total resection (>90%) rates range from 16% to 87%, and subtotal resection rates (>70%) range from 62% to 100%. A sophisticated understanding of the surgical anatomy of the insular region and its relationship to the adjacent MCA and its perforating vessels has enabled neurosurgeons to achieve maximal resection without catastrophically impacting neurologic status.

It is well known that maximal resection of gliomas (including LGGs and HGGs) guarantees longer overall survival (OS) and progression-free survival (PFS), and this surgical strategy can be applied intuitively to insular gliomas. However, studies demonstrating a concrete association between the extent of resection and survival have been very rare, and most previous surgical series have focused on functional outcome rather than survival and progression.

Only 2 studies (Simon and colleagues[14] and Sanai and colleagues[5]) have conducted detailed survival analysis and prognostic factor assessment including extent of resection in the surgical management of insular gliomas. Simon and colleagues[14] enrolled 94 patients with LGGs (36%) and HGGs (64%). In their series, the 5-year OS and PFS rates for World Health Organization (WHO) grade 2 gliomas were 68% and 58%, respectively. Notably, the rates for anaplastic oligodendrogliomas were 83 and 80%, respectively. The median OS and PFS of patients with anaplastic astrocytomas were 61 and 51 months, respectively. These survival results are markedly better than those of historical controls.[35–38] Moreover, they demonstrated that patient age, tumor histopathology, Yasargil type 5 with frontal lobe involvement, and degree of resection were all significant prognostic factors for OS and PFS by multivariate analysis.

The recent work of Sanai and colleagues[5] was the largest such study. They enrolled 104 patients, including 60% with LGGs and 40% with HGGs. Of note, they analyzed both tumor location and extent of resection in detail, and they proposed a classification in which the location of the tumor was divided into 4 zones: zone 1, anterior–superior; zone 2, posterior–superior; zone 3, posterior–inferior; and zone 4, anterior–inferior. They demonstrated that zone 1 is associated with the highest median extent of resection, and the insular quadrant anatomy was found to be predictive of the extent of resection. In their work, patients with LGGs resected over 90% had a 5-year OS rate of 100%, whereas those with lesions resected less than 90% had a 5-year OS rate of 84%. In the same context, patients with HGGs resected over 90% had a 2-year OS rate of 91%, whereas those with lesions resected less than 90% had a 2-year OS rate of 75%. Finally, they concluded that the extent of resection was a significant predictor of OS and PFS after surgery for insular LGGs and HGGs.

NEUROLOGIC DEFICITS AND FUNCTIONAL OUTCOME

Although the evidence that maximal resection guarantees longer OS and PFS is convincing, neurosurgeons face several obstacles to removing insular tumors radically, because radical resection can induce prominent neurologic complications after surgery. Thus, even in the pioneering surgical series (see **Table 2**), immediate and permanent neurologic complication rates reached 14% to 59% and 0% to 20%, respectively. These complications consisted of hemiparesis, facial palsy, dysphasia, and dysarthria. Postoperative neurologic complications are caused by the direct injury of functional peri-insular neural tissue and vascular compromise, especially that of perforating vessels of the MCA.

Splitting and retraction injuries of the frontal operculum in the dominant hemisphere cause Broca dysphasia with dysnomia, and damage to the horizontal fibers of the arcuate fasciculus near the superior peri-insular sulcus or to the uncinate fasciculus near the inferior peri-insular sulcus causes conduction aphasia, impaired perception, and short-term memory deficits.[39] The external capsule is a vulnerable structure during the medial dissection of insular gliomas, and injury to this region results in semantic paraphasias.[39,40] The corona radiata, with its motor and sensory fibers, is also vulnerable when on the superior edge of the tumor. Inadvertent dissection deep into the superior peri-insular sulcus can directly disrupt these fibers, and damage to the lateral fibers results in sensorimotor impairment of the upper limbs and face. Damage to the medial fibers results in sensori-motor impairment of the lower limbs.[11,18]

Perforating vessels likely to be involved in prominent neurologic deficits after insular region surgery include the lateral lenticulostriate arteries and the long perforators of M2. The lateral lenticulostriate arteries originating from the M1 trunk supply the internal capsule and course along the medial side of insular tumors. Because injury to these vessels results in a dense hemiplegia, defining the first lateral lenticulostriate artery is an essential step during inferomedial dissection of the tumor. Moreover, Duffau[13] indicates that gross total removal of a tumor is impossible if the tumor involves the region medial to these vessels and encases them. The long perforating vessels arise from the M2 segment in the upper portion of the insula and supply the corona radiate. Injury to these vessels by means of dissection of the superior portion of the tumor results in the previously mentioned hemiparesis.

Previous authors suggested several sophisticated techniques for avoiding such neurovascular injuries. Lang and colleagues[18] used specific methods (including wide sylvian dissection) to identify the base of the peri-insular sulcus and the superior and inferior dissection planes of the tumor. They performed subpial dissection of the tumor with preservation of all the large perforating arteries from the posterior M2 segment and awake craniotomy with brain stimulation. In contrast, Sanai and colleagues[5] used the transcortical approach to avoid any injury to or iatrogenic spasming of the MCA and its perforating vessels. Duffau[13] recommended a multiple stage surgical approach in the case of tumor removal involving the medial portion over the lateral lenticulostriate arteries or the posterior part of the insula. He noted that an initially incomplete surgery could generate a functional remapping of the residual parts, and a second surgery could be safer in terms of neurologic outcome.

The intraoperative functional monitoring is also important for achieving favorable functional outcome with these sophisticated surgical techniques. Berger and his colleagues were the leading neurosurgeons of the intraoperative functional monitoring and described the intraoperative language and sensorimotor mapping using cortico–subcortical electrical stimulation for glioma resection.[5,41] They applied a bipolar electrode with an interelectrode distance of 5 mm, delivering biphasic current to the cerebral cortex as well as the subcortical area. This monitoring was performed under general anesthesia with a nondominant-side tumor and under awake anesthesia with a dominant-side tumor for monitoring sensorimotor and language functions. Once functional areas had been identified, transcortical incisions above and below the sylvian fissure were created through nonfunctional cortex, taking care to maintain at least a 1 cm margin from any functional site.[5]

NONSURGICAL MANAGEMENT ALTERNATIVES

Due to the risk of neurologic complications associated with radical surgery for insular gliomas, some authors have reported alternative treatment methods for these tumors.[42,43] Mehrkens and colleagues[42] evaluated the long-term outcome of interstitial radiosurgery with I-125 for WHO grade 2 astrocytomas. In that study, 55 consecutive patients underwent interstitial radiosurgery with I-125 by permanent or temporary implant after a stereotactic biopsy. The 5-year OS and PFS rates of the patients were 55% and 41%, respectively, and the 10-year OS and PFS rates were 28% and 20%, respectively. Although the patients had no postoperative neurologic morbidities, 26% of them experienced transient and progressive radiogenic complications, and the 1-year overall complication rate was 18%. Radiogenic complications were significantly associated with a tumor diameter over 3.5 cm.

SUMMARY

The primary goals of the management of insular gliomas are oncological control of the tumor by maximal resection and functional preservation by avoiding neurologic complications. A sophisticated understanding of the anatomic and functional characteristics of the neurovascular structures adjacent to the insular region and of the insula itself and an intraoperative functional mapping using cortico–subcortical electrical stimulation can help neurosurgeons achieve these goals in the treatment of insular gliomas.

REFERENCES

1. Signorelli F, Guyotat J, Elisevich K, et al. Review of current microsurgical management of insular gliomas. Acta Neurochir (Wien) 2010;152(1):19–26.
2. Yasargil MG, von Ammon K, Cavazos E, et al. Tumours of the limbic and paralimbic systems. Acta Neurochir (Wien) 1992;118(1–2):40–52.
3. Shelley BP, Trimble MR. The insular lobe of Reil—its anatamico-functional, behavioural and neuropsychiatric attributes in humans—a review. World J Biol Psychiatry 2004;5(4):176–200.
4. Ture U, Yasargil DC, Al-Mefty O, et al. Topographic anatomy of the insular region. J Neurosurg 1999; 90(4):720–33.
5. Sanai N, Polley MY, Berger MS. Insular glioma resection: assessment of patient morbidity, survival, and tumor progression. J Neurosurg 2010;112(1):1–9.
6. Makris N, Goldstein JM, Kennedy D, et al. Decreased volume of left and total anterior insular lobule in schizophrenia. Schizophr Res 2006;83(2–3):155–71.
7. Guenot M, Isnard J. Epilepsy and insula. Neurochirurgie 2008;54(3):374–81 [in French].
8. Isnard J, Guenot M, Sindou M, et al. Clinical manifestations of insular lobe seizures: a stereoelectroencephalographic study. Epilepsia 2004; 45(9):1079–90.
9. Ebeling U, Kothbauer K. Circumscribed low grade astrocytomas in the dominant opercular and insular region: a pilot study. Acta Neurochir (Wien) 1995; 132(1–3):66–74.
10. Zentner J, Meyer B, Stangl A, et al. Intrinsic tumors of the insula: a prospective surgical study of 30 patients. J Neurosurg 1996;85(2):263–71.
11. Hentschel SJ, Lang FF. Surgical resection of intrinsic insular tumors. Neurosurgery 2005;57(Suppl 1): 176–83 [discussion: 176–83].
12. Moshel YA, Marcus JD, Parker EC, et al. Resection of insular gliomas: the importance of lenticulostriate artery position. J Neurosurg 2008;109(5):825–34.
13. Duffau H. A personal consecutive series of surgically treated 51 cases of insular WHO grade II glioma: advances and limitations. J Neurosurg 2009;110(4):696–708.
14. Simon M, Neuloh G, von Lehe M, et al. Insular gliomas: the case for surgical management. J Neurosurg 2009;110(4):685–95.
15. Vanaclocha V, Saiz-Sapena N, Garcia-Casasola C. Surgical treatment of insular gliomas. Acta Neurochir (Wien) 1997;139(12):1126–34 [discussion: 1134–5].
16. Stummer W, Reulen HJ, Meinel T, et al. Extent of resection and survival in glioblastoma multiforme: identification of and adjustment for bias. Neurosurgery 2008;62(3):564–76 [discussion: 564–76].
17. Ture U, Yasargil MG, Al-Mefty O, et al. Arteries of the insula. J Neurosurg 2000;92(4):676–87.
18. Lang FF, Olansen NE, DeMonte F, et al. Surgical resection of intrinsic insular tumors: complication avoidance. J Neurosurg 2001;95(4):638–50.
19. Pignatti F, van den Bent M, Curran D, et al. Prognostic factors for survival in adult patients with cerebral low-grade glioma. J Clin Oncol 2002;20(8): 2076–84.
20. Kim YH, Kim CH, Kim JS, et al. Resection frequency map after awake resective surgery for non-lesional neocortical epilepsy involving eloquent areas. Acta Neurochir (Wien) 2011;153(9):1739–49.
21. Duffau H, Capelle L. Preferential brain locations of low-grade gliomas. Cancer 2004;100(12):2622–6.
22. Roux FE, Ibarrola D, Tremoulet M, et al. Methodological and technical issues for integrating functional magnetic resonance imaging data in a neuronavigational system. Neurosurgery 2001;49(5):1145–56 [discussion: 1156–7].
23. Barba C, Barbati G, Minotti L, et al. Ictal clinical and scalp-EEG findings differentiating temporal lobe epilepsies from temporal 'plus' epilepsies. Brain 2007;130(Pt 7):1957–67.
24. Ostrowsky K, Isnard J, Ryvlin P, et al. Functional mapping of the insular cortex: clinical implication in temporal lobe epilepsy. Epilepsia 2000;41(6): 681–6.
25. Dobesberger J, Ortler M, Unterberger I, et al. Successful surgical treatment of insular epilepsy with nocturnal hypermotor seizures. Epilepsia 2008;49(1):159–62.

26. Neuloh G, Pechstein U, Schramm J. Motor tract monitoring during insular glioma surgery. J Neurosurg 2007;106(4):582–92.

27. Penfield W, Faulk ME Jr. The insula; further observations on its function. Brain 1955;78(4):445–70.

28. Bancaud J. [Clinical symptomatology of epileptic seizures of temporal origin]. Rev Neurol (Paris) 1987;143(5):392–400 [in French].

29. Klein M, Engelberts NH, van der Ploeg HM, et al. Epilepsy in low-grade gliomas: the impact on cognitive function and quality of life. Ann Neurol 2003; 54(4):514–20.

30. Meyers CA, Hess KR. Multifaceted end points in brain tumor clinical trials: cognitive deterioration precedes MRI progression. Neuro Oncol 2003;5(2):89–95.

31. Schramm J, Aliashkevich AF. Temporal mediobasal tumors: a proposal for classification according to surgical anatomy. Acta Neurochir (Wien) 2008; 150(9):857–64 [discussion: 864].

32. Makela JP, Forss N, Jaaskelainen J, et al. Magnetoencephalography in neurosurgery. Neurosurgery 2006;59(3):493–510 [discussion: 510–1].

33. Signorelli F, Guyotat J, Isnard J, et al. The value of cortical stimulation applied to the surgery of malignant gliomas in language areas. Neurol Sci 2001; 22(1):3–10.

34. Kim CH, Chung CK, Koo BB, et al. Changes in language pathways in patients with temporal lobe epilepsy: diffusion tensor imaging analysis of the uncinate and arcuate fasciculi. World Neurosurg 2011;75(3–4):509–16.

35. Cairncross G, Berkey B, Shaw E, et al. Phase III trial of chemotherapy plus radiotherapy compared with radiotherapy alone for pure and mixed anaplastic oligodendroglioma: Intergroup Radiation Therapy Oncology Group Trial 9402. J Clin Oncol 2006; 24(18):2707–14.

36. Kristof RA, Neuloh G, Hans V, et al. Combined surgery, radiation, and PCV chemotherapy for astrocytomas compared to oligodendrogliomas and oligoastrocytomas WHO grade III. J Neurooncol 2002; 59(3):231–7.

37. van den Bent MJ, Carpentier AF, Brandes AA, et al. Adjuvant procarbazine, lomustine, and vincristine improves progression-free survival but not overall survival in newly diagnosed anaplastic oligodendrogliomas and oligoastrocytomas: a randomized European Organisation for Research and Treatment of Cancer phase III trial. J Clin Oncol 2006;24(18): 2715–22.

38. Kim YH, Park CK, Cho WH, et al. Temozolomide during and after radiation therapy for WHO grade III gliomas: preliminary report of a prospective multicenter study. J Neurooncol 2011;103(3):503–12.

39. Duffau H, Peggy Gatignol ST, Mandonnet E, et al. Intraoperative subcortical stimulation mapping of language pathways in a consecutive series of 115 patients with grade II glioma in the left dominant hemisphere. J Neurosurg 2008;109(3):461–71.

40. Duffau H, Thiebaut de Schotten M, Mandonnet E. White matter functional connectivity as an additional landmark for dominant temporal lobectomy. J Neurol Neurosurg Psychiatry 2008;79(5):492–5.

41. Sanai N, Mirzadeh Z, Berger MS. Functional outcome after language mapping for glioma resection. N Engl J Med 2008;358(1):18–27.

42. Mehrkens JH, Kreth FW, Muacevic A, et al. Long term course of WHO grade II astrocytomas of the Insula of Reil after I-125 interstitial irradiation. J Neurol 2004;251(12):1455–64.

43. Shankar A, Rajshekhar V. Radiological and clinical outcome following stereotactic biopsy and radiotherapy for low-grade insular astrocytomas. Neurol India 2003;51(4):503–6.

The Rise and Fall of "Biopsy and Radiate": A History of Surgical Nihilism in Glioma Treatment

Seunggu J. Han, MD[a], Michael E. Sughrue, MD[b],*

KEYWORDS

- Surgery • Glioma • Resection

COMMONLY HELD VIEWS ABOUT GLIOMA TREATMENT

Infiltrating gliomas, defined as World Health Organization grade II through IV astrocytic or oligodendoglial neoplasms, are known to all with even casual exposure to their clinical history as invariably multiply recurrent and eventually fatal, albeit at grade-specific rates, despite lesionectomy, adjuvant radiotherapy, and chemotherapy.[1–3] Despite generations of effort, the outcome for these lesions has improved only marginally, and the cure rate remains dismally low.[3] The future of glioma therapy is in the laboratory, and eventually some molecular-based therapy will be developed that will be the ultimate solution for this terrible disease, because surgery clearly is not.[4] In many cases, aggressive surgery is ill-advised, pointless, and harmful. In these cases, biopsy and radiation alone serves as an acceptable alternative to surgery, despite the dismal prognosis with this approach.

The paragraph above summarizes how many surgeons and oncologists view treatment of gliomas. Many of these views are handed down between clinicians, yet given that there are not definitive class 1 studies demonstrating most of these statements, we feel these views are worth a critical reassessment. This article summarizes much of what been taught regarding glioma treatment and, more specifically, glioma surgery. Unquestionably, a great deal of published data support this ideology, not the least of which are from the collective experience of many who have treated patients using this paradigm. The purpose of the article is not to entirely discount these ideas, but rather to critically address the scientific and clinical foundations on which these approaches are based. A review of the scientific studies supporting the commonly held beliefs about gliomas shows that these nihilistic ideas regarding gliomas are based on overgeneralizations of older historical studies that have been applied to the greater concept of what gliomas are, how they behave, and what should be done to treat them.

NIHILISM IN GLIOMA SURGERY

High-grade gliomas, notably glioblastoma, behave extremely aggressively. Regardless of grade, they have a high rate of recurrence and progression to higher grades, such as glioblastoma, and are ultimately fatal in most patients.[5] These tumors notoriously infiltrate normal brain, meaning that surgical resection generally involves removal of functional

Financial Disclosure: The author declares that he is not involved in any other relationships with companies that make products related to this study.
[a] Department of Neurological Surgery, University of California, San Francisco, 505 Parnassus Avenue, M779, San Francisco, CA 94117, USA
[b] Department of Neurological Surgery, Comprehensive Brain Tumor Center, University of Oklahoma, 1000 North Lincoln Boulevard, Suite 400, Oklahoma City, OK 73104-5023, USA
* Corresponding author.
E-mail address: mes261@columbia.edu

tissue. Hence, these tumors are difficult to remove completely, especially when neoplastic cells spread widely throughout the brain.[6] Given these challenges, many neurosurgeons still (despite evidence to the contrary) choose to avoid this risk by instead biopsying these tumors and then radiating them.

IS NIHILISM JUSTIFIED?
The Hemispherectomy Experience

A common belief is that, regardless of radiographic appearance, gliomas disseminate widely and have often microscopically infiltrated even across to the contralateral hemisphere at initial presentation. Thus, many claim that gliomas are incurable.[4,7] As support, many authors refer back to early studies attempting to cure glioblastoma with hemispherectomy. The recurrence rates despite this approach are cited as the ultimate proof that surgery cannot definitively treat these tumors.

The most prominent report by Dandy[8] in *JAMA* in 1928 described the approach in five patients. Two of these patients died of early postsurgical complications and one was still alive at last follow-up. The remaining two patients died of recurrent tumors 3 months and 3.5 years after surgery, respectively. The patient who died at 3 months was noted to have disease extending into the basal ganglia that was intentionally not resected.[8] The patient who lived 3.5 years was in a coma at presentation and lived well beyond the present mean life expectancy despite no adjuvant therapy, which was not available in 1928.

The only other notable report, which was published in 1949, is of five patients who underwent surgery at the Cleveland Clinic.[9] One of these patients died from early postoperative complications; two died of a recurrent tumor 15 months and 3 years after surgery; one died 4 years after surgery from a traumatic brain injury; and one lived at least 10 years after surgery. After this article was published, reports about hemispherectomy in glioma become fewer, and the latest report identified was in 1975, in which the patient died from a contralateral meningioma.[10]

Given this paucity of evidence, particularly the lack of any current evidence, one cannot say what hemispherectomy would do for patients with glioma, and what it would accomplish if tried today when applied in the context of existing management paradigms. Given that most of these reports are 60 years to 80 years old and predate MRI and CT, many important facts about these patients are unknown, most notably whether these tumors were bilaterally disseminated at diagnosis, making hemispherectomy a suboptimal option. Information regarding radiographic extent of resection is also not available for these patients. 5-Aminolevulinic acid (5-ALA) certainly was not used, because operating microscopes with or without fluorescent filters were not available to visualize it. None of these patients received radiotherapy or chemotherapy. No repeat surgeries were performed for recurrence, because there was no way to detect it until the patient was near death. Many of these patients could have died of the siderosis that occurred frequently with old techniques of hemispherectomy, because no insight into this problem was available at the time, and detailed postmortems looking for this problem were not performed on many of these patients. Furthermore, the histopathologic diagnostic criteria of gliomas have changed several times since these reports. No control cohort is available with any meaningful relevance to contemporary therapy, and therefore perhaps all of these patients experience recurrence, but after many more years.

Thus, one of the key pieces of evidence dismissing glioma surgery as futile is from from decades-old case series of five or fewer patients who were managed using outdated surgical techniques, outdated diagnostic techniques, and outdated adjuvant treatment paradigms. In addition, these patients were diagnosed using outdated criteria, and had inadequate follow-up according to today's standards of evidence in surgical studies. This fact is stunning when considering the large number of patients who are denied full aggressive surgical treatment for gliomas based partly on these outdated studies.

The Tumor Cell Dissemination Story

Grade II through IV astrocytomas and oligodendrogliomas are known as infiltrating gliomas based on their long observed tendency to spread widely throughout the brain far beyond the primary site of disease. This finding was first documented by Bailey and Cushing,[11] 1926, and was most fastidiously documented by Scherer[12] in a report in 1940. In this frequently cited autopsy study of 120 patients with gliomas, Scherer concludes that, except for ependymomas, "infiltrative growth must be regarded as characteristic of the enormous majority of gliomatous tumors." He then concludes that "complete extirpation is not possible." He notes that, even in this study of postmortem gliomas, bilateral involvement with tumor was observable in only 30% of these cases.

Certainly, several autopsy studies subsequent to Scherer have shown that these tumors can spread widely, to the point that this propensity of gliomas to migrate throughout the brain in some cases is beyond debate.[13–15] The autopsy-based literature has failed, however, in a fallacy of extension. More specifically, many clinicians have concluded that because evidence shows that many gliomas demonstrate widespread microcellular dissemination at the end stage (ie, the subjects in most postmortem studies), this implies that all gliomas are widely disseminated at diagnosis, including lower-grade astrocytomas. Furthermore, it implies that these distant microcellular satellite cells are the source of the tumor that ultimately kills the patient. In this belief system, leaving the tumor behind seems perfectly reasonable, because aggressive treatment would be futile if more tumor is always extending beyond the margins of the resection.

The most prescient argument against this belief system is an observation practitioners are all familiar with, namely that most glioma recurrences, especially with low grades, occur near or within the previous resection cavity.[16,17] Studies have shown that approximately 76% of glioblastoma recurrences occur within 2 cm of the surgical resection margin.[17] This finding argues strongly that the problem with the current surgical paradigm is inadequate control of tumor at the margins, rather than the presence of distant disease, in most patients treated. Thus, the issue for most failures is inherently inadequate margins of resection, not far-flung satellite cells. This theory is further strengthened by studies showing that radiotherapy margins could be successfully reduced from whole-brain fields to fields extending just 2 cm beyond the resection bed,[5] suggesting that infiltration is largely by cells just beyond the edge of MRI-guided tumor resection cavity that cause recurrence. The radiation oncology world figured out many years ago that the problem is usually at the margins and not the whole brain.

To further show that the issue for most of these tumors, at least initially, is local treatment failure, the authors refer to four well-executed, influential, and frequently cited studies from the CT/MRI era showing the existence of infiltrating tumor cells beyond the area of radiographic tumor involvement. Although frequently cited as evidence of the futility of aggressive glioma surgery by those who have not read them closely with a critical eye, these studies in fact show that the problem is probably one of inadequate resection margins in many cases.

Salazar and Rubin, 1976
Salazar and Rubin[14] reported an autopsy study of 42 patients with glioblastoma who died shortly after diagnosis (meaning not altered by treatment), including 35 supratentorial tumors, 6 intratentorial tumors, and 2 spinal tumors. They concluded that 29 of 35 patients had tumor that extended outside the clinically expected boundary of the tumor. Of these 35 tumors, 9 had spread to the contralateral hemisphere, only 4 had spread to infratentorial structures, and 4 had spread from peripheral brain to deep structures not anticipated clinically. Of the 29 peripherally located glioblastomas, 6 crossed to the other hemisphere, 4 invaded the deep structures, and 2 invaded the infratentorial brain. Although they do not publish whether any of these patients were duplicated in these classes, the findings imply that, at worst, 48% of these patients with rapidly fatal glioblastomas had anatomic characteristics that would make aggressive surgical resection undesirable. The findings also fail to account for the fact that the study was performed on patients diagnosed in the 1950s and 1960s, when these tumors were generally caught much closer to end stage than is likely common in contemporary practice. Thus, even in the worst case scenario, many of these tumors are still not as widely disseminated as seems to be suggested in the nihilistic view.

Burger and colleagues, 1983
In perhaps one of the most interesting studies of this group, Burger and colleagues[15] focused on analyses of surgical specimens and autopsies in 20 patients with untreated high-grade gliomas (5 cases), lesions in patients experiencing remission who died of other diseases (3 cases), and recurrent tumors (12 cases), correlating pathologic findings with imaging characteristics.[15] They found that in untreated glioblastoma, although cells were present outside the area of imaging abnormality, no evidence of tumor cells could be found beyond 3 cm outside of tumor center, nor any tumor cells in the contralateral hemisphere. Similarly, lesions in remission did not show any evidence of widespread dissemination. Only at recurrence did the investigators note tumor cells spread far beyond the primary tumor site, but they also noted that the greatest concentration of tumor cells was seen locally. Together with the previous study, this suggests again that widespread dissemination is an end-stage, not primary, trait of glioblastomas in most cases.

Kelly and colleagues, 1987
By far the most influential study on this topic (cited more than 400 times) was that of Kelly and his team[18] at New York University. In this landmark study, they performed serial stereotactic biopsies both inside and outside of the tumor volume, thus obtaining 195 biopsy specimens in 40 patients, including 8 grade IV tumors, 7 grade III tumors, 17 low-grade astrocytomas, and 8 low-grade oligodendrogliomas. By doing so, they

were able to correlate MRI and CT findings with histologic specimens, and this study is widely cited as providing proof that MRI and CT underestimate the true extent of tumor involvement. More importantly, it showed that T2 changes, previously thought to be edema from the tumor, were often also tumor tissue.

This important study is frequently cited, but how many people have critically reviewed the numbers in this study is unclear, because these numbers show that regardless of grade, MRI does not miss many tumor cells. For example, of the 117 biopsies containing infiltrating tumor cells, only 18 (15%) were found in regions with a normal T1 signal. Higher sensitivity was found for T2 images, with 5 of 128 (4%) specimens with infiltrating tumor cells found in regions with a normal T2 signal. Thus, although tumor infiltration outside the area of tumor tissue does occur, critical analysis of this important data set shows that regardless of tumor grade, if the areas of abnormal T2 signal are resected, most of the infiltrating cells are removed in most patients. Furthermore, taking a slight margin is likely removing an even higher number of cells. Thus, in defining this report in a binary fashion, instead of a probabilistic one, many practitioners justified discontinuing glioma surgery.

Pallud and colleagues, 2010

Similar to the study by Kelly and colleagues,[18] Pallud and colleagues[19] reported on 16 patients with low-grade oligodendrogliomas studied with serial stereotactic biopsies performed using a rigorous paradigm. They increased their histologic yield through using mindbomb homolog 1 (MIB-1) labeling to identify mitotic cells that may have been missed by simple histology. The investigators show that although tumor cells are frequently found outside the MRI region, they are seldom found far from it in these low-grade tumors. More specifically, they did not find evidence that MIB-1–positive cells are located outside of a 2-cm perimeter around the tumor at a higher rate than in normal brain. Thus, the investigators concluded that low-grade oligodendrogliomas are locally infiltrative to approximately 2 cm but are probably not widely disseminated at initial diagnosis. This idea of the local 2- to 3-cm margin of tumor infiltration is similar to the observation of Burger and colleagues,[15] who found that these tumors are frequently locally infiltrative at diagnosis.

IS AN AGGRESSIVE SURGICAL PHILOSOPHY WARRANTED?

Based on the earlier discussion, the authors suggest that one can safely conclude that, although many gliomas are widely disseminated at end stage, sparse evidence suggests that they are always widely disseminated far beyond the imaging-defined tumor borders at initial diagnosis. At the very least, one can reasonably hypothesize that some patients present with localized lesions at diagnosis. Beyond just a simple lack of evidence, reason exists to also disbelieve that these gliomas are widely disseminated in initial stages. First, recurrent disease is classically seen as local recurrence at the margins, with multifocal disease and cerebrospinal fluid dissemination much less common. More importantly, cells distant from the primary tumor at diagnosis would lie outside of conventional radiotherapy fields, and thus distant foci would be expected to grow faster than more proximally located cells. The fact that, despite this, most recurrences occur in the margins of the lesionectomy cavity suggests that the wide-flung cells are not what kills patients with glioma, but rather the inadequately treated margins.

Furthermore, associating widespread invasion and dissemination with early-stage tumors is simply incompatible with current understanding of cancer biology, because these tumors usually need to acquire several mutations to gain those abilities, which takes time and possibly exposure to DNA-altering therapies, such as radiation and alkylating chemotherapy.[20] Regardless, with any tumor, one can logically hypothesize that outward radial spread from the primary tumor mass should lead to a decreasing probability of finding a cancer cell with increasing distance from the primary site. In other words, even if the tumor had invasive properties uniformly at initial presentation, it takes time for tumor cells to reach distant sites, and thus the probability of finding a cancer cell infiltrating seemingly normal brain is likely not equal for distant sites and the margins.

In addition, a growing body of evidence shows that aggressive lesionectomy is superior to subtotal lesionectomy and biopsy. Class 1 evidence includes the randomized experience with 5-ALA–guided resections, which showed that gross total resection conferred improved survival compared with less-aggressive lesionectomy.[21] Additionally, the landmark trial by Stupp and colleagues[3] reporting a survival benefit with temozolomide and radiotherapy over radiotherapy alone showed a 6-month survival benefit with surgery over biopsy alone in both arms of the trial, although the study did not aim to address this comparison. Meta-analyses of class 2 and 3 data have suggested that aggressive surgery confers a survival benefit regardless of grade.[2] Similarly, two recent well-executed retrospective volumetric studies have shown a survival benefit for patients with glioblastoma receiving aggressive complete or near-complete resections compared with less-aggressive resections.[22,23] A large study of low-grade astrocytomas similarly showed a stepwise improvement in 8-year survival for patients with greater than 90% resection compared with those with lesser resections (91% vs 60%).[24] In addition to extending survival, complete removal has been shown to improve seizure control in both retrospective studies and meta-analyses.[25,26] Thus, although not a cure, aggressive lesionectomy improves survival and renders biopsy and radiation alone an archaic strategy for treating most of these patients.

IS THE RISK WORTH IT?

The predominant reason surgeons provide for not aggressively attacking these tumors, and instead promoting the option of biopsy and radiation, is that they wish to avoid hurting the patient with surgery, especially because glioma is thought to be incurable. Although no studies have directly compared the quality of life between the two treatment paradigms, what follows are a list of reasons why aggressive surgery, even in many high-risk brain areas, is worth the risk in most cases.

- Most importantly, patients have the right to be offered the option of living longer (even if only slightly longer) with a deficit versus dying earlier with longer retention of function (of course with the possibility that the tumor will cause a deficit). By not even offering patients the option of aggressive resection, practitioners are making the decision for them.
- Many of the deficits surgeons are afraid to cause will happen eventually if the tumor is allowed to grow. These patients eventually stop coming to the clinic and die at home, reinforcing the idea that conservative treatment helped the patient.
- Many deficits caused by surgery improve or resolve with time and rehabilitation. Deficits caused by tumors generally get worse over time.
- Functional deficits can often be avoided with intraoperative mapping and other functional mapping.
- Often areas that practitioners are sure will cause a deficit if removed do not cause this deficit. The brain has the ability to reorganize its cortical regions over time, and sometimes this is to the patient's advantage.
- No adjuvant therapy is more likely to work on a huge tumor burden than on a small one. Thus, although not a cure, removing more cells likely improves the efficacy of these adjuvant treatments.
- Function is routinely sacrificed without a great deal of debate in several life-threatening conditions to prolong life, making aggressive glioma surgery not without precedent, such as
  o Limb amputation for gangrene, cancer,
  o Liver transplant requiring immunosuppression for liver cancer,
  o Total proctocolectomy with ostomy in patients with familial adenomatous polyposis,
  o Esophagectomy for esophageal cancer,
  o Pneumonectomy for lung cancer,
  o Large disfiguring skin resection for aggressive skin cancers,
  o Conditions such as orbital exenteration and mandibulectomy for aggressive nasopharyngeal and skull base malignancies, and
  o Sacrectomy for chordoma.
- Functional loss is considered an acceptable risk by some in the pursuit of gross total resection for several benign intracranial tumors. These losses include
  o Facial nerve palsy in vestibular schwannoma,[27–43]
  o Cranial neuropathy in skull base meningiomas,[44]
  o Carotid sacrifice and bypass for cavernous sinus meningiomas,[45,46] and
  o Sagittal sinus sacrifice and bypass for parasagittal meningiomas.[45,47]

MARGINS IN GLIOMA SURGERY

The idea of treating the margins in these tumors has been around in radiation oncology for some time, yet has never entered the neurosurgical stream of consciousness. Part of this is nihilism; people simply do not wish to push the resection beyond the imaging boundaries of the tumor for something they view is a pointless effort, especially in light of the widely held belief that even hemispherectomy has failed. Additionally, there is likely inadequate awareness that most of the tumor cells are located within 2- to 3- cm margins of the tumor. Thus, few attempts have been made to see what surgically removing gliomas with a wide margin, followed by adjuvant therapy, could accomplish, especially if that margin takes the surgeon near or into the speech or motor areas. Certainly, some cases exist in which a 3-cm margin is not worth the risk; however, the appropriate boundaries for aggressive surgery have not been studied in any significant detail, because most practitioners think that tumor cells are present all over the brain in these cases and therefore it does not make a difference.

The authors could identify two studies in which the idea of aggressively removing brain in excess of the MRI-defined lesion barrier was formally addressed. One was the 1984 study by Laws and colleagues,[48] which showed a survival benefit for patients with gliomas treated with a lobectomy over lesionectomy. Unfortunately, this interesting finding was not further fleshed out in an analysis segregating these patients by grade, so whether this is a true finding is unclear. A more recent and more convincing effort was published last year by Yordanova and colleagues,[4] who showed that using intraoperative mapping techniques to push the resection margin up to eloquent brain regions obtained a supramaximal resection with margins. Although the follow-up is modest, they reported that all patients achieved their normal preoperative neurologic function and that none experienced malignant transformation with a median follow-up of approximately 3 years (range, 1–10 years). This finding provides preliminary support for the thesis that, given that most of the infiltrating tumor cells are within 2 to 3 cm of the tumor, aggressive local therapy is the most effective approach to at least significantly reducing the number of cells an adjuvant therapy must kill.

Thus, although whether excising the primary mass with a margin will help is unclear, one can reasonably assume that in many cases it will help, or at least be better than what is currently done, which fails in nearly every case. In this paradigm, the newly diagnosed glioma is viewed as a probability function, wherein the probability of cell infiltration decreases as a function of distance from the visible tumor tissue. Certainly, this approach is consistent with the existing histologic data for many patients.

FUNDAMENTAL PROBLEMS WITH NIHILISM FOR PATIENTS WITH GLIOMA

Regardless of the uniqueness of gliomas, they still are a solid tumor, and the basic tenets of oncology still apply. Most notably, because a neoplasm is a heterogenous collection of different cell populations, an inherent percentage of cells in any given tumor are resistant, or less sensitive, to any adjuvant therapy, including radiotherapy, conventional chemotherapy, and targeted molecular therapy.[49] Despite a heterogeneous population of cells, no cell population in gliomas is resistant to surgical removal. Thus, surgical cytoreduction is the cornerstone of most successful therapies for any cancer; it dramatically reduces the number of cells that need to be destroyed by adjuvant therapy, and

thus reduces the chance of encountering a resistant cell population. Few success stories in solid tumor oncology do not begin with gross total resection of the primary lesion as a starting point. Breast, colon, lung, pancreas, stomach, ovary, and nasopharyngeal cancers and melanoma represent a few examples in which the critical role of cytoreductive surgery has been vividly shown.

Why does nihilism hurt us as tumor surgeons and researchers? Why does it hurt patients? Quite simply, it causes otherwise intelligent clinicians to follow a nonsensical treatment paradigm, thinking they are doing the patient a favor by leaving a highly malignant tumor growing in their brain, and to just treat it with a therapy that is known to have only marginal benefit in most cases.[50] It stops oncologists as a group from trying to improve techniques for removing these tumors from difficult areas, such as the thalamus, insula, and caudate,[51] because it makes it alright to quit on these patients as a specialty; "The cure will come from the laboratory.[7]"

Perhaps the cure will come from the laboratory in this lifetime; however, in the meantime, the authors argue that nihilism hurts practitioners' progress as scientists and surgeons. It has cast a cloud of doubt on every negative glioma therapy study to date, because it has forced many therapies targeting a single pathway, yielding partial benefits in simple animal studies, to take on the millions of cells in visible tumor masses, instead of the much smaller number of cells left behind by an aggressive resection with wide margins (again, the foundation of an oncologic resection). Undoubtedly, many otherwise promising drugs have been relegated to the dustbin of history after being tested on inadequately resected tumors. Secondly, nihilism has collectively allowed suboptimal glioma surgeries. With the view that glioma resection is marginally pointless, practitioners as a group reconcile with mediocrity in glioma surgery. Any tumor specialist knows exactly to what this statement refers. Practitioners have all seen cases in which 20% resection has been performed for a right frontal glioma, or tumors that have been biopsied and radiated at another center that is entirely outside eloquent tissue. Many practitioners operating on gliomas do not use microscopic visualization for these cases, even when working on tumors around delicate structures such as the middle cerebral artery, simply because they do not plan on going near these structures. Glioma surgery for many is macrosurgery, because in their eyes total removal is not a goal. Large residual tumors are common. None of these acts of sloppy thinking or sloppy surgery would be well regarded with surgery for vestibular schwannoma, yet this attitude is tolerated with glioma surgery, because many think glioma surgery does not make a difference.

CONCLUSION: THE FUTURE OF GLIOMA SURGERY

The common belief is that the cure for gliomas will come from the laboratory. Intuition suggests that these therapies are unlikely to work in a paradigm in which surgeons leave behind large amounts of tumor, hoping that the adjuvant therapy will take care of the remainder. As the neurosurgical community gradually arises out of the nihilistic sleep of the "biopsy and radiate" years and realizes that, barring a miracle cure, the only hope for gliomas therapy lies in treating small residual tumors, it will be increasingly important to approach this new era with an open mind. The authors encourage surgeons to take glioma surgery more seriously than in the past, and believe that the next natural, yet critical, step is to define the boundaries of an acceptable risk/benefit ratio in well-controlled cohorts on whom surgery is performed using modern techniques and who are treated using modern adjuvant paradigms. Surgical techniques for difficult gliomas must be refined in much the same methodical, anatomic way that meningioma surgery and vestibular schwannoma surgery have been. In short, glioma is a devastating disease, and little can be accomplished by giving up on it.

REFERENCES

1. Berger MS, Deliganis AV, Dobbins J, et al. The effect of extent of resection on recurrence in patients with low grade cerebral hemisphere gliomas. Cancer 1994;74(6):1784–91.
2. Sanai N, Berger MS. Glioma extent of resection and its impact on patient outcome. Neurosurgery 2008; 62(4):753–64 [discussion: 264–6].
3. Stupp R, Mason WP, van den Bent MJ, et al. Radiotherapy plus concomitant and adjuvant temozolomide for glioblastoma. N Engl J Med 2005;352(10): 987–96.
4. Yordanova YN, Moritz-Gasser S, Duffau H. Awake surgery for WHO Grade II gliomas within "noneloquent" areas in the left dominant hemisphere: toward a "supratotal" resection. J Neurosurg 2011; 115(2):232–9.
5. Laperriere N, Zuraw L, Cairncross G. Radiotherapy for newly diagnosed malignant glioma in adults: a systematic review. Radiother Oncol 2002;64(3): 259–73.
6. Berger MS, Rostomily RC. Low grade gliomas: functional mapping resection strategies, extent of resection, and outcome. J Neurooncol 1997;34(1):85–101.
7. Silbergeld DL, Chicoine MR. Isolation and characterization of human malignant glioma cells from histologically normal brain. J Neurosurg 1997;86(3):525–31.
8. Dandy W. Removal of the right cerebral hemisphere for certain tumors with hemiplegia: preliminary report. JAMA 1928;90(11):823–5.
9. Bell E, Karnosh L. Cerebral hemispherectomy: report of a case ten years after operation. J Neurosurg 1949;6(4):285–93.
10. Wilson PJ, Ashley DJ. Meningioma after contralateral hemispherectomy for malignant glioma: case report. J Neurol Neurosurg Psychiatry 1975;38(5): 493–9.
11. Bailey P, editor. A classification of the tumors of the glioma group on a histogenetic basis with a correlated study of prognosis. Philadelphia: JB Lippincott; 1926.
12. Scherer HJ. The forms of growth in gliomas and their practical significance. Brain 1940;63(1):1–34.
13. Marsh JS. The necropsy incidence of glioblastoma multiforme; with reference to its age and sex occurrence in a series of four hundred and twenty-three intracranial gliomas verified at autopsy. Bull Los Angel Neuro Soc 1956;21(1):27–9.
14. Salazar OM, Rubin P. The spread of glioblastoma multiforme as a determining factor in the radiation treated volume. Int J Radiat Oncol Biol Phys 1976; 1(7–8):627–37.
15. Burger PC, Dubois PJ, Schold SC Jr, et al. Computerized tomographic and pathologic studies of the untreated, quiescent, and recurrent glioblastoma multiforme. J Neurosurg 1983;58(2):159–69.
16. Gaspar LE, Fisher BJ, Macdonald DR, et al. Supratentorial malignant glioma: patterns of recurrence and implications for external beam local treatment. Int J Radiat Oncol Biol Phys 1992;24(1):55–7.
17. Wallner KE, Galicich JH, Krol G, et al. Patterns of failure following treatment for glioblastoma multiforme and anaplastic astrocytoma. Int J Radiat Oncol Biol Phys 1989;16(6):1405–9.
18. Kelly PJ, Daumas-Duport C, Kispert DB, et al. Imaging-based stereotaxic serial biopsies in untreated intracranial glial neoplasms. J Neurosurg 1987;66(6):865–74.
19. Pallud J, Varlet P, Devaux B, et al. Diffuse low-grade oligodendrogliomas extend beyond MRI-defined abnormalities. Neurology 2010;74(21):1724–31.
20. Talmadge JE, Fidler IJ. AACR centennial series: the biology of cancer metastasis: historical perspective. Cancer Res 2010;70(14):5649–69.
21. Stummer W, Pichlmeier U, Meinel T, et al. Fluorescence-guided surgery with 5-aminolevulinic acid for resection of malignant glioma: a randomised controlled multicentre phase III trial. Lancet Oncol 2006;7(5):392–401.
22. Sanai N, Polley MY, McDermott MW, et al. An extent of resection threshold for newly diagnosed glioblastomas. J Neurosurg 2011;115(1):3–8.

23. Lacroix M, Abi-Said D, Fourney DR, et al. A multivariate analysis of 416 patients with glioblastoma multiforme: prognosis, extent of resection, and survival. J Neurosurg 2001;95(2):190–8.

24. Smith JS, Chang EF, Lamborn KR, et al. Role of extent of resection in the long-term outcome of low-grade hemispheric gliomas. J Clin Oncol 2008; 26(8):1338–45.

25. Chang EF, Potts MB, Keles GE, et al. Seizure characteristics and control following resection in 332 patients with low-grade gliomas. J Neurosurg 2008;108(2):227–35.

26. Englot DJ, Berger MS, Barbaro NM, et al. Predictors of seizure freedom after resection of supratentorial low-grade gliomas. J Neurosurg 2011;115(2):240–4.

27. Sughrue ME, Kaur R, Rutkowski MJ, et al. Extent of resection and the long-term durability of vestibular schwannoma surgery. J Neurosurg 2011;114(5): 1218–23.

28. Jian BJ, Sughrue ME, Kaur R, et al. Implications of cystic features in vestibular schwannomas of patients undergoing microsurgical resection. Neurosurgery 2011;68(4):874–80 [discussion: 879–80].

29. Sughrue ME, Kaur R, Rutkowski MJ, et al. A critical evaluation of vestibular schwannoma surgery for patients younger than 40 years of age. Neurosurgery 2010;67(6):1646–53 [discussion: 1653–4].

30. Sughrue ME, Yang I, Rutkowski MJ, et al. Preservation of facial nerve function after resection of vestibular schwannoma. Br J Neurosurg 2010;24(6):666–71.

31. Bloch O, Sughrue ME, Kaur R, et al. Factors associated with preservation of facial nerve function after surgical resection of vestibular schwannoma. J Neurooncol 2011;102(2):281–6.

32. Sughrue ME, Yang I, Aranda D, et al. Hearing preservation rates after microsurgical resection of vestibular schwannoma. J Clin Neurosci 2010;17(9): 1126–9.

33. Sughrue ME, Kaur R, Kane AJ, et al. Intratumoral hemorrhage and fibrosis in vestibular schwannoma: a possible mechanism for hearing loss. J Neurosurg 2011;114(2):386–93.

34. Sughrue ME, Kane AJ, Kaur R, et al. A prospective study of hearing preservation in untreated vestibular schwannomas. J Neurosurg 2011;114(2):381–5.

35. Sughrue ME, Kaur R, Kane AJ, et al. The value of intraoperative facial nerve electromyography in predicting facial nerve function after vestibular schwannoma surgery. J Clin Neurosci 2010;17(7):849–52.

36. Sughrue ME, Yang I, Han SJ, et al. Non-audiofacial morbidity after Gamma Knife surgery for vestibular schwannoma. Neurosurg Focus 2009;27(6):E4.

37. Yeung AH, Sughrue ME, Kane AJ, et al. Radiobiology of vestibular schwannomas: mechanisms of radioresistance and potential targets for therapeutic sensitization. Neurosurg Focus 2009;27(6):E2.

38. Sughrue ME, Yang I, Aranda D, et al. Beyond audiofacial morbidity after vestibular schwannoma surgery. J Neurosurg 2011;114(2):367–74.

39. Sughrue ME, Yeung AH, Rutkowski MJ, et al. Molecular biology of familial and sporadic vestibular schwannomas: implications for novel therapeutics. J Neurosurg 2011;114(2):359–66.

40. Yang I, Sughrue ME, Han SJ, et al. A comprehensive analysis of hearing preservation after radiosurgery for vestibular schwannoma. J Neurosurg 2010; 112(4):851–9.

41. Sughrue ME, Yang I, Aranda D, et al. The natural history of untreated sporadic vestibular schwannomas: a comprehensive review of hearing outcomes. J Neurosurg 2010;112(1):163–7.

42. Yang I, Sughrue ME, Han SJ, et al. Facial nerve preservation after vestibular schwannoma Gamma Knife radiosurgery. J Neurooncol 2009;93(1):41–8.

43. Yang I, Aranda D, Han SJ, et al. Hearing preservation after stereotactic radiosurgery for vestibular schwannoma: a systematic review. J Clin Neurosci 2009;16(6):742–7.

44. Langevin CJ, Hanasono MM, Riina HA, et al. Lateral transzygomatic approach to sphenoid wing meningiomas. Neurosurgery 2010;67(2 Suppl Operative): 377–84.

45. Sindou M, Mazoyer JF, Fischer G, et al. Experimental bypass for sagittal sinus repair. Preliminary report. J Neurosurg 1976;44(3):325–30.

46. Liu JK, Couldwell WT. Interpositional carotid artery bypass strategies in the surgical management of aneurysms and tumors of the skull base. Neurosurg Focus 2003;14(3):e2.

47. Sindou M, Hallacq P. Venous reconstruction in surgery of meningiomas invading the sagittal and transverse sinuses. Skull Base Surg 1998;8(2):57–64.

48. Laws ER Jr, Taylor WF, Clifton MB, et al. Neurosurgical management of low-grade astrocytoma of the cerebral hemispheres. J Neurosurg 1984;61(4):665–73.

49. Axtell AE, Lee MH, Bristow RE, et al. Multi-institutional reciprocal validation study of computed tomography predictors of suboptimal primary cytoreduction in patients with advanced ovarian cancer. J Clin Oncol 2007;25(4):384–9.

50. Kreth FW, Warnke PC, Scheremet R, et al. Surgical resection and radiation therapy versus biopsy and radiation therapy in the treatment of glioblastoma multiforme. J Neurosurg 1993;78(5):762–6.

51. Bernstein M, Hoffman HJ, Halliday WC, et al. Thalamic tumors in children. Long-term follow-up and treatment guidelines. J Neurosurg 1984;61(4): 649–56.

The Use of Motor Mapping to Aid Resection of Eloquent Gliomas

Bryan D. Choi, AB[a,b,*], Ankit I. Mehta, MD[a],
Kristen A. Batich, BA[b], Allan H. Friedman, MD[a],
John H. Sampson, MD, PhD, MHSc[a,b]

KEYWORDS

- Neurosurgery • Brain mapping • Glioma • Motor cortex

One of the oldest and still most important forms of treatment available for patients with glioma is surgery. Even in the contemporary milieu of multimodal regimens, including radiotherapy and chemotherapy, glioma resection remains a mainstay, given its central role in establishing a histologic diagnosis and in relieving symptoms of mass effect by mechanical cytoreduction.[1] In addition, mounting clinical data reinforce the conventional notion that a greater extent of resection can improve outcomes and prolong life expectancy.[2–6]

As is the case for all solid tumors, the advantages of surgical resection for glioma must also be balanced with the potential risks of operative morbidity, and, as such, a great deal of focus in neurosurgical oncology is placed on minimizing collateral damage to surrounding eloquent brain.

Central to performing minimally morbid surgery is a thorough understanding of neuroanatomy and physiology in the region of interest. Given that primary central nervous system (CNS) tumors are highly infiltrative, display variable gross appearance, and may incorporate functional brain, the measures and observations that are used to plan a surgical approach must be diverse and must possess great precision. To that end, functional brain mapping allows the pursuance of safer operations with more aggressive surgical resections; these techniques include "gold standard" procedures such as direct electrical stimulation as well as newer, less invasive imaging technologies that can be integrated into preoperative planning processes as well as intraoperative decision making.

The first region of the brain to be mapped was the motor cortex. Many strategies to refine surgical approaches have been developed to minimize damage to motor cortex and motor fibers. Although similar principles have since been applied to the preservation of sensory, language, and memory functions, the mapping of motor pathways in the context of intracranial malignancy is a unique entity and thus poses a distinct set of risks and challenges. As reviewed herein, the history and background of motor mapping techniques are discussed, along with the current state of functional motor mapping in neurosurgical oncology and the potential implications of complementary technologies on the surgical management of patients with glioma.

EARLY WORK ON THE MOTOR CORTEX

Cerebral localization of function is one of the most fascinating and controversial topics in neurologic history. The first observation that control over motor function could be lateralized in the brain dates back to the fifth century BC, when the ancient Greek physician Hippocrates noted that unilateral cerebral injury results in contralateral paralysis.[7] Over the next 2 millennia, there was little written

[a] Division of Neurosurgery, Department of Surgery, Duke University Medical Center, 200 Trent Drive, Room 4517, Busse Building, Durham, NC 27710, USA
[b] Department of Pathology, Duke University Medical Center, Box 3712, Durham, NC 27710, USA
* Corresponding author. Department of Pathology, Duke University Medical Center, Box 3712, Durham, NC 27710.
E-mail address: bryan.choi@duke.edu

Neurosurg Clin N Am 23 (2012) 215–225
doi:10.1016/j.nec.2012.01.013

to explain this phenomenon. Interest in cerebral physiology instead seemed to be fixated on a philosophic discussion of the brain as "the seat of the soul." It was not until the early nineteenth century that this focus began to shift toward a more localized or segmental view of brain functions, largely due to theories of phrenology set forth by Franz Joseph Gall (1758–1828). Although Gall was heavily criticized by those who believed his work to be pseudoscience and damaging to religion, he was nevertheless instrumental in altering thinking in the field.

The latter part of the nineteenth century fostered a series of seminal clinical discoveries related to specific localization of function in the cortex, beginning with John Hughlings Jackson's assertion in 1864 that "the convolutions of the brain must contain nervous arrangements representing movements."[8] In 1870, the German neurologist Gustav Fritsch and an anatomist Eduard Hitzig[9] performed the first experiment demonstrating that topographically restricted electrical stimuli could be applied to the mammalian cerebral cortex to elicit corresponding contralateral movements. Although perhaps less well recognized, these findings were shortly followed by the first recorded experience with direct electrical stimulation of the human brain by Robert Bartholow in 1874,[10] who, inspired by localized testing on animal brains by contemporary David Ferrier, attempted to elicit sensory and motor responses by applying wires to the exposed dura of a patient who had a hole in her skull caused by a cancerous ulcer.

The earliest maps that depicted specific localization of motor control in the human cortex were based on findings from Ferrier's work with monkeys, in which recordings of movements in response to cortical stimulation were grossly transferred to an outline of the human brain. These maps, along with a map developed by the surgeon Horsley,[11] which was also based on experiments on monkeys and limited observations in humans, were the first of their kind to be included in Gray's Anatomy in 1887.

In 1901, Harvey Cushing, at an early stage in his career, began to map the primate motor cortex with Charles Sherrington and by 1909 had published numerous reports on his experience with intraoperative faradic stimulation in patients being operated under local anesthesia, thus confirming somatotopy of the human cortex along the precentral and postcentral gyri.[12–14] Advances in functional cortical localization were also enhanced significantly by Otfrid Foerster,[8] who, through close collaboration with Oskar and Cécile Vogt, developed a broader, more complex human cortical map from the observations he made during surgeries for patients with epilepsy. In 1928, Wilder Penfield[15] traveled to Germany, which marked the beginning of his collaborative work with Foerster. Over the next decade, Penfield performed extensive intraoperative investigations that would ultimately shape the modern understanding of cortical organization; synthesizing data from more than 163 craniotomies, Penfield eventually simplified his findings in a proverbial homunculus cartoon to convey the relative cortical representation of various anatomic parts.

With a special emphasis on mapping, the pioneers in cortical localization tended to perceive the brain as a collection of discrete functional areas. The original observations of Sherrington and Cushing suggested that the motor cortex is delimited within a narrow precentral strip, a legacy that can still be appreciated in modern anatomy textbooks; however, this degree of localization has perhaps been overemphasized in spite of abundant scientific evidence to support the finding that sensorimotor function is in fact broader and has overlapping cortical representations. Regardless, over the past 150 years, the advancements made by forefathers in neurosurgery initiated an exponential increase in the understanding of cortical representations; the original mapping techniques used by Penfield and others, which involved continuous stimulation for 1 to 6 seconds with a 60-Hz line frequency,[16] set a standard for performing intraoperative neurophysiologic examinations based on the electrical excitability of the human brain, and many original principles of electrocortical stimulation (ECS) remain largely unchanged in current practice.

PRINCIPLES OF DIRECT CORTICAL STIMULATION

The application of ECS as a tool for functional manipulation is based on the resting membrane potential of a neuron, which varies between −60 and −100 mV because of the asymmetrical distribution of charges across the lipid layers of the cell membrane. When the membrane is depolarized (in this case, via local application of an electrode), an action potential is generated. Membrane depolarization is a binary event that, once triggered, exhibits consistent characteristics regardless of the stimulation parameters.

The first and primary concern for ECS is safety, given that electrical stimulation to the cerebral parenchyma can lead to neural damage through multiple possible mechanisms. In addition to the direct effects of power dissipation (ie, heat) on surrounding tissues, prolonged application of electrical current may also result in the toxic accumulation of negative charge at the cathode and electrode dissolution products at the anode.[17]

To address this risk, biphasic impulses are recommended, which compensate for relative depolarization and hyperpolarization of pericathodic and perianodic tissues.[18] In addition, rectangular impulses are used to offset the phenomenon of accommodation, which otherwise occurs when membrane potentials depolarize gradually.

Perhaps the greatest risk of ECS is the induction of seizure. After stimulation, neurons are transiently refractory for 0.6 to 2.0 minutes, after which they enter a short phase of hyperexcitability and are thus at greater risk for unintentional depolarization; in one study, prolonged 60-Hz stimulation produced clinical or subclinical seizures in more than 20% of patients.[19] Most such events are minor or self-limiting, and some have found that the seizures can be terminated more quickly by application of cold Ringer lactate to the cortex.[20] Furthermore, owing to its overall safety, it has been demonstrated that in the absence of epileptiform activity, repeated stimulation with impulses of the magnitude used for motor mapping do not induce permanent histologic changes in the human cortex,[21] and functionality returns to normal levels almost immediately after removal of the stimulus.

Aside from safety, the most valuable characteristics for any method of ECS are reproducibility and precision. Electrical stimuli are characterized in detail by plotting their ability to elicit a tissue response (in this case, neuron excitability). The ideal stimulus, with regard to intensity and duration, at which an action potential is triggered with minimal energy input is termed chronaxis. Chronaxis, by definition, is the shortest duration of an effective electrical stimulus that is equal to twice the minimum strength required for neuronal excitation (rheobasis).[22] These parameters are inherently dependent on the impedance of the tissue being stimulated, which in turn can vary significantly as a function of anesthesia and local pathologic condition, such as tumor.

Factors that affect the precision of depolarizing impulses and thus the spatial resolution of ECS include electrode size and spacing, the type of electrodes that are used, and the current level. Although 2 electrodes are always necessary for producing a current, stimulation is considered to be monopolar when a single electrode is localized to the target tissue and the second grounding electrode is placed at some distance from the site of stimulation.[23,24] Although some assert that the placement of a monopolar electrode is physically unambiguous and thus more precise, pathway of the current from a monopolar source may be less predictable than that from the bipolar approach, in which both the cathode and anode are located close to the target tissue and evoked changes are confined to an elliptical area based on the electrodes.[25–28] However, most recent evidence suggests that this perception of bipolar stimulation may not be completely accurate because the threshold of activation in the region of the cortex between electrodes has been demonstrated to be significantly greater than the areas directly beneath the anode and cathode.[29] There is a relative dearth of literature directly comparing bipolar with monopolar stimulation; however, findings suggest that bipolar mapping is more sensitive in localizing functionality for certain areas such as the premotor frontal cortex.[30] Despite evolving interest in the use of monopolar cortical stimulation for mapping,[24,31,32] bipolar electrodes nonetheless remain standard and tend to be generally preferred in practice.

Current Density Distribution Generated by ECS

Despite the extensive use of ECS both clinically and experimentally, there are relatively few data available concerning what specific cells or parts of cells in the CNS are being activated.[33,34] Although surgeons may generally have a greater interest in the behavioral consequences of stimulation, studies should be communicated in such a way to allow interpretation of findings on a cellular level. Because of uncertainties in tissue properties and geometry, the various numerical models that have been developed to describe the relationship between current density and distance from an electrode are expected to represent only crude predictions. Generally, it is thought that the amount of current applied to a given neuron is directly proportional to the square of the distance between the neuron and the electrode tip.[35] Models that predict distribution of local potential are based on the solution of the Laplace equation:

$$\nabla(\sigma \nabla V) = 0$$

where V is the scalar potential, σ is the conductivity, and ∇ is the gradient vector. Assuming uniform conductivity,

$$\sigma\left(\frac{\partial^2 V}{\partial x^2} + \frac{\partial^2 V}{\partial y^2} + \frac{\partial^2 V}{\partial z^2}\right) = 0$$

with boundary conditions (1) $V = V_o$ and (2) the derivative of the scalar potential is zero at all other points. In this way, the electric fields and current density can be derived as

$$E = -\nabla V$$

$$J = \sigma E$$

where E is the electric field and J is the current density.[27]

The lowest current threshold sites for evoking motor responses from the cortex have been demonstrated to be between layers II and V of the cortex, and, as such, most unit activity is likely encountered when current is applied to layers II, III, and V (ie, the laminae that contain pyramidal cells).[34] On applying an electrical stimulus to the gray matter, recent studies have suggested that axons, but not cell bodies, are primarily activated; however, this area continues to be an active area of research.[36]

ECS MAPPING AND IDENTIFICATION OF ROLANDIC CORTEX

Few modifications have been made to Penfield's original method for mapping the functional motor cortex by ECS.[37–42] Mapping of the motor cortex can occur in the presence or absence of general anesthesia without muscle relaxants; however, in the case in which the patient is awake, both muscle activation and inhibition can be investigated, as negative motor phenomena may assist in the identification of associative areas.[43] In typical present day practice, bipolar electrodes are applied to the cortex, delivering a biphasic square wave pulse between contacts spaced approximately 5 mm apart. During stimulation, cortical areas that correspond to movements are notated and spared during resection; to supplement gross observation, electromyographic (EMG) recordings can also be monitored to increase sensitivity for detecting even low-amplitude muscle responses or when mapping under general anesthesia.[19,44] Motor evoked potentials as measured by EMG may be especially useful when using high-frequency monopolar stimulation or when performing continuous monitoring as with the train of 5 techniques.[45]

Because gliomas may invade cortical as well as subcortical structures, functional boundaries along pathways running in the white matter must also be determined.[46–48] Direct electrical stimulation can also be used in these areas to successfully identify and spare descending white motor tracts.[49–51] Although relatively fewer studies specifically address the subject of identifying deep fibers during tumor resection, recent literature suggests that when both cortical and subcortical sites are delineated with direct stimulation, the boundaries of resection can be safely identified with an acceptable risk of postoperative morbidity. The caveat is that electrical stimulation does not predict deficits secondary to stroke from injury of perforating blood vessels. Stroke occurs more commonly in the white than in the gray matter.

Identification of the Central Sulcus Using Phase Reversal of Somatosensory Evoked Potentials

Through an indirect approach, the central sulcus can be identified by phase reversal of somatosensory evoked potentials (SEP-PR), a method that was first described in surgeries for patients with epilepsy by Goldring and colleagues[52,53] in the 1970s. Since then, several studies have demonstrated the utility of SEP-PR in cortical mapping during tumor resection.[23,54–64] The concept of phase reversal is based on the perceived direction of an afferent neural volley's dipole as detected from the postcentral or precentral sulcus; that is to say, a somatosensory potential recorded from the sensory cortex is the mirror image of the potential detected from the motor cortex. This phenomenon is related to the orientation of pyramidal cells located in the postcentral sulcus, such that somatosensory evoked potentials are negative posteriorly and positive anteriorly.

The physical coordinates that correspond to the point of phase reversal are determined intraoperatively by a strip electrode placed perpendicularly to the approximated central sulcus. After peripheral nerve stimulation, somatosensory evoked potentials are assessed, and the strip grid is adjusted until clear phase reversal of the N20/P20 peak is observed between a pair of electrodes, indicating that the primary motor and sensory cortical areas are located anteriorly and posteriorly, respectively. Using these techniques, SEP-PR localizes the central sulcus, with a success rate greater than 90%, with only occasional failures attributed to the influence of edema or lesions on mass effect and inaccurate placement of the strip grid.[23,62,65] Electrodes may also be placed directly on the surface of the brain for more general purposes. Although traditionally used for defining epileptogenic foci, electrocorticography has recently been suggested as a possible method for motor mapping, based on perceptible changes in power across higher spectral frequencies, also termed the χ-index.[66] Noninvasive electroencephalography has also been shown to provide high-quality signals for high gamma power changes during motor activity.[67]

When combined with ECS, the application of SEP-PR for intraoperative localization has demonstrated a clear impact on preserving function in the resection of low-grade glioma.[50,68,69] Direct cortical stimulation yields excellent spatial resolution, and the predictive value of these techniques for mapping functional motor cortex is well characterized. Several limitations persist, however, and perhaps the most obvious drawback of these approaches is their inherent invasiveness and requirement for a craniotomy, factors that preclude their use in preoperative evaluation and planning.

Transcranial Stimulation

Transcranial magnetic stimulation (TMS) refers to the use of a magnetic field applied across the scalp and cranium to create a corresponding perpendicular electric field, which can then be used to stimulate or inhibit neuronal activity. This technique is closely related to earlier attempts at transcranial electrical stimulation; however, TMS is generally favored because of the untoward effects that direct current has when passing through superficial tissues and associated pain receptors.[70] Broadly, transcranial approaches possess the significant advantage of generating anatomofunctional information without the need for invasive technique.[71] A growing body of literature suggests that TMS before tumor resection correlates with intraoperative ECS mapping and may be a reliable tool for preoperative mapping of motor function.[72–74]

Like ECS, TMS stimulates specific regions of the brain and thus carries the risk of causing seizures on repetitive pulsing.[75] Furthermore, as with all methods that attempt to map functionality solely based on the causal relationship between stimulation and motor response, TMS and ECS may not comprehensively identify other supportive areas involved in performance, areas which may only be elicited when a patient is subject to a behavioral paradigm.

OBSERVATIONAL MAPPING TECHNIQUES

The development of newer, less invasive approaches to functional mapping has provided neurosurgeons with an unprecedented array of options to use both as alternatives and adjuncts to traditional methods of direct cortical stimulation. When combined with data from intraoperative ECS, perioperative functional neuroimaging has the potential to greatly enhance the general understanding of both neuroanatomical and physiologic associations that a specific lesion might have with surrounding eloquent brain. Moreover, such imaging modalities possess the additional capacity to define regions of the brain that may only be recruited during a motor task, areas which might otherwise be difficult to determine solely based on direct activation through stimulation.

Functional imaging for motor mapping is rapidly gaining traction in the clinical setting, and several forms of technology are currently available, each of which relies on detection of specific types of alterations and the various physiologic properties thereof. The multitude of neuroimaging modalities being developed toward this end include functional magnetic resonance imaging (fMRI), positron emission tomography (PET), magnetoencephalography (MEG), and diffusion tensor imaging (DTI); a description of each is presented in the later discussion and also briefly summarized in **Table 1**.

fMRI

Concomitant with neuronal activity is an increase of blood flow through local cerebral vessels. These changes in cerebral blood flow can be visualized by a method of fMRI that measures blood oxygen level–dependent (BOLD) variations in the area of interest. Because the ratio of oxyhemoglobin to deoxyhemoglobin increases as blood perfusion meets neuronal demand and because this change leads to perceptible elevation in T2 signal, data from BOLD analyses can be used to identify an area of the brain that is active during a particular task as a ratio over control levels observed at rest.[76,77] A map of BOLD activity is then superimposed on a conventional MRI scan to reveal detailed location of the signal relative to the adjacent neuroanatomy.

Depending on the magnitude and rate of neuronal depolarization, signal as measured by fMRI has been shown to vary proportionally[78,79] with a typical spatial resolution of 2 to 5 mm[80];

Table 1
Summary of motor mapping techniques

Modality	Type	Spatial Resolution	Temporal Resolution	Invasiveness
ECS	Stimulation	■ ■ ■	■ ■ ■	■ ■ ■
TMS	Stimulation	■	■ ■ ■	■ ■
PET	Observation	■	■	■ ■
fMRI	Observation	■ ■	■ ■	■
MEG	Observation	■ ■	■ ■ ■	■
DTI	Observation	■ ■	■ ■	■

however, these data may be confounded by technical limitations, including motion-related artifacts and predominant signal from macrovascular venous drainage.[81] Furthermore, because fMRI does not directly detect neuronal activity, instead relying on changes in cerebral blood flow as a surrogate, factors that disrupt normal hemodynamic physiology (eg, lesions, medication, general attentiveness) may ultimately reduce the specificity of analysis and lead to misinterpretation of the acquired data. Early studies suggested that fMRI, when used alone to map functional regions (ie, without support from intraoperative ECS), might be associated with higher incidences of new postoperative neurologic deficits.[82] Conversely, several centers have validated fMRI against ECS in the identification of motor areas with nearly universal agreement between the 2 modalities.[83–86]

Despite the fact that indications and parameters for the use of fMRI are still developing, the role of fMRI in neurosurgical oncology has rapidly expanded, given that it provides many advantages; these include its completely noninvasive nature, ease of acquirement, and its specific ability to localize neuronal activation in deep cortical sulci or other areas that may not be readily accessible by standard cortical stimulation. In current practice, fMRI is successfully integrated as an adjunctive mapping modality in most neuro-oncological cases[87]; for example, one recent prospective study reported that inclusion of fMRI findings in the surgical plan altered treatment approaches and increased the extent of tumor resection for more than 40% of patients.[88] One major shortcoming of fMRI is that it does not map white matter pathways.

PET

Much like fMRI, PET also has the capability to assess changes in cerebral blood flow as a surrogate for neuronal activation and can similarly be used to map motor areas before tumor resection.[89–91] Imaging with PET, however, relies on the administration of a radioactive tracer, such as ^{15}O in the form of $H_2^{15}O$, the relative abundance of which indicates an area of increased cerebral perfusion. Radioactive molecules can also be administered in the form of fluorodeoxyglucose F 18, a glucose analogue that, once injected, is retained by tissues with high metabolic activity (ie, tissues found in tumors or, for the purposes of functional mapping, areas of the brain that are activated during task performance).[92]

One possible advantage accompanying PET is the ability to grade a tumor and simultaneously perform motor mapping during a single session.[93]

As an imaging modality, PET scanning continues to develop. However, its general clinical use is hindered by technical drawbacks, including poor signal-to-noise ratio, moderate spatiotemporal resolution, and undesirable, albeit low level, radiation exposure. Nevertheless, a broad range of emerging applications for this technology exists, and successful attempts at integration into neuronavigational guidance systems have recently been demonstrated.[94]

MEG

On performing a behavioral paradigm or motor task, synchronized neuronal currents in the cerebrum induce the production of weak orthogonal magnetic fields, which can then be recorded by a biomagnetometer as an MEG signal. Because data during MEG are measured extracranially, the actual location of electrical activity must be estimated based on models that take into account prior knowledge of functional cerebral anatomy. This requirement leads to some inherent ambiguity and thus variable resolution depending on the model used; however, several studies report a generally high degree of correlation for MEG mapping with intraoperative ECS,[44,95–98] and coregistration of these technologies has been integrated into stereotactic databases to support preoperative planning and intraoperative neuronavigation in multiple settings.[99–102]

Perhaps the most demanding aspect of MEG technology is that the magnitude of signal derived from ionic flow within brain tissue is exceedingly weak. Therefore, great efforts must be made to minimize influence of external sources, including the earth's natural geomagnetism and other magnetic fields that are produced by standard hospital equipment. The need for specialized personnel and heavily shielded rooms makes the purchase and maintenance of an MEG apparatus extremely costly, thereby restricting its current availability and hampering its implementation in common practice.

Anisotropic DTI

Recent developments in DTI have made it possible to visualize the trajectory of subcortical white matter bundles, as well as to obtain data regarding the potential effects of proximal neoplasms on the integrity of these tracts. The diffusion of water molecules throughout the cerebrum is anisotropic (ie, flow is directionally dependent) and is greatest along vectors tangential rather than perpendicular to axon fibers.[103] As a molecule of water moves along a neural fiber, MRI is used to derive the direction of maximum diffusivity, which in turn is used to determine the orientation of the major principle axis of white matter tracts traversing each voxel.

Disruption of normal anisotropic patterns can be detected in the presence of a tumor because of the effects that neoplastic lesions have on water molecule diffusivity. Signals, as evaluated by DTI, can be altered either in intensity or position, and variations in these parameters may suggest different pathologies. For example, a decreased signal with normal direction and location is thought to indicate vasogenic edema, whereas displaced or complete loss of anisotropy may correspond to mass effect or obliteration of white matter anatomy by direct tumor infiltration.[104]

Because DTI does not independently provide functional data per se, its use in motor mapping is often in conjunction with ECS[105] or fMRI.[106–110] This coregistration allows the neurosurgeon to approximate fibers spatially that are associated with cortical areas and other eloquent tissues involved in motion or task execution. In current practice, structural data from diffuse tensor analyses are more commonly used in the preoperative setting; however, a few recent studies have integrated DTI with intraoperative neuronavigational systems with some success.[111,112]

Although DTI is the only available technology specifically designed to image white matter, its widespread clinical use has been hindered by certain technical limitations including poor signal-to-noise ratio and spatial resolution.[113] Furthermore, although DTI reliably visualizes major subcortical structures with relative ease, some reports suggest that it is a less consistent imaging modality for other areas, including the optic tract, fornix, and tapetum.[104]

SURGICAL CONSIDERATIONS FOR FUNCTIONAL MOTOR MAPPING

As discussed earlier, various complementary techniques are available for use in motor mapping, each of which uses a separate set of electrophysiologic principles, thus yielding distinct types of data to assist in the preparation and execution of an operative approach. The clinical use of these technologies is increasing dramatically in neurooncology, thus meeting the need to tailor treatment according to anatomofunctionality that can be significantly altered because of the presence of space-occupying lesions in and around the area of interest. It has been shown, for example, that motor-associated cortex may be unpredictably displaced by tumors located in perirolandic areas, either as a result of direct mass effect or from cortical plasticity associated with compensatory cerebral reorganization of function in and around the lesion.[107,114]

Although combinatorial imaging for preoperative motor mapping clearly possesses multiple applications, perhaps the greatest challenge in optimizing the information gleaned from these studies is the concept of brain shift. Because of mechanical and physiologic strain that occurs during a neurosurgical operation (eg, edema, cerebrospinal fluid and blood loss, body position), the position of the brain can change significantly, leading to anatomic discrepancies with preoperative imaging of more than 1 cm within the first hour of surgery.[115–118] Moreover, these changes have been shown to variably affect cortical anatomy and deeper subcortical structures, further hindering extrapolation of preoperative data to intraoperative relevance.[119] Given the dynamic character of peritumoral cortical organization, strategies have been developed to combine intraoperative imaging with preoperative data to account brain shift phenomena[120]; however, despite these advances, the classical method of direct intraoperative mapping with ECS still remains paramount.

SUMMARY

The landscape of technologies available to assist in the planning and execution of safe maximal tumor resection is rapidly expanding. Although the traditional approach of motor mapping by direct ECS is still the most widely applied technique, the clinical use of newer, less invasive imaging modalities such as fMRI and DTI is currently evolving and has in many cases been successfully implemented with varying degrees of validation; similar advances are also being explored in the mapping of sensory, language, and cognitive functions with promises of enhancing care and improving outcome after surgery. In the future, it will fall to neurosurgeons to gain familiarity with these widely complementary sources; the rapid synthesis and interpretation of such abundant and highly processed material will be necessary to realize its great potential and to translate benefits directly to patient care.

REFERENCES

1. Shapiro WR. Treatment of neuroectodermal brain tumors. Ann Neurol 1982;12:231–7.
2. Sanai N, Berger MS. Glioma extent of resection and its impact on patient outcome. Neurosurgery 2008;62:753–64 [discussion: 264–6].
3. Ammirati M, Vick N, Liao YL, et al. Effect of the extent of surgical resection on survival and quality of life in patients with supratentorial glioblastomas

and anaplastic astrocytomas. Neurosurgery 1987; 21:201–6.

4. Ciric I, Ammirati M, Vick N, et al. Supratentorial gliomas: surgical considerations and immediate postoperative results. Gross total resection versus partial resection. Neurosurgery 1987;21:21–6.

5. Hirakawa K, Suzuki K, Ueda S, et al. Multivariate analysis of factors affecting postoperative survival in malignant astrocytoma. Importance of DNA quantification. J Neurooncol 1984;2:331–40.

6. Yordanova YN, Moritz-Gasser S, Duffau H. Awake surgery for WHO Grade II gliomas within "nonelo-quent" areas in the left dominant hemisphere: toward a "supratotal" resection. Clinical article. J Neurosurg 2011;115:232–9.

7. Ballance C. A glimpse into the history of the surgery of the brain. Lancet 1922;1:111–6.

8. Foerster O. The motor cortex in man in the light of Hughlings Jackson's doctrines. Brain 1936;59: 135–59.

9. Fritsch G, Hitzig E. Electric excitability of the cere-brum (Uber die elektrische erregbarkeit des gros-shirns). Epilepsy Behav 2009;15:123–30.

10. Harris LJ, Almerigi JB. Probing the human brain with stimulating electrodes: the story of Roberts Bartholow's (1874) experiment on Mary Rafferty. Brain Cogn 2009;70:92–115.

11. Horsley V. Remarks on ten consecutive cases of operations upon the brain and cranial cavity to illustrate the details and safety of the method em-ployed. Br Med J 1887;1:863–5.

12. Thomas HM, Cushing H. Removal of a subcortical cystic tumor at a second-stage operation without anesthesia. JAMA 1908;50:847–56.

13. Cushing H. A note upon the faradic stimulation of the postcentral gyrus in conscious patients. Brain 1909;32:44–53.

14. Cushing H. III. Partial hypophysectomy for acro-megaly: with remarks on the function of the hypophysis. Ann Surg 1909;50:1002–17.

15. Penfield W, Boldrey E. Somatic motor and sensory representation in the cerebral cortex of man as studied by electrical stimulation. Brain 1937;60: 389–443.

16. Penfield W, Perot P. The brain's record of auditory and visual experience. A final summary and discus-sion. Brain 1963;86:595–696.

17. Agnew WF, McCreery DB. Considerations for safety in the use of extracranial stimulation for motor evoked potentials. Neurosurgery 1987;20: 143–7.

18. Jayakar P. Physiological principles of electrical stimulation. Adv Neurol 1993;63:17–27.

19. Yingling CD, Ojemann S, Dodson B, et al. Identifi-cation of motor pathways during tumor surgery facilitated by multichannel electromyographic recording. J Neurosurg 1999;91:922–7.

20. Sartorius CJ, Berger MS. Rapid termination of intra-operative stimulation-evoked seizures with applica-tion of cold Ringer's lactate to the cortex. Technical note. J Neurosurg 1998;88:349–51.

21. Gordon B, Lesser RP, Rance NE, et al. Parameters for direct cortical electrical stimulation in the human: histopathologic confirmation. Electroence-phalogr Clin Neurophysiol 1990;75:371–7.

22. Jayakar P, Alvarez LA, Duchowny MS, et al. A safe and effective paradigm to functionally map the cortex in childhood. J Clin Neurophysiol 1992;9:288–93.

23. Cedzich C, Taniguchi M, Schafer S, et al. Somato-sensory evoked potential phase reversal and direct motor cortex stimulation during surgery in and around the central region. Neurosurgery 1996;38: 962–70.

24. Taniguchi M, Cedzich C, Schramm J. Modification of cortical stimulation for motor evoked potentials under general anesthesia: technical description. Neurosurgery 1993;32:219–26.

25. Haglund MM, Ojemann GA, Hochman DW. Optical imaging of epileptiform and functional activity in human cerebral cortex. Nature 1992;358:668–71.

26. Haglund MM, Ojemann GA, Blasdel GG. Optical imaging of bipolar cortical stimulation. J Neurosurg 1993;78:785–93.

27. Nathan SS, Sinha SR, Gordon B, et al. Determina-tion of current density distributions generated by electrical stimulation of the human cerebral cortex. Electroencephalogr Clin Neurophysiol 1993;86: 183–92.

28. Phillips CG, Porter R. Unifocal and bifocal stimula-tion of the motor cortex. J Physiol 1962;162:532–8.

29. Wongsarnpigoon A, Grill WM. Computer-based model of epidural motor cortex stimulation: effects of electrode position and geometry on activation of cortical neurons. Clin Neurophysiol 2012;123(1): 160–72.

30. Kombos T, Suess O, Kern BC, et al. Comparison between monopolar and bipolar electrical stimula-tion of the motor cortex. Acta Neurochir (Wien) 1999;141:1295–301.

31. Suess O, Suess S, Brock M, et al. Intraoperative electrocortical stimulation of Brodman area 4: a 10-year analysis of 255 cases. Head Face Med 2006;2:20.

32. Ng WH, Ochi A, Rutka JT, et al. Stimulation threshold potentials of intraoperative cortical motor mapping using monopolar trains of five in pedi-atric epilepsy surgery. Childs Nerv Syst 2010;26: 675–9.

33. Ranck JB Jr. Which elements are excited in electri-cal stimulation of mammalian central nervous system: a review. Brain Res 1975;98:417–40.

34. Tehovnik EJ. Electrical stimulation of neural tissue to evoke behavioral responses. J Neurosci Methods 1996;65:1–17.

35. Tehovnik EJ, Tolias AS, Sultan F, et al. Direct and indirect activation of cortical neurons by electrical microstimulation. J Neurophysiol 2006;96:512–21.

36. Nowak LG, Bullier J. Axons, but not cell bodies, are activated by electrical stimulation in cortical gray matter. II. Evidence from selective inactivation of cell bodies and axon initial segments. Exp Brain Res 1998;118:489–500.

37. Berger MS, Kincaid J, Ojemann GA, et al. Brain mapping techniques to maximize resection, safety, and seizure control in children with brain tumors. Neurosurgery 1989;25:786–92.

38. Ebeling U, Schmid UD, Reulen HJ. Tumour-surgery within the central motor strip: surgical results with the aid of electrical motor cortex stimulation. Acta Neurochir (Wien) 1989;101:100–7.

39. Ebeling U, Schmid UD, Ying H, et al. Safe surgery of lesions near the motor cortex using intra-operative mapping techniques: a report on 50 patients. Acta Neurochir (Wien) 1992;119:23–8.

40. Kombos T, Suess O, Ciklatekerlio O, et al. Monitoring of intraoperative motor evoked potentials to increase the safety of surgery in and around the motor cortex. J Neurosurg 2001;95:608–14.

41. Kombos T, Suess O, Funk T, et al. Intra-operative mapping of the motor cortex during surgery in and around the motor cortex. Acta Neurochir (Wien) 2000;142:263–8.

42. Berger MS, Ojemann GA, Lettich E. Neurophysiological monitoring during astrocytoma surgery. Neurosurg Clin N Am 1990;1:65–80.

43. Luders HO, Dinner DS, Morris HH, et al. Cortical electrical stimulation in humans. The negative motor areas. Adv Neurol 1995;67:115–29.

44. Sutherling WW, Crandall PH, Darcey TM, et al. The magnetic and electric fields agree with intracranial localizations of somatosensory cortex. Neurology 1988;38:1705–14.

45. Szelenyi A, Langer D, Beck J, et al. Transcranial and direct cortical stimulation for motor evoked potential monitoring in intracerebral aneurysm surgery. Neurophysiol Clin 2007;37:391–8.

46. Lang FF, Olansen NE, DeMonte F, et al. Surgical resection of intrinsic insular tumors: complication avoidance. J Neurosurg 2001;95:638–50.

47. Peraud A, Meschede M, Eisner W, et al. Surgical resection of grade II astrocytomas in the superior frontal gyrus. Neurosurgery 2002;50:966–75 [discussion: 75–7].

48. Coenen VA, Krings T, Mayfrank L, et al. Three-dimensional visualization of the pyramidal tract in a neuronavigation system during brain tumor surgery: first experiences and technical note. Neurosurgery 2001;49:86–92 [discussion: 92–3].

49. Carrabba G, Fava E, Giussani C, et al. Cortical and subcortical motor mapping in rolandic and perirolandic glioma surgery: impact on postoperative morbidity and extent of resection. J Neurosurg Sci 2007;51:45–51.

50. Duffau H, Capelle L, Denvil D, et al. Usefulness of intraoperative electrical subcortical mapping during surgery for low-grade gliomas located within eloquent brain regions: functional results in a consecutive series of 103 patients. J Neurosurg 2003;98: 764–78.

51. Keles GE, Lundin DA, Lamborn KR, et al. Intraoperative subcortical stimulation mapping for hemispherical perirolandic gliomas located within or adjacent to the descending motor pathways: evaluation of morbidity and assessment of functional outcome in 294 patients. J Neurosurg 2004;100:369–75.

52. Goldring S. A method for surgical management of focal epilepsy, especially as it relates to children. J Neurosurg 1978;49:344–56.

53. Goldring S, Gregorie EM. Surgical management of epilepsy using epidural recordings to localize the seizure focus. Review of 100 cases. J Neurosurg 1984;60:457–66.

54. Aiba T, Seki Y. Intraoperative identification of the central sulcus: a practical method. Acta Neurochir Suppl (Wien) 1988;42:22–6.

55. Allen A, Starr A, Nudleman K. Assessment of sensory function in the operating room utilizing cerebral evoked potentials: a study of fifty-six surgically anesthetized patients. Clin Neurosurg 1981;28:457–81.

56. Allison T. Scalp and cortical recordings of initial somatosensory cortex activity to median nerve stimulation in man. Ann N Y Acad Sci 1982;388:671–8.

57. Allison T. Localization of sensorimotor cortex in neurosurgery by recording of somatosensory evoked potentials. Yale J Biol Med 1987;60:143–50.

58. Allison T, McCarthy G, Wood CC, et al. Human cortical potentials evoked by stimulation of the median nerve. I. Cytoarchitectonic areas generating short-latency activity. J Neurophysiol 1989;62:694–710.

59. Desmedt JE, Cheron G. Somatosensory evoked potentials in man: subcortical and cortical components and their neural basis. Ann N Y Acad Sci 1982;388:388–411.

60. Firsching R, Klug N, Borner U, et al. Lesions of the sensorimotor region: somatosensory evoked potentials and ultrasound guided surgery. Acta Neurochir (Wien) 1992;118:87–90.

61. Grundy BL. Intraoperative monitoring of sensory-evoked potentials. Anesthesiology 1983;58:72–87.

62. Wood CC, Spencer DD, Allison T, et al. Localization of human sensorimotor cortex during surgery by cortical surface recording of somatosensory evoked potentials. J Neurosurg 1988;68:99–111.

63. Woolsey CN, Erickson TC, Gilson WE. Localization in somatic sensory and motor areas of human cerebral cortex as determined by direct recording of evoked potentials and electrical stimulation. J Neurosurg 1979;51:476–506.

64. Romstock J, Fahlbusch R, Ganslandt O, et al. Localisation of the sensorimotor cortex during surgery for brain tumours: feasibility and waveform patterns of somatosensory evoked potentials. J Neurol Neurosurg Psychiatry 2002;72:221–9.

65. King RB, Schell GR. Cortical localization and monitoring during cerebral operations. J Neurosurg 1987;67:210–9.

66. Miller KJ, denNijs M, Shenoy P, et al. Real-time functional brain mapping using electrocorticography. Neuroimage 2007;37:504–7.

67. Darvas F, Scherer R, Ojemann JG, et al. High gamma mapping using EEG. Neuroimage 2010; 49:930–8.

68. Duffau H, Lopes M, Arthuis F, et al. Contribution of intraoperative electrical stimulations in surgery of low grade gliomas: a comparative study between two series without (1985-96) and with (1996-2003) functional mapping in the same institution. J Neurol Neurosurg Psychiatry 2005;76:845–51.

69. Ojemann G, Ojemann J, Lettich E, et al. Cortical language localization in left, dominant hemisphere. An electrical stimulation mapping investigation in 117 patients. J Neurosurg 1989;71:316–26.

70. Merton PA, Morton HB. Stimulation of the cerebral cortex in the intact human subject. Nature 1980; 285:227.

71. Barker AT, Jalinous R, Freeston IL. Non-invasive magnetic stimulation of human motor cortex. Lancet 1985;1:1106–7.

72. Picht T, Schmidt S, Brandt S, et al. Preoperative functional mapping for rolandic brain tumor surgery: comparison of navigated transcranial magnetic stimulation to direct cortical stimulation. Neurosurgery 2011;69:581–8 [discussion: 8].

73. Forster MT, Hattingen E, Senft C, et al. Navigated transcranial magnetic stimulation and functional magnetic resonance imaging: advanced adjuncts in preoperative planning for central region tumors. Neurosurgery 2011;68:1317–24 [discussion: 24–5].

74. Krings T, Buchbinder BR, Butler WE, et al. Stereotactic transcranial magnetic stimulation: correlation with direct electrical cortical stimulation. Neurosurgery 1997;41:1319–25 [discussion: 25–6].

75. Sack AT, Linden DE. Combining transcranial magnetic stimulation and functional imaging in cognitive brain research: possibilities and limitations. Brain Res Brain Res Rev 2003;43:41–56.

76. Ogawa S, Lee TM, Kay AR, et al. Brain magnetic resonance imaging with contrast dependent on blood oxygenation. Proc Natl Acad Sci U S A 1990;87:9868–72.

77. Fox PT, Raichle ME. Focal physiological uncoupling of cerebral blood flow and oxidative metabolism during somatosensory stimulation in human subjects. Proc Natl Acad Sci U S A 1986;83: 1140–4.

78. Heeger DJ, Huk AC, Geisler WS, et al. Spikes versus BOLD: what does neuroimaging tell us about neuronal activity? Nat Neurosci 2000;3:631–3.

79. Logothetis NK, Pauls J, Augath M, et al. Neurophysiological investigation of the basis of the fMRI signal. Nature 2001;412:150–7.

80. Yoo SS, Talos IF, Golby AJ, et al. Evaluating requirements for spatial resolution of fMRI for neurosurgical planning. Hum Brain Mapp 2004;21:34–43.

81. Gati JS, Menon RS, Ugurbil K, et al. Experimental determination of the BOLD field strength dependence in vessels and tissue. Magn Reson Med 1997;38:296–302.

82. Roux FE, Boulanouar K, Ranjeva JP, et al. Usefulness of motor functional MRI correlated to cortical mapping in rolandic low-grade astrocytomas. Acta Neurochir (Wien) 1999;141:71–9.

83. Majos A, Tybor K, Stefanczyk L, et al. Cortical mapping by functional magnetic resonance imaging in patients with brain tumors. Eur Radiol 2005;15:1148–58.

84. Roux FE, Boulanouar K, Ibarrola D, et al. Functional MRI and intraoperative brain mapping to evaluate brain plasticity in patients with brain tumours and hemiparesis. J Neurol Neurosurg Psychiatry 2000; 69:453–63.

85. Yousry TA, Schmid UD, Jassoy AG, et al. Topography of the cortical motor hand area: prospective study with functional MR imaging and direct motor mapping at surgery. Radiology 1995;195:23–9.

86. Roessler K, Donat M, Lanzenberger R, et al. Evaluation of preoperative high magnetic field motor functional MRI (3 Tesla) in glioma patients by navigated electrocortical stimulation and postoperative outcome. J Neurol Neurosurg Psychiatry 2005;76: 1152–7.

87. Lee CC, Ward HA, Sharbrough FW, et al. Assessment of functional MR imaging in neurosurgical planning. AJNR Am J Neuroradiol 1999;20:1511–9.

88. Petrella JR, Shah LM, Harris KM, et al. Preoperative functional MR imaging localization of language and motor areas: effect on therapeutic decision making in patients with potentially resectable brain tumors. Radiology 2006;240:793–802.

89. Schreckenberger M, Spetzger U, Sabri O, et al. Localisation of motor areas in brain tumour patients: a comparison of preoperative [18F]FDG-PET and intraoperative cortical electrostimulation. Eur J Nucl Med 2001;28:1394–403.

90. Vinas FC, Zamorano L, Mueller RA, et al. [15O]-water PET and intraoperative brain mapping: a comparison in the localization of eloquent cortex. Neurol Res 1997;19:601–8.

91. Fried I, Nenov VI, Ojemann SG, et al. Functional MR and PET imaging of rolandic and visual cortices for neurosurgical planning. J Neurosurg 1995;83:854–61.

92. Tai YF, Piccini P. Applications of positron emission tomography (PET) in neurology. J Neurol Neurosurg Psychiatry 2004;75:669–76.

93. Alavi JB, Alavi A, Chawluk J, et al. Positron emission tomography in patients with glioma. A predictor of prognosis. Cancer 1988;62:1074–8.

94. Pirotte B, Acerbi F, Lubansu A, et al. PET imaging in the surgical management of pediatric brain tumors. Childs Nerv Syst 2007;23:739–51.

95. Gallen CC, Schwartz BJ, Bucholz RD, et al. Presurgical localization of functional cortex using magnetic source imaging. J Neurosurg 1995;82:988–94.

96. Kamada K, Takeuchi F, Kuriki S, et al. Functional neurosurgical simulation with brain surface magnetic resonance images and magnetoencephalography. Neurosurgery 1993;33:269–72 [discussion: 72–3].

97. Rezai AR, Hund M, Kronberg E, et al. Introduction of magnetoencephalography to stereotactic techniques. Stereotact Funct Neurosurg 1995;65:37–41.

98. Castillo EM, Simos PG, Wheless JW, et al. Integrating sensory and motor mapping in a comprehensive MEG protocol: clinical validity and replicability. Neuroimage 2004;21:973–83.

99. Rezai AR, Hund M, Kronberg E, et al. The interactive use of magnetoencephalography in stereotactic image-guided neurosurgery. Neurosurgery 1996;39:92–102.

100. McDonald JD, Chong BW, Lewine JD, et al. Integration of preoperative and intraoperative functional brain mapping in a frameless stereotactic environment for lesions near eloquent cortex. Technical note. J Neurosurg 1999;90:591–8.

101. Ganslandt O, Fahlbusch R, Nimsky C, et al. Functional neuronavigation with magnetoencephalography: outcome in 50 patients with lesions around the motor cortex. J Neurosurg 1999;91:73–9.

102. Schulder M, Maldjian JA, Liu WC, et al. Functional image-guided surgery of intracranial tumors located in or near the sensorimotor cortex. J Neurosurg 1998;89:412–8.

103. Moseley ME, Cohen Y, Kucharczyk J, et al. Diffusion-weighted MR imaging of anisotropic water diffusion in cat central nervous system. Radiology 1990;176:439–45.

104. Jellison BJ, Field AS, Medow J, et al. Diffusion tensor imaging of cerebral white matter: a pictorial review of physics, fiber tract anatomy, and tumor imaging patterns. AJNR Am J Neuroradiol 2004;25:356–69.

105. Berman JI, Berger MS, Mukherjee P, et al. Diffusion-tensor imaging-guided tracking of fibers of the pyramidal tract combined with intraoperative cortical stimulation mapping in patients with gliomas. J Neurosurg 2004;101:66–72.

106. Kamada K, Houkin K, Takeuchi F, et al. Visualization of the eloquent motor system by integration of MEG, functional, and anisotropic diffusion-weighted MRI in functional neuronavigation. Surg Neurol 2003;59:352–61 [discussion: 61–2].

107. Krings T, Topper R, Willmes K, et al. Activation in primary and secondary motor areas in patients with CNS neoplasms and weakness. Neurology 2002;58:381–90.

108. Moller-Hartmann W, Krings T, Coenen VA, et al. Preoperative assessment of motor cortex and pyramidal tracts in central cavernoma employing functional and diffusion-weighted magnetic resonance imaging. Surg Neurol 2002;58:302–7 [discussion: 8].

109. Parmar H, Sitoh YY, Yeo TT. Combined magnetic resonance tractography and functional magnetic resonance imaging in evaluation of brain tumors involving the motor system. J Comput Assist Tomogr 2004;28:551–6.

110. Witwer BP, Moftakhar R, Hasan KM, et al. Diffusion-tensor imaging of white matter tracts in patients with cerebral neoplasm. J Neurosurg 2002;97:568–75.

111. Nimsky C, Ganslandt O, Fahlbusch R. Implementation of fiber tract navigation. Neurosurgery 2006;58:ONS-292–303 [discussion: ONS–4].

112. Nimsky C, Ganslandt O, Merhof D, et al. Intraoperative visualization of the pyramidal tract by diffusion-tensor-imaging-based fiber tracking. Neuroimage 2006;30:1219–29.

113. Hunsche S, Moseley ME, Stoeter P, et al. Diffusion-tensor MR imaging at 1.5 and 3.0 T: initial observations. Radiology 2001;221:550–6.

114. Duffau H. Lessons from brain mapping in surgery for low-grade glioma: insights into associations between tumour and brain plasticity. Lancet Neurol 2005;4:476–86.

115. Nabavi A, Black PM, Gering DT, et al. Serial intraoperative magnetic resonance imaging of brain shift. Neurosurgery 2001;48:787–97 [discussion: 97–8].

116. Nimsky C, Ganslandt O, Cerny S, et al. Quantification of, visualization of, and compensation for brain shift using intraoperative magnetic resonance imaging. Neurosurgery 2000;47:1070–9 [discussion: 9–80].

117. Nimsky C, Ganslandt O, Hastreiter P, et al. Intraoperative compensation for brain shift. Surg Neurol 2001;56:357–64 [discussion: 64–5].

118. Hata N, Nabavi A, Wells WM 3rd, et al. Three-dimensional optical flow method for measurement of volumetric brain deformation from intraoperative MR images. J Comput Assist Tomogr 2000;24:531–8.

119. Reinges MH, Nguyen HH, Krings T, et al. Course of brain shift during microsurgical resection of supratentorial cerebral lesions: limits of conventional neuronavigation. Acta Neurochir (Wien) 2004;146:369–77 [discussion: 77].

120. Archip N, Clatz O, Whalen S, et al. Non-rigid alignment of pre-operative MRI, fMRI, and DT-MRI with intra-operative MRI for enhanced visualization and navigation in image-guided neurosurgery. Neuroimage 2007;35:609–24.

Characteristics and Treatment of Seizures in Patients with High-Grade Glioma: A Review

Dario J. Englot, MD, PhD[a,b,*], Mitchel S. Berger, MD[a,c],
Edward F. Chang, MD[a,b], Paul A. Garcia, MD[a,d]

KEYWORDS

- Anaplastic astrocytoma • Epilepsy • High-grade glioma
- Glioblastoma • Seizure

High-grade gliomas (HGGs), including anaplastic astrocytoma (AA) and glioblastoma multiforme (GBM), are the most common primary tumors of the central nervous system.[1,2] Despite medical and surgical advances, the prognosis of patients with HGGs remains poor, with a median survival of approximately 22 months for AA and 12 months for GBM, even after surgery, irradiation, and chemotherapy.[2–4] Seizures are common in these patients, affecting between 25% and 60% of individuals with HGGs, and they are frequently the presenting symptom.[5–9] Tumor-related epilepsy affects patients' quality of life significantly, causes cognitive deterioration, and may result in significant morbidity.[5,10–13] However, the importance of seizure control in patients with HGG remains underappreciated because most neuro-oncologic studies and practices focus primarily on tumor progression and the overall survival. An understanding of the underlying risk factors and treatment options for seizures in patients with HGG is critical in their evaluation and treatment. This review briefly discusses the potential mechanistic underpinnings and predictors of seizures in HGGs, and focuses primarily on important therapeutic considerations.

PREDICTORS, MECHANISMS, AND CHARACTERISTICS OF EPILEPSY IN PATIENTS WITH HGG

The predilection for seizures in patients with brain tumor has long been recognized, and was described by Hughlings Jackson in 1882.[14] Across various clinical series, 25% to 60% of individuals with HGGs experience seizures, suggesting that brains harboring these lesions possess a strong predisposition to epileptogenicity,[5,10–13] but seizures are not equally common among different types of gliomas. The highest rates of epilepsy are

This article has not been previously published in whole or in part or submitted elsewhere for review.
The authors have no conflicts of interest to disclose.

[a] UCSF Epilepsy Center, University of California, San Francisco, 505 Parnassus Avenue, Box 0138, San Francisco, CA 94143, USA
[b] Department of Neurological Surgery, University of California, San Francisco, 505 Parnassus Avenue, Box 0112, San Francisco, CA 94143-0112, USA
[c] UCSF Brain Tumor Research Center, University of California, San Francisco, 505 Parnassus Avenue, Box 0112, San Francisco, CA 94143-0112, USA
[d] Department of Neurology, University of California, San Francisco, 505 Parnassus Avenue, Box 0138, San Francisco, CA 94143, USA
* Corresponding author. Department of Neurological Surgery, University of California, San Francisco, 505 Parnassus Avenue, Box 0112, San Francisco, CA 94143-0112.
E-mail address: EnglotDJ@neurosurg.ucsf.edu

observed in patients with low-grade gliomas (LGGs) (World Health Organization [WHO] grade I–II), whereas among patients with HGGs, seizures are more common in patients with AAs (WHO grade II) than in those with GBMs (WHO grade IV).[15–17] Smaller tumors and those growing less quickly are associated with higher rates of seizures than large tumors and rapidly growing lesions.[5–9,17,18] Although the reason for this trend is not known, proposed explanations include the predilection of HGG for white matter locations, the possibility that rapid growth might preclude the development of epileptogenesis, and the prospect that some patients with HGG do not survive long enough to develop epilepsy.[17–19]

HGGs located in superficial cortical areas are most likely to produce seizures,[17,20–23] as are tumors centered in the temporal or frontal lobes or the insula.[17,20,21,24–26] Lee and colleagues[17] analyzed tumor location in 124 glioma patients with seizures, and mapped aggregate tumor location using a summed-statistic image, as depicted in **Fig. 1**. These investigators also found that many HGGs causing seizures were located in the temporal lobe, followed by the frontal lobe. The inherent epileptogenicity of mesial temporal structures making seizures more likely in the temporal region is a possibility.[27,28] Furthermore, Spencer and colleagues[29,30] have suggested that "dual pathology," including any combination of foreign-tissue lesions, cortical dysgenesis, gliosis, or hippocampal sclerosis, further drives epileptogenesis in tumoral temporal lobe epilepsy. Some investigators have found

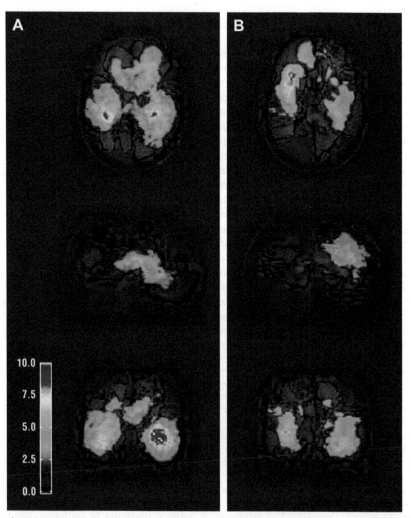

Fig. 1. Summed-statistic image showing the aggregate location of 124 tumors. At each voxel, the number of patients presenting with tumors is calculated. Maps are generated from the sum of the binary tumor masks for high-grade (*A*) and low-grade (*B*) gliomas. (*From* Lee JW, Wen PY, Hurwitz S, et al. Morphological characteristics of brain tumors causing seizures. Arch Neurol 2010;67:339; with permission.)

a lower likelihood of seizures in de novo GBMs than those having progressed from known LGGs,[8,18] and others have noted that seizures may sometimes precede radiographic evidence of malignant tumor transformation.[31] It is perhaps not surprising that epilepsy is more common in patients with multifocal disease than in those with a solitary tumor.[8]

Although the molecular pathophysiology of epileptogenicity in gliomas remains incompletely understood, several contributory mechanisms have been proposed. Peritumoral changes, such as hypoxia, neurotransmitter alterations, and blood-brain barrier disruption, have all been observed in parenchyma adjacent to brain tumors, and may contribute to epileptogenicity in patients with HGG.[32–36] Furthermore, although neurons are traditionally credited with seizure initiation, increasing evidence suggests that astrocytes also likely contribute to the induction and maturation of epileptogenesis.[37] Bordey and Sontheimer[38] observed that astrocytes from seizure foci in patients with temporal lobe epilepsy consistently express faster-activating sodium channels and diminished potassium buffering compared with normal cells. Downregulation of glutamine synthetase, an enzyme known to be deficient in sclerotic hippocampi of patients with temporal lobe epilepsy[39] and in brains of animal epilepsy models,[40] has also been observed in astrocytes of patients with HGG.[37] Thus, glutamate accumulation may represent another molecular contribution to seizure generation in patients with HGG. Although the process of epileptogenesis is known to occur over time, rapid ictogenesis may arise in the absence of epileptogenesis with acute pathophysiologic phenomena seen in gliomas, such as hemorrhage, edema, and electrolytic changes, thus causing early seizures in some patients.[18]

Seizure semiology with HGGs is variable, and may resemble seizure characteristics seen in defined anatomic epilepsy syndromes, but typically includes simple- and complex-partial seizures.[5,8] Secondary generalization is also not infrequent, and status epilepticus may occur.[5,8] Given the significant risk of epilepsy in these patients, seizures should be high on the differential diagnosis when a patient harboring a known HGG presents with altered mental status or novel sensorimotor symptoms.

SURGICAL AND ADJUVANT TREATMENT OF HGGS ASSOCIATED WITH EPILEPSY

Although several groups have studied seizure outcomes in the surgical treatment of LGGs,[15,22,41] only one study to the authors' knowledge has specifically examined predictors of seizure freedom in the surgical resection of HGGs.[5] Chaichana and colleagues[5] retrospectively analyzed 648 patients with surgically resected HGG, of whom 24% presented with seizures. Preoperative seizures were observed to be more common in younger patients, as well as with AA (compared with GBM), and with cortically based and temporal lobe lesions. Twelve months after surgical resection (gross total in 33%), 77% of patients with preoperative seizures were seizure free (Engel class I),[33] whereas only 5% experienced no improvement in seizures (Engel class IV). Seizure freedom was somewhat less common in patients who suffered from uncontrolled epilepsy before surgery, although 56% of these individuals also achieved seizure freedom postoperatively. The investigators also noted that individuals with parietal lobe lesions were least likely to achieve seizure freedom postoperatively. Seizure recurrence in patients initially seizure-free after surgery was independently associated with tumor recurrence. These results suggest that seizure freedom can be achieved in the resection of HGGs, even in some patients with medically refractory epilepsy, and thus should represent an important goal in the surgical treatment of these patients. Nevertheless, given the limitations of retrospective study design and the lack of confirmatory investigations, further studies in this area are important.

In patients with LGG, various investigators have reported that gross-total resection predicts a higher likelihood of postoperative seizure freedom.[15,22,41] Chaichana and colleagues[5] did not observe a similar relationship between resection extent and seizure outcome in HGGs, and, to the author's knowledge no other studies have investigated this question in HGGs. Similarly, although the use of intraoperative electrocorticography in LGG resection has been advocated to delineate epileptic cortex surrounding the tumor,[41,42] this has not been studied in HGGs. Thus, although there is mounting evidence suggesting that extent of resection may influence patient survival in HGGs,[43,44] it is unknown whether this factor also affects seizure outcome.

There is some evidence that chemotherapy or radiotherapy may also positively affect the seizure burden in patients with brain tumors. In a small case series, Chalifoux and Elisevich[45] describe a significant seizure reduction in unresected patients with HGG after ionizing radiation treatment, with benefit extending beyond the early postradiation period.[45] Similar positive effects on seizure frequency have been described in patients with LGG after radiotherapy[46] or chemotherapy with temozolomide.[47] Antitumor therapy by surgery, cranial radiation, or chemotherapy may all contribute to reduced seizure burden in patients with glioma.[48] Although more prospective data are important in evaluating the possible effects of chemotherapy and radiotherapy on seizure profiles, adjuvant antineoplastic therapy should not be considered antiepileptic treatment.

ANTIEPILEPTIC MEDICATIONS IN PATIENTS WITH HGG

Although surgery and adjuvant antitumor therapies improve the overall and progression-free survival in patients with HGG, they very rarely result in a cure. Antiepileptic drugs (AEDs) are therefore the mainstay of seizure treatment in these patients, and understanding the approach, efficacy, and serious side effects of AED treatment is critically important in reducing patient morbidity and improving patients' quality of life. Some investigators have reported that although seizures are less common in patients with HGGs than in those with LGGs, they may be more difficult to control in patients with malignant lesions.[18]

The general approach to AED treatment in patients with glioma, as in all patients with epilepsy, is to first use a single AED at the lowest dose that effectively controls seizures, followed by additional trials of serial monotherapy versus polytherapy as necessary.[48–50] Common first-line agents used in glioma-related epilepsy include valproic acid and phenytoin,[49–51] and more recently levetiracetam has been proposed as monotherapy for tumoral epilepsy.[48,49,52,53] Topiramate and lamotrigine are also sometimes used as initial first-line monotherapy.[48] Van Breemen and colleagues[50] advocate for valproic acid as an efficacious first-line AED in patients with glioma who also have epilepsy, reporting a 79% responder rate and seizure freedom in 52% of patients with monotherapy. Valproic acid is also the most commonly used agent in children with focal epilepsy,[54] and a recent phase I study suggests that it is well tolerated in pediatric patients with brain tumor, with phase II results pending.[51] Phenytoin is also frequently used as initial monotherapy, and in one study it was associated with 730 (median) seizure-free days in patients with glioma suffering from at least 1 seizure.[49] More recently, monotherapy with the newer agent levetiracetam has been reported to be efficacious in this population, with benefits over valproic acid and phenytoin, including the ability to forgo the monitoring of serum level, a lower incidence of toxicity, and the lack of significant drug interactions.[48,49,52,53] However, none of these studies were performed with the rigor required for inclusion in a Cochrane review on the topic.[55] The only study meeting the Cochrane

meta-analysis criteria was an unblinded, randomized trial of phenytoin continuation versus change to levetiracetam at the time of surgery.[56] This study showed similar efficacy and side effects for both arms with a suggestion of more balance problems in the phenytoin arm. As a possible confounder, more patients dropped out of the levetiracetam arm and were not included in the analysis.[56]

When AED monotherapy fails to adequately control seizures in patients with glioma, there is disagreement over whether to trial a second agent as monotherapy or to add an adjunct medication, provided the absence of significant side effects with the initial AED. Although a common approach is to attempt 1 or 2 serial monotherapy trials as necessary, reserving polytherapy for refractory cases,[49] other practitioners have advocated add-on therapy immediately after initial drug failure. Van Breemen and colleagues[50] report encouraging results with the addition of levetiracetam to valproic acid, and Newton and colleagues[57] observed a 90% rate of benefit and 59% rate of seizure freedom when adding levetiracetam to a patient's existing regimen. Based on these varied approaches to patients who fail initial monotherapy, a randomized, controlled trial of serial monotherapy versus polytherapy comparing various agents in tumoral epilepsy is certainly warranted.

Side effects and toxicity of AED are critical considerations in patients with HGG, particularly given the importance of quality of life in this almost universally terminal illness. AEDs are associated with significant adverse effects,[58–60] including cognitive deficits,[61–63] and first-generation medications may result in a higher incidence of side effects in patients with glioma than in other epileptics.[6,49,64] In a large European survey of patients with epilepsy, Baker and colleagues[65] found that 31% of individuals changed their AED at least once in the past year because of side effects, and 44% were worried about possible side effects related to AEDs. Other researchers have shown that adverse AED effects have the single greatest influence on quality of life in patients with controlled seizures,[66] and that patients would prefer to pay more for medications with improved side-effect profiles.[67]

Although phenytoin is commonly used, given the favorable efficacy it is associated with a significant number of drug interactions, and its common dose–related side effects (disequilibrium and drowsiness) are often poorly tolerated by patients with brain tumors. Additional side effects include rash, drowsiness, dizziness, and hirsutism, with Stevens-Johnson syndrome being the most feared adverse event.[49] Moreover, monitoring of serum level is necessary, and toxic levels frequently occur in the therapeutic dose range because of zero-order kinetics.[49] Along with carbamazepine and oxcarbazepine, phenytoin may cause leukopenia, necessitating the monitoring of blood count during initial treatment.[68,69] Valproic acid has a lower incidence of adverse effects, but can result in thrombocytopenia, and the monitoring of serum level can be challenging because of the variable pharmacokinetics.[68,69] The second-generation AEDs, although not necessarily associated with greater efficacy than first-generation medications, may in some circumstances possess improved tolerability.[49] Monitoring of levels is not necessary with these newer agents, as many are not metabolized by the hepatic P450 system, and significant drug interactions are rare.[49] Levetiracetam is renally excreted and typically well tolerated, with infrequent side effects including somnolence, nausea/vomiting, headache, and insomnia.[53] Two recent studies of levetiracetam in patients with glioma cited little or no medication discontinuation secondary to adverse effects.[52,53]

Another important consideration of AED treatment in patients with HGG is the potential for interaction with chemotherapy. CYP3A4 enzyme-inducing AEDs, such as phenytoin, carbamazepine, and oxcarbazepine, may increase the clearance of drugs metabolized by the P450 system, including numerous chemotherapeutic agents (including thiotepa, taxanes, irinotecan, imatinib, gefitinib, temsirolimus, erlotinib, tipifarnib, and vorinostat), as well as corticosteroids such as dexamethasone, which are frequently prescribed to reduce peritumoral edema.[49,70–75] This may be less of a concern with valproic acid, a weak CYP3A4 inducer, and noninducing agents such as levetiracetam and lamotrigine, and potential chemotherapeutic interactions with topiramate require further study.[75] Not all AED interactions with chemotherapeutic agents are deleterious. Bobustuc and colleagues[76] recently observed that levetiracetam may inhibit the expression of the DNA-repair enzyme O^6-methylguanine-DNA methyltransferase in vitro, and therefore sensitize glioma cells to the alkylating agent temozolomide. Furthermore, Jaeckle and colleagues[77] reviewed data from patients with HGG treated with enzyme-inducing anticonvulsants (used largely for prophylaxis), finding paradoxically that patients treated with these drugs survived longer than those who did not undergo treatment, this increase in survival being independent of seizure activity. It is not clear whether this observation was due to an effect on chemotherapy, an effect on the tumor directly, or a confounding variable not accounted for in their detailed multivariate analysis. In general, epilepsy providers must be aware of these potential drug interactions between AEDs and chemotherapy, to ensure optimal coordination of antiepileptic and neuro-oncologic treatment in patients with HGG.

A final question is whether to initiate prophylactic AED therapy in the patient with HGG who has not had a seizure. Various investigators have advocated for prophylaxis in patients with brain tumors, citing efficacy in preventing seizures, despite the risk of adverse effects of medication.[78–80] In 1996, a randomized controlled trial of valproic acid prophylaxis in adults with brain tumors showed that patients receiving the prophylactic AED actually had a nonsignificantly higher rate of seizures compared with those taking placebo.[81] Subsequently, the American Academy of Neurology recommended against long-term prophylactic AEDs in patients who are newly diagnosed with brain tumor,[6] and a meta-analysis of the relevant literature provided further evidence that AEDs should not be used prophylactically.[82] One exception is that AED prophylaxis may be considered for 1 week following surgical resection, given the higher incidence of postoperative seizures during this time,[6,83–87] although even the evidence supporting this practice remains inconclusive.[88] Thus, while prophylactic AEDs remain commonly prescribed in patients with HGGs and other tumors,[18,89–91] the preponderance of evidence and clinical guidelines recommend strongly against this practice, and the use of perioperative AEDs will require further scrutiny.

SUMMARY AND RECOMMENDATIONS

HGGs are the most common primary brain tumor and are often associated with seizures, particularly with lesions involving the temporal or frontal neocortex. Seizure control is a critical but often underappreciated goal in the treatment of patients harboring these malignant lesions. Although surgical resection of HGGs may reduce the seizure burden in these individuals, insufficient evidence exists regarding the surgical factors that contribute to seizure freedom. The authors' recommendation based on the recognized impact of seizures on the quality of life in patients with HGG is that patients with medically intractable seizures be considered for a palliative resection guided by electrocorticography and functional mapping. Many patients treated at their center have benefited from this approach. Similarly, although other antitumoral treatments such as chemotherapy and irradiation may improve a patient's seizure profile, these adjunctive treatments should not be considered as antiepileptic

Table 1
Factors affecting anticonvulsant choice in patients with HGG

Avoid or adjust dose with chemotherapy	DPH, CBZ, VPA, OXC
Avoid with bone marrow suppression	DPH, CBZ, VPA
Avoid with mood or thought disorder	LEV, TPM, ZON
Avoid with SIADH	OXC, CBZ
Avoid if immediate effect required	LMT, TPM
Avoid if cost is an issue (no generics)	PGB, LAC

Abbreviations: CBZ, carbamazepine; DPH, phenytoin; LAC, lacosamide; LEV, levetiracetam; LMT, lamotrigine; OXC, oxcarbazepine; PGB, pregabalin; SIADH, syndrome of inappropriate antidiuretic hormone; TPM, topiramate; VPA, sodium valproate; ZON, zonisamide.

therapy. AEDs remain the mainstay of seizure treatment in patients with HGG, and antiepileptic medication should be started after a tumor-related seizure, but should not be used prophylactically in the absence of seizure activity. Although Class I evidence is not available to guide the management of AED in patients who present with seizures, the authors offer the following practical suggestions: (1) because many patients undergo chemotherapy, it is preferable to choose a medicine that does not affect chemotherapy levels or exacerbate chemotherapy-induced bone marrow suppression (**Table 1**); (2) because patients presenting anew are not otherwise protected from seizures, medications with a slow titration are usually not acceptable (see **Table 1**); and (3) newer medications without generic equivalents or obvious advantages over other medications should not be first-line choices (see **Table 1**). Based on these criteria, levetiracetam and zonisamide seem to be ideal medications for initiating treatment. Both can be started at a dose known to be effective (for levetiracetam, 500 mg twice daily, and zonisamide, 100 mg/d). Failure to respond sufficiently to initial treatment warrants referral for subspecialty seizure care. Although HGG remains almost universally a terminal illness, seizure control is a critical goal in the treatment of these patients, given the deleterious effects of epilepsy on patients' quality of life.

REFERENCES

1. Kleihues P, Burger PC, Scheithauer BW. The new WHO classification of brain tumours. Brain Pathol 1993;3:255–68.

2. DeAngelis LM. Brain tumors. N Engl J Med 2001; 344:114–23.

3. Curran WJ Jr, Scott CB, Horton J, et al. Recursive partitioning analysis of prognostic factors in three Radiation Therapy Oncology Group malignant glioma trials. J Natl Cancer Inst 1993;85:704–10.

4. Buckner JC. Factors influencing survival in high-grade gliomas. Semin Oncol 2003;30:10–4.

5. Chaichana KL, Parker SL, Olivi A, et al. Long-term seizure outcomes in adult patients undergoing primary resection of malignant brain astrocytomas. Clinical article. J Neurosurg 2009;111:282–92.

6. Glantz MJ, Cole BF, Forsyth PA, et al. Practice parameter: anti-convulsant prophylaxis in patients with newly diagnosed brain tumors. Report of the Quality Standards Subcommittee of the American Academy of Neurology. Neurology 2000;54:1886–93.

7. Herman ST. Epilepsy after brain insult: targeting epileptogenesis. Neurology 2002;59:S21–6.

8. Moots PL, Maciunas RJ, Eisert DR, et al. The course of seizure disorders in patients with malignant gliomas. Arch Neurol 1995;52:717–24.

9. Pasquier B, Peoc HM, Fabre-Bocquentin B, et al. Surgical pathology of drug-resistant partial epilepsy. A 10-year-experience with a series of 327 consecutive resections. Epileptic Disord 2002;4:99–119.

10. Jacoby A, Wang W, Vu TD, et al. Meanings of epilepsy in its sociocultural context and implications for stigma: findings from ethnographic studies in local communities in China and Vietnam. Epilepsy Behav 2008;12:286–97.

11. Sizoo EM, Braam L, Postma TJ, et al. Symptoms and problems in the end-of-life phase of high-grade glioma patients. Neurol Oncol 2010;12: 1162–6.

12. van Breemen MS, Wilms EB, Vecht CJ. Epilepsy in patients with brain tumours: epidemiology, mechanisms, and management. Lancet Neurol 2007;6: 421–30.

13. Sheth RD. Adolescent issues in epilepsy. J Child Neurol 2002;17(Suppl 2):2S23–22S27.

14. Jackson J. Localized convulsions from tumors of the brain. Brain 1882;5:364–74.

15. Englot DJ, Berger MS, Barbaro NM, et al. Predictors of seizure-freedom after resection of supratentorial low-grade gliomas. J Neurosurg 2011;115(2): 240–4.

16. Kim OJ, Yong Ahn J, Chung YS, et al. Significance of chronic epilepsy in glial tumors and correlation with surgical strategies. J Clin Neurosci 2004;11: 702–5.

17. Lee JW, Wen PY, Hurwitz S, et al. Morphological characteristics of brain tumors causing seizures. Arch Neurol 2010;67:336–42.

18. Rosati A, Tomassini A, Pollo B, et al. Epilepsy in cerebral glioma: timing of appearance and histological correlations. J Neurooncol 2009;93:395–400.

19. Pace A, Vidiri A, Galie E, et al. Temozolomide chemotherapy for progressive low-grade glioma: clinical benefits and radiological response. Ann Oncol 2003;14:1722–6.

20. Liigant A, Haldre S, Oun A, et al. Seizure disorders in patients with brain tumors. Eur Neurol 2001;45:46–51.

21. Lynam LM, Lyons MK, Drazkowski JF, et al. Frequency of seizures in patients with newly diagnosed brain tumors: a retrospective review. Clin Neurol Neurosurg 2007;109:634–8.

22. Fried I, Kim JH, Spencer DD. Limbic and neocortical gliomas associated with intractable seizures: a distinct clinicopathological group. Neurosurgery 1994;34:815–23 [discussion: 823–4].

23. Penfield W, Erickson T, Tarlov I. Relation of intracranial tumors and symptomatic epilepsy. Arch Neurol Psychiatry 1940;44:300–15.

24. Lund M. Epilepsy in association with intracranial tumor. Acta Psychiatr Neurol Scand Suppl 1952;81:1–149.

25. Zaatreh MM, Firlik KS, Spencer DD, et al. Temporal lobe tumoral epilepsy: characteristics and predictors of surgical outcome. Neurology 2003;61:636–41.

26. Zaatreh MM, Spencer DD, Thompson JL, et al. Frontal lobe tumoral epilepsy: clinical, neurophysiologic features and predictors of surgical outcome. Epilepsia 2002;43:727–33.

27. Engel J Jr, Bragin A, Staba R, et al. High-frequency oscillations: what is normal and what is not? Epilepsia 2009;50:598–604.

28. Delgado-Escueta AV, Ward AA Jr, Woodbury DM, et al. New wave of research in the epilepsies. Adv Neurol 1986;44:3–55.

29. Fish DR, Spencer SS. Clinical correlations: MRI and EEG. Magn Reson Imaging 1995;13:1113–7.

30. Spencer S, Huh L. Outcomes of epilepsy surgery in adults and children. Lancet Neurol 2008;7:525–37.

31. Rossi R, Figus A, Corraine S. Early presentation of de novo high grade glioma with epileptic seizures: electroclinical and neuroimaging findings. Seizure 2010;19:470–4.

32. Haglund MM, Berger MS, Kunkel DD, et al. Changes in gamma-aminobutyric acid and somatostatin in epileptic cortex associated with low-grade gliomas. J Neurosurg 1992;77:209–16.

33. Engel J, Van Ness P, Rasmussen T, et al. Outcome with respect to epileptic seizures. In: Engel J, editor. Surgical treatment of the epilepsies. 2nd edition. New York: Raven Press; 1993. p. 609–21.

34. Ruda R, Trevisan E, Soffietti R. Epilepsy and brain tumors. Curr Opin Oncol 2010;22:611–20.

35. Shamji MF, Fric-Shamji EC, Benoit BG. Brain tumors and epilepsy: pathophysiology of peritumoral changes. Neurosurg Rev 2009;32:275–84 [discussion: 284–76].

36. Kim JH, Guimaraes PO, Shen MY, et al. Hippocampal neuronal density in temporal lobe epilepsy with and without gliomas. Acta Neuropathol 1990;80:41–5.

37. Rosati A, Marconi S, Pollo B, et al. Epilepsy in glioblastoma multiforme: correlation with glutamine synthetase levels. J Neurooncol 2009;93:319–24.

38. Bordey A, Sontheimer H. Properties of human glial cells associated with epileptic seizure foci. Epilepsy Res 1998;32:286–303.

39. Eid T, Thomas MJ, Spencer DD, et al. Loss of glutamine synthetase in the human epileptogenic hippocampus: possible mechanism for raised extracellular glutamate in mesial temporal lobe epilepsy. Lancet 2004;363:28–37.

40. Laming PR, Cosby SL, O'Neill JK. Seizures in the Mongolian gerbil are related to a deficiency in cerebral glutamine synthetase. Comp Biochem Physiol C 1989;94:399–404.

41. Chang EF, Potts MB, Keles GE, et al. Seizure characteristics and control following resection in 332 patients with low-grade gliomas. J Neurosurg 2008;108:227–35.

42. Awad IA, Rosenfeld J, Ahl J, et al. Intractable epilepsy and structural lesions of the brain: mapping, resection strategies, and seizure outcome. Epilepsia 1991;32:179–86.

43. Sanai N, Berger MS. Glioma extent of resection and its impact on patient outcome. Neurosurgery 2008;62:753–64 [discussion: 264–6].

44. Sanai N, Polley MY, McDermott MW, et al. An extent of resection threshold for newly diagnosed glioblastomas. J Neurosurg 2011;115(1):3–8.

45. Chalifoux R, Elisevich K. Effect of ionizing radiation on partial seizures attributable to malignant cerebral tumors. Stereotact Funct Neurosurg 1996;67:169–82.

46. Rogers LR, Morris HH, Lupica K. Effect of cranial irradiation on seizure frequency in adults with low-grade astrocytoma and medically intractable epilepsy. Neurology 1993;43:1599–601.

47. Sherman JH, Moldovan K, Yeoh HK, et al. Impact of temozolomide chemotherapy on seizure frequency in patients with low-grade gliomas. J Neurosurg 2011;114(6):1617–21.

48. Vecht CJ, Wilms EB. Seizures in low- and high-grade gliomas: current management and future outlook. Expert Rev Anticancer Ther 2010;10:663–9.

49. Merrell RT, Anderson SK, Meyer FB, et al. Seizures in patients with glioma treated with phenytoin and levetiracetam. J Neurosurg 2010;113:1176–81.

50. van Breemen MS, Rijsman RM, Taphoorn MJ, et al. Efficacy of anti-epileptic drugs in patients with gliomas and seizures. J Neurol 2009;256:1519–26.

51. Su JM, Li XN, Thompson P, et al. Phase 1 study of valproic acid in pediatric patients with refractory solid or CNS tumors: a children's oncology group report. Clin Cancer Res 2011;17:589–97.

52. Rosati A, Buttolo L, Stefini R, et al. Efficacy and safety of levetiracetam in patients with glioma: a clinical prospective study. Arch Neurol 2010;67: 343–6.

53. Usery JB, Michael LM 2nd, Sills AK, et al. A prospective evaluation and literature review of levetiracetam use in patients with brain tumors and seizures. J Neurooncol 2010;99:251–60.

54. Loscher W. Basic pharmacology of valproate: a review after 35 years of clinical use for the treatment of epilepsy. CNS Drugs 2002;16:669–94.

55. Kerrigan S, Grant R. Anti-epileptic drugs for treating seizures in adults with brain tumours. Cochrane Database Syst Rev 2011;8:CD008586.

56. Lim DA, Tarapore P, Chang E, et al. Safety and feasibility of switching from phenytoin to levetiracetam monotherapy for glioma-related seizure control following craniotomy: a randomized phase II pilot study. J Neurooncol 2009;93:349–54.

57. Newton HB, Goldlust SA, Pearl D. Retrospective analysis of the efficacy and tolerability of levetiracetam in brain tumor patients. J Neurooncol 2006;78: 99–102.

58. Marks WJ Jr, Garcia PA. Management of seizures and epilepsy. Am Fam Physician 1998;57:1589–600, 1603–4.

59. Cramer JA, Mintzer S, Wheless J, et al. Adverse effects of anti-epileptic drugs: a brief overview of important issues. Expert Rev Neurother 2010;10:885–91.

60. Cascino GD. When drugs and surgery don't work. Epilepsia 2008;49(Suppl 9):79–84.

61. Sisodiya SM, Lin WR, Harding BN, et al. Drug resistance in epilepsy: expression of drug resistance proteins in common causes of refractory epilepsy. Brain 2002;125:22–31.

62. Taphoorn MJ, Klein M. Cognitive deficits in adult patients with brain tumours. Lancet Neurol 2004;3: 159–68.

63. Wagner GL, Wilms EB, Van Donselaar CA, et al. Levetiracetam: preliminary experience in patients with primary brain tumours. Seizure 2003;12:585–6.

64. Batchelor TT, Byrne TN. Supportive care of brain tumor patients. Hematol Oncol Clin North Am 2006;20:1337–61.

65. Baker GA, Jacoby A, Buck D, et al. Quality of life of people with epilepsy: a European study. Epilepsia 1997;38:353–62.

66. Auriel E, Landov H, Blatt I, et al. Quality of life in seizure-free patients with epilepsy on monotherapy. Epilepsy Behav 2009;14:130–3.

67. Lloyd A, McIntosh E, Price M. The importance of drug adverse effects compared with seizure control for people with epilepsy: a discrete choice experiment. Pharmacoeconomics 2005;23:1167–81.

68. Blackburn SC, Oliart AD, Garcia Rodriguez LA, et al. Anti-epileptics and blood dyscrasias: a cohort study. Pharmacotherapy 1998;18:1277–83.

69. Tohen M, Castillo J, Baldessarini RJ, et al. Blood dyscrasias with carbamazepine and valproate: a pharmacoepidemiological study of 2,228 patients at risk. Am J Psychiatry 1995;152:413–8.

70. Brown PD, Krishnan S, Sarkaria JN, et al. Phase I/II trial of erlotinib and temozolomide with radiation therapy in the treatment of newly diagnosed glioblastoma multiforme: North Central Cancer Treatment Group Study N0177. J Clin Oncol 2008;26: 5603–9.

71. Drappatz J, Schiff D, Kesari S, et al. Medical management of brain tumor patients. Neurol Clin 2007;25:1035–71, ix.

72. Galanis E, Jaeckle KA, Maurer MJ, et al. Phase II trial of vorinostat in recurrent glioblastoma multiforme: a north central cancer treatment group study. J Clin Oncol 2009;27:2052–8.

73. Raymond E, Brandes AA, Dittrich C, et al. Phase II study of imatinib in patients with recurrent gliomas of various histologies: a European Organisation for Research and Treatment of Cancer Brain Tumor Group Study. J Clin Oncol 2008;26:4659–65.

74. Michelucci R. Optimizing therapy of seizures in neurosurgery. Neurology 2006;67:S14–8.

75. Pursche S, Schleyer E, von Bonin M, et al. Influence of enzyme-inducing anti-epileptic drugs on trough level of imatinib in glioblastoma patients. Curr Clin Pharmacol 2008;3:198–203.

76. Bobustuc GC, Baker CH, Limaye A, et al. Levetiracetam enhances p53-mediated MGMT inhibition and sensitizes glioblastoma cells to temozolomide. Neuro Oncol 2010;12:917–27.

77. Jaeckle KA, Ballman K, Furth A, et al. Correlation of enzyme-inducing anti-convulsant use with outcome of patients with glioblastoma. Neurology 2009;73: 1207–13.

78. North JB, Penhall RK, Hanieh A, et al. Phenytoin and postoperative epilepsy. A double-blind study. J Neurosurg 1983;58:672–7.

79. Franceschetti S, Binelli S, Casazza M, et al. Influence of surgery and anti-epileptic drugs on seizures symptomatic of cerebral tumours. Acta Neurochir (Wien) 1990;103:47–51.

80. Forsyth PA, Weaver S, Fulton D, et al. Prophylactic anticonvulsants in patients with brain tumour. Can J Neurol Sci 2003;30:106–12.

81. Glantz MJ, Cole BF, Friedberg MH, et al. A randomized, blinded, placebo-controlled trial of divalproex sodium prophylaxis in adults with newly diagnosed brain tumors. Neurology 1996;46:985–91.

82. Sirven JI, Wingerchuk DM, Drazkowski JF, et al. Seizure prophylaxis in patients with brain tumors: a meta-analysis. Mayo Clin Proc 2004;79:1489–94.

83. Matthew E, Sherwin AL, Welner SA, et al. Seizures following intracranial surgery: incidence in the first post-operative week. Can J Neurol Sci 1980;7: 285–90.

84. Kuijlen JM, Teernstra OP, Kessels AG, et al. Effectiveness of anti-epileptic prophylaxis used with supratentorial craniotomies: a meta-analysis. Seizure 1996;5: 291–8.

85. Lee ST, Lui TN, Chang CN, et al. Prophylactic anticonvulsants for prevention of immediate and early postcraniotomy seizures. Surg Neurol 1989;31:361–4.

86. Kvam DA, Loftus CM, Copeland B, et al. Seizures during the immediate postoperative period. Neurosurgery 1983;12:14–7.

87. Telfeian AE, Philips MF, Crino PB, et al. Postoperative epilepsy in patients undergoing craniotomy for glioblastoma multiforme. J Exp Clin Cancer Res 2001;20:5–10.

88. De Santis A, Villani R, Sinisi M, et al. Add-on phenytoin fails to prevent early seizures after surgery for supratentorial brain tumors: a randomized controlled study. Epilepsia 2002;43:175–82.

89. Lwu S, Hamilton MG, Forsyth PA, et al. Use of peri-operative anti-epileptic drugs in patients with newly diagnosed high grade malignant glioma: a single center experience. J Neurooncol 2010; 96:403–8.

90. Riva M, Salmaggi A, Marchioni E, et al. Tumour-associated epilepsy: clinical impact and the role of referring centres in a cohort of glioblastoma patients. A multicentre study from the Lombardia Neurooncology Group. Neurol Sci 2006;27:345–51.

91. Siomin V, Angelov L, Li L, et al. Results of a survey of neurosurgical practice patterns regarding the prophylactic use of anti-epilepsy drugs in patients with brain tumors. J Neurooncol 2005;74:211–5.

Pathology: Commonly Monitored Glioblastoma Markers: EFGR, EGFRvIII, PTEN, and MGMT

Joaquin Q. Camara-Quintana, BS, Ryan T. Nitta, PhD,
Gordon Li, MD*

KEYWORDS

• EGFR • EGFRvIII • PTEN • MGMT • Glioblastoma

In 1926, Bailey and Cushing established the first widely accepted classification scheme of astrocytic neoplasms.[1] Since then, neuropathologists have worked to improve this classification system to guide clinicians with diagnostic and prognostic information. Recent advances and discoveries in immunocytochemistry markers, radiographic imaging modalities, and genetic/molecular markers have helped further characterize these tumors. Many of these advances have not yet changed the management of astrocytic neoplasms. Nevertheless, they have provided a wealth of information and continue to challenge current understanding of tumor biology and patient management while providing insight into possible novel therapeutic strategies.

The most common astrocytoma, glioblastoma (GB), is also the most malignant primary brain tumor in adults.[2] There are 2 types of GBs distinguished by their origin and molecular phenotype: primary (de novo) and secondary tumors. De novo cases represent the majority (>90%) of GB patients and develop rapidly over the course of weeks, presenting as a grade IV tumor. Secondary GBs present as lower-grade gliomas (grade II or III) and eventually progress to grade IV. Regardless of its classification, once a diagnosis of GB has been made, the overall median survival time for patients treated with surgery and concomitant radiation plus temozolomide, followed by adjuvant temozolomide, is approximately 15 months.[3]

It is still unclear which molecular and cellular alterations transform a normal cell into tumorigenic GB cells. Previous research has begun to identify and elucidate the molecular pathways that are often perturbed in GBs. These signaling pathways can be therapeutically beneficial because they not only help identify and classify glioma tumors but also may provide novel targets for therapy. This article highlights and reviews 4 important GB molecular markers: epidermal growth factor receptor (EGFR), EGFR variant III (EGFRvIII), phosphatase and tensin homolog deleted on chromosome 10 (PTEN), and O^6-methylguanine-DNA methyltransferase (MGMT).

EGFR
Background on EGFR

EGFR is a cell surface transmembrane tyrosine kinase (TK) receptor that belongs to a family of 4 related receptors: ErbB1/EGFR, ErbB2/Neu/Her2, ErbB3/Her3, and ErbB4/Her4.[4] All members of this family contain 3 basic components: an extracellular ligand-binding domain, a transmembrane portion, and an intracellular TK domain.[5] Upon the binding of a ligand, the receptor transforms from an inactive monomer into a catalytically active homodimer that autophosphorylates its own C-terminal tyrosines.[6] This dimerization stabilizes the active receptor confirmation and generates a docking site for proteins to be phosphorylated

Disclosures: No conflicts of interest.
Department of Neurosurgery, Stanford University, 1201 Welch Road, MSLS p309, Stanford, CA 94305, USA
* Corresponding author.
E-mail address: gordonli@stanford.edu

Neurosurg Clin N Am 23 (2012) 237–246
doi:10.1016/j.nec.2012.01.011

by the now-active TK domain. Activation of EGFR leads to phosphorylation of downstream proteins, including phosphatidylinositol 3-kinase (PI3K), AKT, RAS, RAF, and mitogen-activated protein kinases. These downstream proteins have been associated with cell division, migration, adhesion, differentiation, and apoptosis, making EGFR an important player in tumorigenicity.[7]

EGFR signaling has been implicated in the pathogenesis of many human cancers, including head and neck, ovarian, cervical, bladder, esophageal, gastric, breast, endometrial, colorectal, and GB.[8,9] Often, EGFR expression or activity is enhanced in tumors through gene amplification, aberrant activity through autocrine overproduction of the receptor ligands, or mutations to the *EGFR* gene. In GBs, EGFR is overexpressed in approximately 40% to 50% of cases, and clinical and research studies show that tumors with overexpressed or amplified *EGFR* exhibit worse prognosis, increased tumor aggressiveness, and resistance to therapeutic treatments.[4] Furthermore, in vitro studies have shown increased resistance to radiation therapy in immortalized GB cell lines stably transduced with EGFR.[10,11] *EGFR* gene amplification is 5-fold higher in primary GBs compared with secondary tumors, and EGFR overexpression occurs in approximately 60% of primary cases, although this is found only in 10% of secondary GBs.[12]

Because aberrant EGFR activity plays an important role in malignant transformation, new therapeutic strategies have been developed targeting this gene. For instance, small-molecule TK inhibitors and monoclonal antibodies (mAbs) have been studied in clinical trials. Recently, newer treatments, including RNA-based therapies, ligand-toxin conjugates, and radioimmunoconjugates, have had promising preclinical results.[13–19]

EGFR Inhibitors Targeting the ATP-Binding Pocket

One of the earliest and most common methods of inhibiting EGFR is the use of small molecules that bind to the ATP-binding pocket of the TK domain, thereby preventing autophosphorylation and subsequent activation of the signal mechanism. Imatinib and lapatinib are two examples of molecular inhibitors of tyrosine kinases (others include erlotinib and gefitinib) that were originally designed to target similar TKs (ABL and HER2, respectively) but were found to also inhibit EGFR. Phase I and II trials investigating these inhibitors in GBs have demonstrated only modest clinical effects.[20,21] Even with small molecules that specifically inhibit EGFR, such as erlotinib and gefitinib, the clinical

results are modest. In a phase II trial, 38 recurrent GB patients were treated with erlotinib monotherapy after radiotherapy. Patients were found to have a median progression-free survival (PFS) of 8 weeks, with only 3% of patients meeting a target goal of PFS at 6 months.[22] A separate, randomized phase II trial of 110 patients with progressive GB after prior radiotherapy showed that only 11.4% of erlotinib-treated patients with recurrent GB had PFS after 6 months compared with 24% of patients in the control arm treated with temozolomide or carmustine (BCNU).[23] No significant difference in overall survival was observed between the 2 treatment arms. When gefinitib was used as the main treatment in a phase II trial, 6-month PFS occurred in 13% of the GB patients with no significant increase in median overall survival compared with historical controls.[24,25] In another phase II trial involving 98 newly diagnosed GB patients treated with adjuvant gefitinib postradiation, the overall survival at 1 year was 54.2% and PFS at 1 year was 16.7%, results that are not significantly different compared with historical controls.[26] In order to enhance the efficacy of gefitinib, a combinational study with an inhibitor to a mammalian target of rapamycin (mTOR) was also conducted. mTOR is located downstream of 2 well-known EGFR substrates, AKT and PI3K, and by combining the 2 inhibitors the goal was to inhibit the PI3K/AKT signaling pathway in concert with EGFR antagonism. In a phase I trial, patients with recurrent, high-grade gliomas treated with gefitinib and sirolimus (an mTOR inhibitor) showed that 44% of the patients achieved either partial response or stable disease, with PFS similar to that in a separate phase II study involving gefitinib treatment alone.[25,27] More recently, the phase II trial of erlotinib plus sirolimus in adults with recurrent GB showed negligible activity.[28] Another study using gefitinib and everolimus treatment in 22 patients with recurrent GB showed 36% of patients with stable disease and 14% with a partial response but only one patient with PFS at 6 months.[29]

Monoclonal Antibodies Blocking EGFR Ligand Binding

Another method of inhibiting EGFR activity is by blocking the ligands that bind to the EGFR (epidermal growth factor, transforming growth factor, heparin-binding epidermal growth factor–like growth factor, amphiregulin, betacellulin, epiregulin, and epigen). mAbs, such as cetuximab and nimotuzumab, were devised to compete with EGF binding and were shown in vitro to decrease the downstream signaling cascade of EGFR.

Cetuximab in preclinical studies was shown to inhibit growth and increase apoptosis in GB cell lines.[30,31] There are conflicting data, however, regarding whether EGFR amplification imparts cetuximab sensitivity.[30,32] In a phase I/II trial (GERT), 17 patients with confirmed GB pathology underwent standard postoperative treatment of radiation and temozolomide, followed by weekly infusions of cetuximab. The median follow-up was 13 months in this group. At 6 months, 81% of patients had PFS, and at 12 months 87% of patients were still alive. In another study, cetuximab was used to treat patients with recurrent high-grade glioma after surgery, radiotherapy, and chemotherapy. Patients were stratified into 2 treatment arms according to EGFR amplification status. A total of 55 patients underwent treatment with cetuximab (28 with and 27 without an increased EGFR copy number). The median duration of PFS was 1.9 months, and the median overall survival was 5 months. The rates of 6-month PFS and overall survival were 10% and 40%, respectively.[33] Lastly, cetuximab has also been tried in a phase II trial in combination with bevacizumab (an mAb that inhibits vascular endothelial growth factor A) and irinotecan (an inhibitor topoisomerase) for patients with primary GBs after tumor progression after radiation therapy and temozolomide treatment. The mean duration of overall survival observed was 29 weeks, with a mean time to tumor progression of 24 weeks. Thirty percent of patients were free of tumor progression at 6 months.[34] Overall, use of cetuximab has shown limited activity in the GB patient population as seen through the results of various phase I/II trials.

Studies using nimotuzumab, which targets the extracellular domain of EGFR, found it to have both antiangiogenic and proapoptotic effects. A phase I trial using nimotuzumab and whole-brain radiation in 28 individuals with newly diagnosed high-grade gliomas after tumor resection (16 with GB) found an objective response rate of 7.9% (defined as either a complete or partial response).[35] Furthermore, the median duration of overall survival observed was 22 months with a median follow-up of 29 months. The results are promising but require further studies, including a randomized control trial to assess efficacy.

In order to generate a better GB therapy, EGFR mAbs were attached to cytotoxic agents and evaluated in clinical trials. mAb-425 (a murine mAb raised against human carcinoma cells that express high levels of EGFR) was conjugated with sodium iodide I 125 and was used to treat high-grade gliomas in a phase II study of 180 patients with either GB or astrocytomas with anaplastic foci.[36] After radiolabeled mAb-425 was administered after surgery and radiation therapy, the median duration of overall survival rates of patients with GB or astrocytomas with anaplastic foci was 13.4 and 50.9 months, respectively.

EGFRvIII
Background on EGFRvIII

There are at least 10 classes of EGFR mutation variants described in gliomas. EGFRvIII is the most common variant of EGFR and is present in approximately 24% to 67% of GBs.[37,38] EGFRvIII results from an in-frame deletion corresponding to exons 2–7 of the EGFR gene, resulting in the deletion of a large portion of the extracellular domain.[39] Despite the loss of the ligand-binding region, EGFRvIII can homodimerize and autophosphorylate, rendering it constitutively active. In vitro studies have demonstrated that EGFRvIII expression can enhance cellular growth and tumorigenicity, indicating that this mutant receptor is oncogenic.[40] The molecular mechanism by which EGFRvIII can transform normal cells into malignant brain tumors is not completely understood, but expression of EGFRvIII was found to correlate with increased activity of PI3K.[41,42]

Clinical studies of EGFRvIII revealed that this mutant EGFR expression is expressed in a variety of tumors, including medulloblastomas, non–small cell lung carcinoma, breast cancer, and GBs.[43] In addition, many in vitro and in vivo studies show that EGFRvIII is specific to tumors and not present in normal cells, making it an intriguing biomarker for cancer. Yet, although its expression is cancer specific, there is currently a debate over the prognostic relevance of EGFRvIII in patients with GB. In some studies, EGFRvIII has not been found an independent prognostic indicator of survival.[44–46] In other studies, however, results have been inconclusive or EGFRvIII found an unfavorable predictor of survival.[47–49] For instance, a recent study showed no significant change in short-term GB survivors in patients with EGFRvIII expression, 0.96 to 1.07 years. In long-term GB survivors, there was a negative correlation in which patients who were EGFRvIII positive had a survival of 1.21 years, whereas EGFRvIII-negative patients survived on average 2.03 years.[50,51] Despite this controversy, EGFRvIII is an attractive target for malignant gliomas and a variety of therapeutics have been developed toward this gene.

Monoclonal Antibodies to EGFRvIII

Because EGFRvIII is expressed on GB and not in normal brain, mAbs have been developed to target and destroy EGFRvIII-expressing tumor cells. Two such antibodies, mAb 806 and mAb Y10, have shown promising preclinical results as evident by a significant reduction in tumor volume in vivo and prolonged length of survival in mice.[52–55] Consistently, EGFRvIII mAbs conjugated to cytotoxic agents decrease glial tumor growth in mice,[56] and radiolabeling of EGFRvIII mAbs increased glial cell death.[57] Although these reports indicate that EGFRvIII mAbs may be an attractive GB therapeutic agent, no clinical trials have been conducted on their efficacy in humans.

EGFRvIII Vaccine Treatment

Another active area of research has been the development of an EGFRvIII vaccine for GB patients. The preclinical studies had promising results that culminated in series of recent clinical trials evaluating active immunization with an EGFRvIII peptide.[58–61] During accrual for the ACTI-VATE study, the Stupp and colleagues[62] study was published and the addition of postoperative temozolomide became standard of care in treatment of GB patients. In response, the ACT II trial was started. Twenty-one patients with newly diagnosed GB who underwent gross total resection followed by concurrent radiotherapy and temozolomide were recruited for treatment with the EGFRvIII peptide vaccine, now called rindopepimut (CDX-110). The median PFS of all patients was 15.2 months, and the overall survival from time of diagnosis was 23.6 months. After adjustment for age and Karnofsky performance status, the risk of death of the vaccinated patients was significantly lower than that observed in the temozolomide-treated historical control group. This trial also evaluated if lymphopenia from temozolomide inhibits the immune response from the peptide vaccination.[63] Patients received either a standard 5-day temozolomide schedule or a daily dose-intensified regimen. Although the dose-intensified group exhibited more profound lymphopenia, those patients mounted a stronger immune response. Histologic samples were available for EGFRvIII expression by immunohistochemical analysis from 12 of 17 recurrent tumors. Eleven of these samples had lost expression of EGFRvIII.

As a result of these promising trials, ACT III was started as a multicenter single-arm trial evaluating the peptide vaccine in 65 patients with newly diagnosed EGFRvIII-positive GBs enrolled after gross total resection and standard chemoradiation. The preliminary results demonstrate a median overall survival of 24.3 months from the initial diagnosis. Furthermore, more than 30% of patients have survived more than 36 months from diagnosis.

ACT IV, a multicenter international, randomized, placebo-controlled trial was verified in January of this year to begin enrolling patients.

PTEN
Background on PTEN

One of the most frequent genes that is either mutated or deleted in tumors is PTEN. PTEN was originally identified in 1997 as a tumor suppressor that was mutated in a variety of cancers, including prostate, breast, and GB.[64] PTEN is a phosphatase that controls the activity of an upstream regulator of PI3K, phosphatidylinositol (3,4,5)-trisphosphate. PTEN plays an important role in regulating cell growth by regulating kinases, such as PI3K, and subsequently AKT.

PTEN Role in GB Cell Lines

Much of what is known about PTEN in GB has been done in cell lines and mouse models. PTEN deletions in astrocytic cell lines were found to have increased proliferation,[65,66] whereas reintroduction of PTEN to GB cell lines deficient in PTEN suppressed proliferation.[66,67] PTEN has also been implicated in migration and invasion, traits particularly notorious in GBs. For instance, PTEN gene deletions in early neural precursors resulted in profound neuronal migration defects.[68,69] Additionally, glioma cells deficient in PTEN demonstrated reduced cell invasiveness when they were treated with PI3K inhibitors or through the overexpression of PTEN. Together these findings demonstrate that PTEN is involved in a variety of cellular processes in GBs, including cell growth, survival, and tumor invasiveness.

Clinical Significance of PTEN in GBs

Clinical studies monitoring PTEN expression in GBs indicated that there could be a correlation between PTEN loss and poorer patient prognosis. Prior studies have shown that pediatric patients with PTEN mutations found in pediatric malignant astrocytomas have a poorer prognosis.[70,71] In adults, loss of chromosome 10q has been found to negatively affect survival for both high-grade gliomas and GB independently.[72–74] Unfortunately, the conclusions drawn from these studies are limited due to small sample size, and further studies must be conducted to conclude whether PTEN loss is a harbinger of poorer outcome. Loss of chromosome 10q occurs more frequently than genetic mutations (70% vs 25%). A study by Zhou and colleagues[75] found that 28% of GBs, 7% of anaplastic astrocytomas, and 0% of low-grade gliomas had PTEN mutations. The lack of PTEN mutations in low-grade gliomas was validated in several other studies and suggests that PTEN loss most likely does not promote a growth advantage early in GB development but could be linked to increased invasiveness.

Although the clinical relevance of PTEN is still unclear, a recent report studying drug efficacy in GB patients indicated that PTEN might be a useful biologic marker. In this study, a correlation between coexpression of EGFRvIII and intact PTEN in recurrent malignant glioma patients was found to predict sensitivity to EGFR inhibitor mono-therapy.[76] Because PTEN expression decreases PI3K activity, then mTOR inhibitors that inhibit the PI3K pathway are expected to function in a similar fashion if used in combination with EGFR inhibitors—both lower PI3K levels. As discussed previously, however, in phase I and II trials, EGFR inhibition (ie, gefitinib) in combination with mTOR inhibitor therapy has not proved effective in GBs.[27,28] It is possible, however, that positive outcomes could have been missed because coexpression of EGFRvIII and intact PTEN was not specifically selected for in the 2 clinical phase trials.

MGMT
Background on MGMT

MGMT is a highly conserved protein involved in DNA repair. The enzyme protects cells against DNA damage by reversing alkylation at the O^6 position of guanine.[77] Specifically, the transfer of an alkyl group to the active site of the enzyme results in the removal of DNA base pairs incorrectly bound to thymidine. If this correction is not made, the cell undergoes apoptosis or cellular senescence.[78] Consequently, the presence of MGMT enhances cell survival after DNA damage.

Clinical Significance of MGMT in GBs

MGMT became clinically relevant in GBs after reports showed some predictive value attributed to the absence of MGMT in patients undergoing chemotherapy with alkylating agents. It was observed that patients with low levels of MGMT derived considerable benefit from BCNU compared with patients with higher levels of MGMT expression.[79,80] In addition, low levels of MGMT protein could predict prolonged PFS in patients with glioma who were treated with temozolomide.[81]

Because there was mounting evidence that MGMT expression predicted GB patient outcome, researchers began studying how this gene is regulated in GBs. Epigenetic methylation at the MGMT promoter region was discovered to decrease transcription of MGMT, thereby making the cells vulnerable to DNA damage and cell death. The process that promotes DNA damage could also make mismatch repair-deficient cells more vulnerable to alkylating agents. Applying this logic, researchers subsequently investigated whether gliomas with increased levels of methylation at the MGMT promoter site were more susceptible to alkylating agents. Silencing the MGMT promoter has been observed in up to 93% of low-grade gliomas[82] and 45% of GBs.[83] These findings suggest that a large percentage of GB patients could be more responsive to chemotherapy if MGMT expression is decreased through methylation.

MGMT Promoter Methylation as a Prognostic Marker for GBs

The strongest support linking MGMT promoter methylation status to prognosis of patients with gliomas came from 2 large randomized clinical trials, the European Organisation for Research and Treatment of Cancer (EORTC) 26981/22981 and the National Cancer Institute of Canada (NCIC) CE.3 trial.[62,83] These trials demonstrated that MGMT promoter methylation was able to predict prolonged PFS in patients treated with te-mozolomide and radiotherapy. The 5-year follow-up data from the EORTC study further confirmed that MGMT methylation was predictive of prognosis in patients with GB.[84] In this study, the median overall survival for MGMT promoter meth-ylated patients treated with radiotherapy and te-mozolomide was 23.4 months versus 15.3 months for those receiving radiotherapy alone. The median overall survival in patients with unme-thylated MGMT promoters was 12.6 months in the radiotherapy plus temozolomide group and 11.8 months for the radiotherapy-alone group.

The heterogeneity of malignant GBs across patients, specifically the heterogeneity of MGMT promoter methylation, requires more attention and research. When this unresolved issue becomes clarified, it will undoubtedly stratify patients into further classes of treatment responders and lead to more distinct prognostic groups. Currently, methylation-specific polymerase chain reaction (MSP) remains the only test that has repeatedly shown predictive and prognostic value in identifying methylated areas in clinical trials.[85] Methylation occurs at CpG islands by epigenetic forces. Tests like MSP can detect the fraction of CpG islands that are methylated at the MGMT promoter site in patients with GBs. More recently, Shah and colleagues,[86] using quantitative bisulfate se-quencing, determined the methylation status of all 97 CpG sites at the MGMT promoter site in tumor samples from 70 newly diagnosed GB patients who subsequently underwent resection and radiation therapy with concurrent temozolomide adjuvant therapy. Of the 70 patients, 39 had 1-year PFS data based on which Shah and colleagues[86] were able to propose a new classification scheme using the methylation patterns observed.

Studies have also begun to show that variability of methylation can lead to affects in survival. For instance, a study by Krex and colleagues[87] showed that 75% of 5-year GB survivors demonstrated MGMT promoter methylation. In another study, patients with more than 29% MGMT methylation (over 12 CpG islands) had significantly better outcomes than those with less methylation.[88] These preliminary studies provide important insights not only into the variability between GB patients that has been known for years but also in regards to the variability between MGMT methylation in patients with respect to treatment responsiveness. Despite this new evidence, the picture remains incomplete and still complex. For instance, there are subsets of GB patients who survive well beyond 5 years who do not possess MGMT methylation, indicating other complex biologic processes and interactions in GB. Nevertheless, methylation of the MGMT promoter region seems an important factor influencing treatment responsiveness.

MGMT promoter methylation has emerged as one of the most important biomarkers of GB with respect to predictive and prognostic value, following the results of EORTC-NCIC clinical trials. Several questions, however, remain: (1) How static is the methylation status throughout temozolomide and radiation treatment? (2) How do variations in the degree of methylation affect outcomes? (3) What ultimately becomes the most sensitive test to analyze methylation status? (4) What other biomarkers along with MGMT further stratify prognosis in patients? and (5) How will this information be managed in clinical practice? (ie, Who will receive therapy and who will be encouraged not to seek treatment despite having a GB?) In the coming years, further insights into the role of MGMT promoter methylation in GB patients will provide answers to these questions, as improving treatment of the devastating disease, GB, continues to make strides.

MGMT Resistance to Temozolomide

Many GB cells develop chemoresistance to temozolomide, and MGMT is thought to play an important factor in GB resistance to temozolomide therapy. GBs that possess high expression of MGMT were found to have higher resistance to temozolomide.[89,90] To combat this resistance, recent studies have begun to use therapeutic agents to suppress, overcome, or sensitize MGMT activity. A recent phase II trial study used the psuedosubstrate O^6-benzylguanine concurrently with temozolomide in recurrent, temozolomide-resistant malignant glioma to overcome the MGMT activity. The investigators were unable to produce significant restoration of temozolomide sensitivity in GBs, however. Other investigators have attempted to overcome MGMT activity by using dose-intensified temozolomide regimens, but thus far, this method has not improved overall survival in these patients.

SUMMARY

To date, EGFR, EGFRvIII, PTEN, and MGMT are the most clinically relevant molecular markers in GB. This article reviews the biology and clinical studies for these markers. There is a great need to find more effective treatments for GB patients afflicted with this highly aggressive and biologically complex disease. As technology improves, more methods will be established to identify new and better diagnostic and prognostic markers. Advances in genomics, proteomics, and molecular understanding of GBs will enable novel therapeutic targets to be identified and tested.

REFERENCES

1. Burger PC, Vogel FS, Green SB, et al. Glioblastoma multiforme and anaplastic astrocytoma. Pathologic criteria and prognostic implications. Cancer 1985; 56(5):1106–11.
2. Louis DN, Ohgaki H, Wiestler OD, et al. The 2007 who classification of tumours of the central nervous system. Acta Neuropathol 2007;114(2):97–109.
3. Wen PY, Kesari S. Malignant gliomas in adults. N Engl J Med 2008;359(5):492–507.
4. Salomon DS, Brandt R, Ciardiello F, et al. Epidermal growth factor-related peptides and their receptors in human malignancies. Crit Rev Oncol Hematol 1995; 19(3):183–232.
5. Wells A. Egf receptor. Int J Biochem Cell Biol 1999; 31(6):637–43.
6. Citri A, Yarden Y. Egf-erbb signalling: towards the systems level. Nat Rev Mol Cell Biol 2006;7(7): 505–16.
7. Hynes NE, Lane HA. Erbb receptors and cancer: the complexity of targeted inhibitors. Nat Rev Cancer 2005;5(5):341–54.
8. Libermann TA, Nusbaum HR, Razon N, et al. Amplification, enhanced expression and possible rearrangement of egf receptor gene in primary human

brain tumours of glial origin. Nature 1985;313(5998): 144–7.

9. Wong AJ, Bigner SH, Bigner DD, et al. Increased expression of the epidermal growth factor receptor gene in malignant gliomas is invariably associated with gene amplification. Proc Natl Acad Sci U S A 1987;84(19):6899–903.

10. Chakravarti A, Chakladar A, Delaney MA, et al. The epidermal growth factor receptor pathway mediates resistance to sequential administration of radiation and chemotherapy in primary human glioblastoma cells in a ras-dependent manner. Cancer Res 2002;62(15):4307–15.

11. Barker FG 2nd, Simmons ML, Chang SM, et al. Egfr overexpression and radiation response in glioblastoma multiforme. Int J Radiat Oncol Biol Phys 2001;51(2):410–8.

12. Watanabe K, Tachibana O, Sata K, et al. Overexpression of the egf receptor and p53 mutations are mutually exclusive in the evolution of primary and secondary glioblastomas. Brain Pathol 1996;6(3): 217–23 [discussion: 23–4].

13. Cohen KA, Liu T, Bissonette R, et al. Dab389egf fusion protein therapy of refractory glioblastoma multiforme. Curr Pharm Biotechnol 2003;4(1): 39–49.

14. Halatsch ME, Schmidt U, Botefur IC, et al. Marked inhibition of glioblastoma target cell tumorigenicity in vitro by retrovirus-mediated transfer of a hairpin ribozyme against deletion-mutant epidermal growth factor receptor messenger rna. J Neurosurg 2000; 92(2):297–305.

15. Liu TF, Hall PD, Cohen KA, et al. Interstitial diphtheria toxin-epidermal growth factor fusion protein therapy produces regressions of subcutaneous human glioblastoma multiforme tumors in athymic nude mice. Clin Cancer Res 2005;11(1):329–34.

16. Lorimer IA, Keppler-Hafkemeyer A, Beers RA, et al. Recombinant immunotoxins specific for a mutant epidermal growth factor receptor: Targeting with a single chain antibody variable domain isolated by phage display. Proc Natl Acad Sci U S A 1996; 93(25):14815–20.

17. Kang CS, Zhang ZY, Jia ZF, et al. Suppression of egfr expression by antisense or small interference rna inhibits u251 glioma cell growth in vitro and in vivo. Cancer Gene Ther 2006;13(5):530–8.

18. Vollmann A, Vornlocher HP, Stempfl T, et al. Effective silencing of egfr with rnai demonstrates non-egfr dependent proliferation of glioma cells. Int J Oncol 2006;28(6):1531–42.

19. Yamazaki H, Kijima H, Ohnishi Y, et al. Inhibition of tumor growth by ribozyme-mediated suppression of aberrant epidermal growth factor receptor gene expression. J Natl Cancer Inst 1998;90(8):581–7.

20. Razis E, Selviaridis P, Labropoulos S, et al. Phase ii study of neoadjuvant imatinib in glioblastoma: evaluation of clinical and molecular effects of the treatment. Clin Cancer Res 2009;15(19):6258–66.

21. Thiessen B, Stewart C, Tsao M, et al. A phase i/ii trial of gw572016 (lapatinib) in recurrent glioblastoma multiforme: clinical outcomes, pharmacokinetics and molecular correlation. Cancer Chemother Pharmacol 2010;65(2):353–61.

22. Raizer JJ, Abrey LE, Lassman AB, et al. A phase ii trial of erlotinib in patients with recurrent malignant gliomas and nonprogressive glioblastoma multiforme postradiation therapy. Neuro Oncol 2010; 12(1):95–103.

23. van den Bent MJ, Brandes AA, Rampling R, et al. Randomized phase ii trial of erlotinib versus temozolomide or carmustine in recurrent glioblastoma: eortc brain tumor group study 26034. J Clin Oncol 2009;27(8):1268–74.

24. Wong ET, Hess KR, Gleason MJ, et al. Outcomes and prognostic factors in recurrent glioma patients enrolled onto phase ii clinical trials. J Clin Oncol 1999;17(8):2572–8.

25. Rich JN, Reardon DA, Peery T, et al. Phase ii trial of gefitinib in recurrent glioblastoma. J Clin Oncol 2004;22(1):133–42.

26. Uhm JH, Ballman KV, Wu W, et al. Phase ii evaluation of gefitinib in patients with newly diagnosed grade 4 astrocytoma: mayo/north central cancer treatment group study n0074. Int J Radiat Oncol Biol Phys 2011;80(2):347–53.

27. Reardon DA, Quinn JA, Vredenburgh JJ, et al. Phase 1 trial of gefitinib plus sirolimus in adults with recurrent malignant glioma. Clin Cancer Res 2006;12(3 Pt 1):860–8.

28. Reardon DA, Desjardins A, Vredenburgh JJ, et al. Phase 2 trial of erlotinib plus sirolimus in adults with recurrent glioblastoma. J Neurooncol 2010; 96(2):219–30.

29. Kreisl TN, Lassman AB, Mischel PS, et al. A pilot study of everolimus and gefitinib in the treatment of recurrent glioblastoma (gbm). J Neurooncol 2009;92(1):99–105.

30. Eller JL, Longo SL, Kyle MM, et al. Anti-epidermal growth factor receptor monoclonal antibody cetuximab augments radiation effects in glioblastoma multiforme in vitro and in vivo. Neurosurgery 2005;56(1): 155–62 [discussion: 62].

31. Patel D, Lahiji A, Patel S, et al. Monoclonal antibody cetuximab binds to and down-regulates constitutively activated epidermal growth factor receptor viii on the cell surface. Anticancer Res 2007; 27(5A):3355–66.

32. Eller JL, Longo SL, Hicklin DJ, et al. Activity of anti-epidermal growth factor receptor monoclonal antibody c225 against glioblastoma multiforme. Neurosurgery 2002;51(4):1005–13 [discussion: 13–4].

33. Neyns B, Sadones J, Joosens E, et al. Stratified phase ii trial of cetuximab in patients with

recurrent high-grade glioma. Ann Oncol 2009;20(9): 1596–603.

34. Hasselbalch B, Lassen U, Hansen S, et al. Cetuximab, bevacizumab, and irinotecan for patients with primary glioblastoma and progression after radiation therapy and temozolomide: a phase ii trial. Neuro Oncol 2010;12(5):508–16.

35. Ramos TC, Figueredo J, Catala M, et al. Treatment of high-grade glioma patients with the humanized anti-epidermal growth factor receptor (egfr) antibody h-r3: report from a phase i/ii trial. Cancer Biol Ther 2006;5(4):375–9.

36. Quang TS, Brady LW. Radioimmunotherapy as a novel treatment regimen: 125i-labeled monoclonal antibody 425 in the treatment of high-grade brain gliomas. Int J Radiat Oncol Biol Phys 2004;58(3):972–5.

37. Humphrey PA, Wong AJ, Vogelstein B, et al. Anti-synthetic peptide antibody reacting at the fusion junction of deletion-mutant epidermal growth factor receptors in human glioblastoma. Proc Natl Acad Sci U S A 1990;87(11):4207–11.

38. Wong AJ, Ruppert JM, Bigner SH, et al. Structural alterations of the epidermal growth factor receptor gene in human gliomas. Proc Natl Acad Sci U S A 1992;89(7):2965–9.

39. Frederick L, Wang XY, Eley G, et al. Diversity and frequency of epidermal growth factor receptor mutations in human glioblastomas. Cancer Res 2000; 60(5):1383–7.

40. Fernandes H, Cohen S, Bishayee S. Glycosylation-induced conformational modification positively regulates receptor-receptor association: a study with an aberrant epidermal growth factor receptor (egfrviii/deltaegfr) expressed in cancer cells. J Biol Chem 2001;276(7):5375–83.

41. Antonyak MA, Moscatello DK, Wong AJ. Constitutive activation of c-jun n-terminal kinase by a mutant epidermal growth factor receptor. J Biol Chem 1998;273(5):2817–22.

42. Moscatello DK, Holgado-Madruga M, Emlet DR, et al. Constitutive activation of phosphatidylinositol 3-kinase by a naturally occurring mutant epidermal growth factor receptor. J Biol Chem 1998;273(1):200–6.

43. Moscatello DK, Holgado-Madruga M, Godwin AK, et al. Frequent expression of a mutant epidermal growth factor receptor in multiple human tumors. Cancer Res 1995;55(23):5536–9.

44. Galanis E, Buckner J, Kimmel D, et al. Gene amplification as a prognostic factor in primary and secondary high-grade malignant gliomas. Int J Oncol 1998;13(4):717–24.

45. Newcomb EW, Cohen H, Lee SR, et al. Survival of patients with glioblastoma multiforme is not influenced by altered expression of p16, p53, egfr, mdm2 or bcl-2 genes. Brain Pathol 1998;8(4):655–67.

46. Waha A, Baumann A, Wolf HK, et al. Lack of prognostic relevance of alterations in the epidermal growth factor receptor-transforming growth factor-alpha pathway in human astrocytic gliomas. J Neurosurg 1996;85(4):634–41.

47. Bouvier-Labit C, Chinot O, Ochi C, et al. Prognostic significance of ki67, p53 and epidermal growth factor receptor immunostaining in human glioblastomas. Neuropathol Appl Neurobiol 1998;24(5):381–8.

48. Etienne MC, Formento JL, Lebrun-Frenay C, et al. Epidermal growth factor receptor and labeling index are independent prognostic factors in glial tumor outcome. Clin Cancer Res 1998;4(10):2383–90.

49. Zhu A, Shaeffer J, Leslie S, et al. Epidermal growth factor receptor: an independent predictor of survival in astrocytic tumors given definitive irradiation. Int J Radiat Oncol Biol Phys 1996;34(4):809–15.

50. Heimberger AB, Hlatky R, Suki D, et al. Prognostic effect of epidermal growth factor receptor and egfr-viii in glioblastoma multiforme patients. Clin Cancer Res 2005;11(4):1462–6.

51. Heimberger AB, Suki D, Yang D, et al. The natural history of egfr and egfrviii in glioblastoma patients. J Transl Med 2005;3:38.

52. Johns TG, Stockert E, Ritter G, et al. Novel monoclonal antibody specific for the de2-7 epidermal growth factor receptor (egfr) that also recognizes the egfr expressed in cells containing amplification of the egfr gene. Int J Cancer 2002;98(3):398–408.

53. Jungbluth AA, Stockert E, Huang HJ, et al. A monoclonal antibody recognizing human cancers with amplification/overexpression of the human epidermal growth factor receptor. Proc Natl Acad Sci U S A 2003;100(2):639–44.

54. Perera RM, Narita Y, Furnari FB, et al. Treatment of human tumor xenografts with monoclonal antibody 806 in combination with a prototypical epidermal growth factor receptor-specific antibody generates enhanced antitumor activity. Clin Cancer Res 2005; 11(17):6390–9.

55. Sampson JH, Crotty LE, Lee S, et al. Unarmed, tumor-specific monoclonal antibody effectively treats brain tumors. Proc Natl Acad Sci U S A 2000;97(13):7503–8.

56. Ochiai H, Archer GE, Herndon JE 2nd, et al. Egfrviii-targeted immunotoxin induces antitumor immunity that is inhibited in the absence of cd4+ and cd8+ t cells. Cancer Immunol Immunother 2008;57(1):115–21.

57. Yang W, Wu G, Barth RF, et al. Molecular targeting and treatment of composite egfr and egfrviii-positive gliomas using boronated monoclonal antibodies. Clin Cancer Res 2008;14(3):883–91.

58. Ciesielski MJ, Kazim AL, Barth RF, et al. Cellular antitumor immune response to a branched lysine multiple antigenic peptide containing epitopes of a common tumor-specific antigen in a rat glioma model. Cancer Immunol Immunother 2005;54(2):107–19.

59. Heimberger AB, Archer GE, Crotty LE, et al. Dendritic cells pulsed with a tumor-specific peptide

induce long-lasting immunity and are effective against murine intracerebral melanoma. Neurosurgery 2002;50(1):158–64 [discussion: 64–6].

60. Heimberger AB, Crotty LE, Archer GE, et al. Epidermal growth factor receptor viii peptide vaccination is efficacious against established intracerebral tumors. Clin Cancer Res 2003;9(11):4247–54.

61. Moscatello DK, Ramirez G, Wong AJ. A naturally occurring mutant human epidermal growth factor receptor as a target for peptide vaccine immunotherapy of tumors. Cancer Res 1997;57(8):1419–24.

62. Stupp R, Mason WP, van den Bent MJ, et al. Radiotherapy plus concomitant and adjuvant temozolomide for glioblastoma. N Engl J Med 2005;352(10): 987–96.

63. Sampson JH, Aldape KD, Archer GE, et al. Greater chemotherapy-induced lymphopenia enhances tumor-specific immune responses that eliminate egfrviii-expressing tumor cells in patients with glioblastoma. Neuro Oncol 2011;13(3):324–33.

64. Li J, Yen C, Liaw D, et al. Pten, a putative protein tyrosine phosphatase gene mutated in human brain, breast, and prostate cancer. Science 1997; 275(5308):1943–7.

65. Fraser MM, Zhu X, Kwon CH, et al. Pten loss causes hypertrophy and increased proliferation of astrocytes in vivo. Cancer Res 2004;64(21):7773–9.

66. Gottschalk AR, Basila D, Wong M, et al. P27kip1 is required for pten-induced g1 growth arrest. Cancer Res 2001;61(5):2105–11.

67. Furnari FB, Huang HJ, Cavenee WK. The phosphoinositol phosphatase activity of pten mediates a serum-sensitive g1 growth arrest in glioma cells. Cancer Res 1998;58(22):5002–8.

68. Backman SA, Stambolic V, Suzuki A, et al. Deletion of pten in mouse brain causes seizures, ataxia and defects in soma size resembling lhermitte-duclos disease. Nat Genet 2001;29(4):396–403.

69. Kwon CH, Zhu X, Zhang J, et al. Pten regulates neuronal soma size: a mouse model of lhermitte-duclos disease. Nat Genet 2001;29(4):404–11.

70. Phillips HS, Kharbanda S, Chen R, et al. Molecular subclasses of high-grade glioma predict prognosis, delineate a pattern of disease progression, and resemble stages in neurogenesis. Cancer Cell 2006;9(3):157–73.

71. Raffel C, Frederick L, O'Fallon JR, et al. Analysis of oncogene and tumor suppressor gene alterations in pediatric malignant astrocytomas reveals reduced survival for patients with pten mutations. Clin Cancer Res 1999;5(12):4085–90.

72. Homma T, Fukushima T, Vaccarella S, et al. Correlation among pathology, genotype, and patient outcomes in glioblastoma. J Neuropathol Exp Neurol 2006;65(9):846–54.

73. Lin H, Bondy ML, Langford LA, et al. Allelic deletion analyses of mmac/pten and dmbt1 loci in gliomas:

relationship to prognostic significance. Clin Cancer Res 1998;4(10):2447–54.

74. Tada K, Shiraishi S, Kamiryo T, et al. Analysis of loss of heterozygosity on chromosome 10 in patients with malignant astrocytic tumors: correlation with patient age and survival. J Neurosurg 2001;95(4):651–9.

75. Zhou XP, Li YJ, Hoang-Xuan K, et al. Mutational analysis of the pten gene in gliomas: molecular and pathological correlations. Int J Cancer 1999; 84(2):150–4.

76. Mellinghoff IK, Wang MY, Vivanco I, et al. Molecular determinants of the response of glioblastomas to egfr kinase inhibitors. N Engl J Med 2005;353(19):2012–24.

77. Mineura K, Izumi I, Watanabe K, et al. Influence of o6-methylguanine-DNA methyltransferase activity on chloroethylnitrosourea chemotherapy in brain tumors. Int J Cancer 1993;55(1):76–81.

78. Gerson SL. Mgmt: its role in cancer aetiology and cancer therapeutics. Nat Rev Cancer 2004;4(4): 296–307.

79. Belanich M, Pastor M, Randall T, et al. Retrospective study of the correlation between the DNA repair protein alkyltransferase and survival of brain tumor patients treated with carmustine. Cancer Res 1996; 56(4):783–8.

80. Jaeckle KA, Eyre HJ, Townsend JJ, et al. Correlation of tumor o6 methylguanine-DNA methyltransferase levels with survival of malignant astrocytoma patients treated with bis-chloroethylnitrosourea: a southwest oncology group study. J Clin Oncol 1998;16(10):3310–5.

81. Hegi ME, Diserens AC, Godard S, et al. Clinical trial substantiates the predictive value of o-6-methylguanine-DNA methyltransferase promoter methylation in glioblastoma patients treated with temozolomide. Clin Cancer Res 2004;10(6):1871–4.

82. Everhard S, Kaloshi G, Criniere E, et al. Mgmt methylation: a marker of response to temozolomide in low-grade gliomas. Ann Neurol 2006; 60(6):740–3.

83. Hegi ME, Diserens AC, Gorlia T, et al. Mgmt gene silencing and benefit from temozolomide in glioblastoma. N Engl J Med 2005;352(10):997–1003.

84. Stupp R, Hegi ME, Mason WP, et al. Effects of radiotherapy with concomitant and adjuvant temozolomide versus radiotherapy alone on survival in glioblastoma in a randomised phase iii study: 5-year analysis of the eortc-ncic trial. Lancet Oncol 2009;10(5):459–66.

85. Weller M, Felsberg J, Hartmann C, et al. Molecular predictors of progression-free and overall survival in patients with newly diagnosed glioblastoma: a prospective translational study of the german glioma network. J Clin Oncol 2009; 27(34):5743–50.

86. Shah N, Lin B, Sibenaller Z, et al. Comprehensive analysis of mgmt promoter methylation: correlation

with mgmt expression and clinical response in gbm. PLoS One 2011;6(1):e16146.

87. Krex D, Klink B, Hartmann C, et al. Long-term survival with glioblastoma multiforme. Brain 2007; 130(Pt 10):2596–606.

88. Dunn J, Baborie A, Alam F, et al. Extent of mgmt promoter methylation correlates with outcome in glioblastomas given temozolomide and radiotherapy. Br J Cancer 2009;101(1):124–31.

89. Hegi ME, Liu L, Herman JG, et al. Correlation of o6-methylguanine methyltransferase (mgmt) promoter methylation with clinical outcomes in glioblastoma and clinical strategies to modulate mgmt activity. J Clin Oncol 2008;26(25):4189–99.

90. Sarkaria JN, Kitange GJ, James CD, et al. Mechanisms of chemoresistance to alkylating agents in malignant glioma. Clin Cancer Res 2008;14(10): 2900–8.

The Role of Adjuvant Radiation Therapy in the Management of High-Grade Gliomas

Joshua J. Wind, MD[a], Richard Young, MD[a],
Ashima Saini, MD[b], Jonathan H. Sherman, MD[a],*

KEYWORDS

- Radiation therapy • Radiosurgery • Glioma • Glioblastoma

High-grade gliomas (HGGs) encompass the most malignant and the most commonly encountered primary brain neoplasms in clinical neuro-oncology practice, with an incidence of 5 cases per 100,000 people.[1] They are commonly defined to include World Health Organization grade III and IV glial-based neoplasms, most frequently glioblastomas, anaplastic astrocytomas, and anaplastic oligodendrogliomas. A multidisciplinary approach to the management of these tumors includes surgical resection when feasible, chemotherapy, and radiation therapy. Each of these treatment components has contributed to increased survival in patients with HGGs, with an improvement in mean survival of 8 to 15 months over the past 40 years.[2]

Radiation therapy has become a standard component of the management of HGGs since the 1970s.[3,4] Advances in the understanding of radiobiology have led to refinements in the delivery methods of radiation, resulting in optimization of radiation therapy in terms of dosage, fractionation schedule, conformality, and treatment modalities. Further development of new radiation technologies such as stereotactic targeting and delivery has allowed physicians to investigate whether focal radiation treatment may improve patient outcomes as well.

RADIOBIOLOGY

The primary physiologic mechanism of radiation therapy is through DNA damage; however, recent advances in the understanding of radiobiology have shown that ionizing radiation triggers a variety of complex and dynamic responses in both normal and neoplastic cells, leading to the concept of the cell damage response.[5] There are 5 core concepts of radiobiology within this concept of the cell damage response (the 5 Rs of radiation): repair, repopulation, reoxygenation, redistribution, and radiosensitivity. These 5 concepts are being further refined at the tissue, cellular and molecular level as our understanding of radiobiology advances.[6]

Repair

The molecular biology of repair includes responses to various different types of cell death, including mitotic death (within 1 to 2 cell cycles), interphase death (death of sensitive cells within hours), apoptotic death (programmed cell death), necrotic death (caused by a pathologic rather than physiologic process), and autophagy. Current studies support that in response to DNA damage, cells trigger elaborate signaling pathways to repair the most lethal DNA damage, including double-stranded DNA breaks and the induction of

Disclosures: Funding Sources: None.
Conflicts of Interest: None.
[a] Department of Neurological Surgery, George Washington University Medical Center, 2150 Pennsylvania Avenue Northwest, Suite 7420, Washington, DC 20037, USA
[b] Department of Radiation Oncology, George Washington University Medical Center, 2300 K Street, NW, Washington, DC 20037, USA
* Corresponding author.
E-mail address: jsherman0620@gmail.com

Neurosurg Clin N Am 23 (2012) 247–258
doi:10.1016/j.nec.2012.01.001
1042-3680/12/$ see front matter © 2012 Elsevier Inc. All rights reserved.

apoptosis. Complicated mechanisms of repair include base excision repair, single-strand repair, homologous and nonhomologous recombination of double-strand DNA breaks, and chromatin remodeling.[6,7] Additional cell death pathways and modulators are manipulated to increase repair, including the p53-dependent apoptosis pathway, survival proteins such as survivin,[7] and epidermal growth factor receptor (EGFR)-mediated signaling for increased repair.[8,9]

Repopulation

Repopulation refers to the ability of neoplastic cells to repopulate after radiation treatment. This repopulation shows a lag period after radiation treatment followed by the triggering of an enhanced regenerative process or accelerated and aggressive repopulation.[10] The onset time of this repopulation is variable, but growth factor signaling has been found to play an important role in accelerated regeneration of cancer stem cells (CSCs) after radiation.

Reoxygenation

Oxygenated neoplastic cells are more sensitive to radiation treatment secondary to the availability of oxygen to participate in the generation of DNA damage via the generation of free radicals. Reoxygenation of hypoxic tumor cell populations is arrested via the cell damage response, with hypoxia-induced genes, EGFR signaling, vascular endothelial growth factor (VEGF) upregulation, and neovascularization. Hypoxia inducible factor 1 also functions in a variety of pathways to create enhanced neoplastic cell survival mechanisms and radioresistance.[11–13]

Redistribution

Redistribution of cells refers to the transition of cells through their natural cell cycle, with differences in their sensitivity to radiation at different points within the cycle. Cells within the mitotic phase are most sensitive to radiation damage, thus conveying radiosensitivity to dividing neoplastic cells over normal cell populations in other phases of the cell cycle. However, ionizing radiation has been shown to trigger cyclin-dependent kinase and EGFR signaling, which interferes with cell cycle progression and results in the arrest of neoplastic cells in relatively radioresistant phases.[7]

Radiosensitivity

Radiosensitivity reflects how cells have different intrinsic genetic sensitivities to radiation and usually reflects the shoulder in cell survival curves that can be manipulated by various radioresistance pathways.[7] The principles of radiobiology described earlier can all be manipulated to convey radioresistance, via enhanced DNA repair, increased repopulation responses, hypoxia, and inhibition of cell cycle redistribution.

Advances in Understanding Radioresistance: The Perivascular Niche, CSCs, and Linear-Quadratic Modeling

The tumor microenvironment, with its heterogeneous cell populations of fibroblasts, endothelial cells, reactive inflammatory cells and microvascular proliferating structures, is crucial to tumor expansion and response to radiation.[14] Ionizing radiation induces a series of events that can lead to a microenvironment favorable to neoplastic growth and radiation resistance. These pathways include a composite of cell loss and damage, gene alteration, induced gene products,[15] immunosuppression, and hypoxia.[8] Recent evidence suggests that the glial microenvironment, also termed the perivascular niche, facilitates expansion and differentiation of brain tumor stem cells.[16] Cell types, such as those listed earlier, are present in the perivascular niche and promote cell damage response and signaling pathways that initiate repair mechanisms resulting in radioresistance. The presence of hypoxia promotes the persistence of stem cells and induces the upregulation of proangiogenic factors such as VEGF. Complex immunosuppressive pathways are activated, including transforming growth factor β 1, which acts to suppress antitumor immune responses, enhance extracellular matrix production, and augment angiogenesis, making neoplastic cells more radioresistant.[17]

The concept of the neural stem cell has also further refined concepts of radiobiology and resistance.[18–20] Recent insights into tumor biology suggest that in many cancers only a small subset of cells, defined as CSCs, have the potential to survive and proliferate indefinitely. This small subpopulation of cells resists the exponential cell kill that is generated during fractionated radiation therapy. Consequently, these CSCs are believed to be a primary reason that HGGs recur and are resistant to known forms of therapy.[21] Research has shown that CD133+ CSCs increase after tumor radiation, conveying radioresistance secondary to increased activation of DNA damage response.[5] Further identification and research of these CSCs is required to determine their role in glioma pathophysiology.

The cumulative impact of the classic concepts of radiobiology as well as new concepts of the perivascular niche and the CSC collectively form the unique response profile of a tumor to radiation as well as the response of normal surrounding tissues. Advances in mathematical modeling of the radiation responses of HGGs have led to the application of the linear-quadratic (LQ) model. The LQ model is used to calculate biologically effective doses (BEDs) to compare various treatment modalities or fractionation schedules.

$$BED = \frac{E}{\alpha} = nd\left(1 + \frac{d}{\alpha/\beta}\right) - \frac{\gamma(T - T_k)}{\alpha}$$

This model can be used to extract BEDs from historical treatment cohorts to compare across radiation modalities and fractionation schemes. In addition, the LQ model can also be used to gain understanding about how specific tumor types respond to radiation and to predict how this response might vary with alterations in fractionation and dosage.[22,23]

[Tags: Radiobiology, repair, repopulation, redistribution, reoxygenation, radioresistance, CSCs, perivascular niche, linear-quadratic model].

DEVELOPMENT OF THE CURRENT RADIATION TREATMENT PARADIGM
Initial Studies and Proof of Efficacy

Radiation therapy was initially observed to provide survival benefit in patients with gliomas in a clinical trial performed in 1967.[24] Subsequently, a randomized controlled trial in 1978 confirmed this survival benefit. In this trial, patients who received treatment with BCNU chemotherapy and radiotherapy displayed a 16-week survival advantage over patients receiving chemotherapy alone (34.5 weeks vs 18.5 weeks, $P = .001$). This trial established the efficacy of radiation treatment in the multimodal therapy for gliomas, with a treatment model of 50 to 60 Gy delivered to the entire brain via 5 fractions per week for 5 to 7 weeks.[4] Subsequent randomized controlled trials have confirmed the survival benefit conveyed by radiation therapy.[25–29]

Effect of Cumulative Radiation Dose on Efficacy

With the knowledge that adjuvant radiation is efficacious, additional studies aimed to address the effect of cumulative radiation dose on survival. These studies displayed an increase in overall survival as the cumulative dose is increased up to 60 Gy.[30,31] As the cumulative dose is increased past 60 Gy to doses up to 70 Gy, no additional survival benefit is identified.[32] In addition, analysis of patient outcomes treated with dose escalation as high as 90 Gy has shown that recurrence still occurs locally, within radiation delivery.[33] Because

of these negative studies, 60-Gy radiation therapy for HGG has remained the standard cumulative dosage.

Effect of Hyperfractionation on Efficacy

Fractionation of radiation therapy represents another variable that has been manipulated in the attempt to optimize outcomes in patients treated with radiation. Hyperfractionation is the use of a larger number of smaller-dosed radiation fractions and can be performed on a standard or accelerated schedule. Hyperfractionation has the positive effects of allowing repair of radiation damage in normal nonneoplastic tissues, redistribution of neoplastic cells to radiosensitive portions of the cell cycle, and reoxygenation of tumor cell populations that renders them more radiosensitive. Hyperfractionation also carries the negative effect of allowing time for the neoplastic cells to repopulate. Standard conventional radiation therapy is currently delivered in a hyperfractionated format, with 30 fractions delivered over 6 weeks.

With the goal of combating fraction-related neoplastic cell repopulation, multiple trials have analyzed the survival outcomes with hyperfractionated radiotherapy into even smaller and more frequent fractions, with most as well as pooled meta-analyses showing no survival advantages (1 smaller trial reported a 10-week survival benefit with further hyperfractionation).[3,34–38] A follow-up Radiation Therapy Oncology Group (RTOG) phase III trial also showed no efficacy from hyperfractionation of 72 Gy delivered in 2 daily fractions of 1.2 Gy over 6 weeks.[39,40]

Effect of Radiation Volume on Efficacy

Analysis of failures from radiation therapy has shown that recurrence occurs locally, within 2 cm of enhancing tumor.[33,41,42] This finding is in contrast to many other malignancies that spread via metastasis or cerebrospinal fluid dissemination. The pattern of local failure has led to investigations of varying radiation volumes, which have guided the transition from whole brain radiation therapy to more regionally focused treatment plans with the goal of maximizing radiation delivery to tumor cells while limiting delivery to normal tissue. A randomized controlled trial reported no survival difference between patients receiving 6020 cGy of whole brain radiation and those receiving 4300 cGy of whole brain radiation plus 1720 cGy delivered to enhancing tumor volume plus a margin of 2 cm.[43] The results of this trial have formed the standard regional delivery of radiation in patients with HGG, as opposed to whole brain radiation that was previously delivered. A recent RTOG phase I study used dose escalation with conformal radiation therapy ranging between 66 and 84 Gy and reported no increase in rates of radiation injury.[44]

[Tags: Glioma, glioblastoma, radiation, whole brain radiation, radiotherapy, dose escalation, fractionation, hyperfractionation].

RADIATION SENSITIZERS

As discussed earlier in relation to radiobiology, there are multiple factors that contribute to the resistance of a neoplasm to radiation treatment. Therefore, multiple radiation sensitizing methods have been investigated as to whether they can increase efficacy of radiation and decrease radiation damage to viable normal brain tissue. The 2 largest radioresistance pathways commonly targeted are DNA repair mechanisms and hypoxia-induced radioresistance.

DNA Damage and Repair-mediated Radiosensitization

Ineffective mismatch repair has been postulated as a mechanism by which radiation may be more effective in treating various neoplasms, and this was confirmed with in vitro and in vivo models.[45–48] In 2005 Stupp and colleagues[49] performed a randomized controlled trial comparing radiotherapy alone against radiotherapy with concomitant temozolomide therapy. Temozolomide depletes the DNA repair enzyme O^6-methylguanine-DNA methyltransferase (MGMT), resulting in mismatched base-pairing, failed DNA replication, and cell death.[50] This trial reported a significant survival benefit of temozolomide, extending median survival by 2.5 months, with minimal toxicity. Additional studies have also shown this survival benefit for temozolomide as part of the standard treatment regimen for HGGs.[49,51,52] The investigators propose the interplay of radiation-induced DNA damage and impaired DNA repair secondary to temozolomide therapy as a synergistic effect leading to the increased survival.[49]

In contrast to limiting innate DNA repair mechanisms, investigators have also studied whether compounds that enhance DNA base-pair damage with radiation might have efficacy as adjuvants to standard therapy. One class of studied agents are the halogenated pyrimidines, such as bromodeoxyuridine, which are substituted for thymidine in dividing cell DNA replication, leading to increased lethality from radiation treatment. However, 2 phase III RTOG trials failed to show any efficacy with bromodeoxyuridine treatment.[53,54]

Oxygen-mediated Radiosensitization

HGGs are known to have regions of hypoxia within the tumor environment, which decreases effectiveness of radiation therapy.[55] Methods for overcoming tumor-related hypoxia include extracorporeal treatments such as hyperbaric oxygen, as well as systemically administered pharmacologic agents.

The concept of hyperbaric oxygenation (HBO) as a method of radiosensitization was initially studied in the 1950s.[56] Studies in HBO have been performed primarily on head and neck cancer and cervical cancer, showing some efficacy with increased rates of radiation injury.[57,58] Khoshi and colleagues[59] published initial results on HBO treatment in HGGs, followed by a nonrandomized trial that reported increased survival in patients treated with adjunct HBO.[60] Other studies have shown the feasibility of HBO therapy in conjunction with radiation therapy.[59,61–64] Despite these results, there are no randomized controlled trials reporting HBO therapy as an efficacious adjunct to radiation therapy. HBO is generally well tolerated; however, it must be delivered in a strict time frame with respect to radiation therapy, making its application difficult in many clinical scenarios. Further investigation is required to assess its efficacy.

Nitroimidazoles such as metronidazole and misonidazole combat hypoxia via oxygen-mimetic mechanisms.[65] They have been investigated as radiosensitizers, with initial increased survival reported in 1976[66]; however, further randomized trials and meta-analyses have failed to show any survival benefit.[3,67,68] Trans-sodium crocetinate (TSC) is an investigational compound that increases blood and tissue oxygenation by its interactions with water and oxygen molecules. This increase in oxygen concentration is proposed as a further mechanism for combating the hypoxic and radioresistant milieu of HGGs. In vivo studies have reported increased oxygen concentrations selectively in tumor tissue via Licox probes (Integra Life Sciences, Plainsboro, NJ) and functional neuroimaging of hypoxia.[69,70] These and other studies have reported radiosensitization of glioblastoma cell lines by treatment with TSC, with an increased mean survival in this animal model.[71,72] Clinical evaluation of TSC is ongoing.

[Tags: Radiosensitizers, hyperbaric oxygen, temozolamide, trans-sodium crocetinate, nitroimidazoles, halogenated pyrimidines].

PREDICTORS OF RESPONSE TO RADIATION THERAPY
Tumor Factors

In an effort to determine whether any factors may be predictive of response to radiation therapy, resected glioma specimens were analyzed via genetic and immunohistochemical studies. This information provides prognostic information to patients as well as helping tailor therapy toward unique tumor populations. Molecular immunology borstel-1 (MIB-1) did not predict survival or response to radiation therapy.[73] Upregulation of EGFR showed equivocal accuracy in predicting prognosis for patients with high-grade glioma,[74] whereas deletion of nuclear factor kappa-B inhibitor alpha (NFKBIA)[75] and an unmethylated MGMT promotor[76,77] were associated with poorer prognosis in patients with high-grade glioma. EGFR pathway manipulation has been implicated in radioresistance in vitro,[78] whereas MGMT promoter methylation status has been shown to be predictive of radiation response in a recent clinical study.[79] Further research is required to stratify HGGs into tumor subsets with clinically significant prognostic and radiation response profiles.

Patient Factors

Recursive partitioning analysis (RPA) of pooled data from several HGG RTOG trials was introduced in 1993, allowing stratification of patients in these trials with significantly different survival curves. The variables in the initial RTOG model with an effect on outcome included age, histology, Karnofsky Performance Status (KPS), mental status and neurologic function, duration of symptoms, extent of resection, and cumulative radiation dose (Table 1).[80] A simplified RPA scheme was introduced in 2010 for patients with glioblastoma, which resulted in 3 classes of patients based on age, KPS, extent of resection, and neurologic function. This simplified model has been validated and shown to provide prognostic information.[81] This newer classification scheme can be seen in Table 2. Median survival for RPA class III (the lowest class for a patient with glioblastoma) was 17.1 months, whereas it was 11.2 months for RPA class IV, and 7.5 months for RPA class V + VI. The patient factors identified in RPA analysis show that pretreatment factors have a significant prognostic significance.

[Tags: MGMT, EGFR, RPA, KPS].

MODIFICATION OF RADIATION DELIVERY TYPES
Methods of Delivering Standard Fractionated Radiotherapy

Before modern imaging techniques, whole brain irradiation was used to deliver radiation to the target tissue as well as all surrounding tissue. Imaging advancements have led to an increased ability to refine tumor shape and volume, thus allowing the evolution of radiation delivery techniques from whole brain irradiation to two-dimensional regional irradiation, to three-dimensional conformal radiotherapy (Fig. 1). The reduction of radiation delivery from whole brain irradiation to regional field delivery is supported by studies reporting no difference in survival with improved performance status.[43,82] Intensity-modulated radiotherapy (IMRT) uses a multileaf collimator to divide the radiation delivery beam into many smaller portions that can be modulated into a desired shape. This strategy allows further

Table 1 RTOG RPA stratification of patients with HGGs	
Class	Definition
I	Age <50 y, anaplastic astrocytoma, and normal mental status
II	Age ≥50 y, KPS 70–100, anaplastic astrocytoma, and at least 3 months from time of first symptoms to initiation treatment
III	Age <50 y, Anaplastic astrocytoma and abnormal mental status Age <50 y, Glioblastoma multiforme and KPS 90–100
IV	Age <50 y, Glioblastoma multiforme, KPS <90 Age ≥50 y, KPS 70–100, anaplastic astrocytoma and 3 months or less from time of first symptoms to start of treatment Age <50 y, glioblastoma multiforme, surgical resection, and good neurologic function
V	Age ≥50 y, KPS 70–100, glioblastoma multiforme, either surgical resection and neurologic function that inhibits the ability to work or biopsy only followed by at least 54.4 Gy of RT Age ≥50 y, KPS <70, normal mental status
VI	Age ≥50 y, KPS <70, abnormal mental status Age ≥50 y, KPS 70–100, glioblastoma multiforme, biopsy only, receiving less than 54.4 Gy of RT

Abbreviation: RT, radiotherapy.

Table 2 Simplified RTOG RPA stratification of glioblastomas	
Class	**Definition**
III	Age <50 y, KPS ≥90
IV	Age <50 y, KPS <90 Age ≥50 y, KPS ≥70, surgical removal with good neurologic function
V + VI	Age ≥50 y, KPS ≥70, surgical removal with poor neurologic function Age ≥50 y, KPS ≥70, no surgical removal Age ≥50 y, KPS <70

restriction of the desired conformal radiation target and minimization of radiation delivery to surrounding tissues.[83] IMRT may decrease rates of radiation toxicity because of improved dose conformality, as reported in a dosimetric study that showed significant reductions in cumulative dose delivery to surrounding sensitive structures such as the spinal cord, optic nerves, eyes, and brainstem.[84]

Stereotactic Radiation Techniques

Stereotactic delivery of radiation allows single or multisession delivery of high doses of radiation, with less radiation delivered to surrounding tissue. Stereotactic radiosurgery (SRS) refers to single-session radiation delivery, whereas stereotactic radiotherapy (SRT) refers to radiation delivery in up to 5 sessions.[85] These delivery methods offer the benefits of shorter or even single-session radiation delivery with decreased risk of radiation injury to surrounding tissue, similar to the highly conformal radiotherapy techniques listed earlier. These techniques are also focal radiation treatments that do not address tumor extending into surrounding tissue outside the radiation treatment field. However, as discussed earlier, most recurrences after radiation therapy occur at the previously treated tumor margin, and less frequently at distant sites.

An RTOG phase II trial studied the use of SRT as a boost of radiation after conventional radiation treatment in patients with residual tumor after surgery. These patients received 4 additional SRT sessions (1 per week) of 5 to 7 Gy per session. This boost therapy was well tolerated, but did not show any survival benefit.[86] Retrospective studies have reported varied survival advantages with this treatment strategy after standard radiotherapy.[87–98] These retrospective studies prompted an RTOG phase III randomized controlled trial with standard treatment compared with patients receiving SRS boost treatment before conventional radiotherapy. This trial reported no benefit in survival or patient quality of life.[99] Although no large phase III trial has examined the application of stereotactic radiation boost therapy after conventional radiotherapy, this RTOG trial led the American Society for the Therapeutic Radiology and Oncology to issue a review that radiosurgery boost followed by conventional radiotherapy does not confer a benefit and is associated with increased toxicity. The investigators further concluded that there was insufficient evidence to support the use of SRS or SRT for patients with malignant glioma at either diagnosis or recurrence.[100]

Charged Particle Therapy

Charged particle therapy (ie, proton beam therapy) offers further evolution on the goals of stereotactic techniques using photons. The Bragg-Peak effect of proton beam treatment creates a sharp fall-off

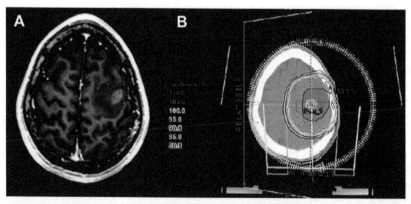

Fig. 1. (A) A preoperative axial T1-weighted magnetic resonance sequence after gadolinium administration in a patient with a left frontal glioblastoma. (B) The postoperative conformal radiation delivery plan after gross total resection.

of radiation after target delivery, allowing even further refinement in conformality with radiation doses of at least 90 cobalt-Gray-equivalent.[101] However, photon-based therapy has shown local failure at dose escalation up to 90 Gy.[33] Therefore, further research is required to evaluate the efficacy of proton beam therapy clinically compared with conventional photon radiation therapy for high-grade gliomas.

[Tags: Radiosurgery, stereotactic, IMRT, conformal radiotherapy, proton beam].

RADIATION THERAPY IN SPECIAL CIRCUMSTANCES
Further Radiation Treatment in Recurrence

High-grade gliomas recur almost universally, and as described earlier the recurrence patterns show that nearly all tumors recur within 2 cm of the primary tumor location. Salvage therapies include repeat surgery, continued or altered systemic chemotherapy administration, or further radiation therapy. Repeat surgical resection has been reported to offer survival benefit in certain selected patients[102]; however, surgery without additional adjuvant therapy may not be effective.[103]

The administration of repeat radiation therapy has been limited by concerns over fear of radiation-related complications associated with increasing radiation doses. Reexamination of radiation toxicity after the advancements of increasing conformal radiation delivery techniques have shown rare cases of radiation necrosis, occurring at doses of more than 100 Gy to normal tissue.[104] Maximum tolerances of critical structures such as the brainstem and optic apparatus are controversial.

The delivery method of repeat radiation therapy can include conformal or IMRT techniques or stereotactic methods. As described earlier, increasing conformality limits the cumulative normal tissue radiation dose and toxicity, suggesting a possible role for stereotactic techniques to minimize toxicity. Studies have reported survival benefit compared with historical controls in SRS,[105] and have attempted to delineate rates of radiation toxicity associated with this type of salvage treatment.[106] On the other hand, fractionated SRT may convey decreased toxicity compared with single-session SRS.[107] Further research is required to determine the optimum method of radiation delivery in recurrent HGGs.

Palliative Radiation Treatment

As described earlier, certain patient characteristics are strongly associated with prognosis and response to various therapies in patients with HGGs. Specifically, older patients tend to

have more aggressive disease and poorer outcomes.[108–110] In addition, the combination of chemotherapy and radiation therapy in elderly patients is associated with significant morbidity.[111] Consequently, patients older than 70 years are generally excluded from randomized trials and are often not treated as aggressively as higher-functioning, younger patients. This more conservative treatment strategy is also true for patients with a poor KPS at the time of presentation. Despite the tendency to treat these patients less aggressively, there is a clear survival benefit to treating patients with radiotherapy as opposed to supportive care.[112] In these specific subsets of patients, some groups have advocated a short course of radiation therapy without concomitant chemotherapy to a total of 40 Gy delivered in 15 fractions over 3 weeks. This treatment modality has shown similar survival to standard radiotherapy schema without a decrease in quality of life.[113]

[Tags: Recurrent glioma, palliative radiation, reirradiation].

SUMMARY

Radiation therapy is an integral part of the multimodality treatment of patients with HGG. An understanding of the radiobiology and mechanisms of radioresistance is critical for clinicians involved in the management of these complex patients. Advances in molecular biology are prompting further investigation into methods to improve the efficacy of chemoradiation in HGGs. Further research in the use of radiation sensitizers may assist clinicians in this regard.

Current radiation therapy schemas for HGGs are supported by multiple clinical trials reporting efficacy in increasing patient survival. Manipulation of radiation delivery in terms of dose escalation, hyperfractionation, and the radiation delivery modality have allowed clinicians to give high doses of radiation to neoplastic cells and progressively limit the cumulative radiation dose to surrounding normal tissues. Despite this situation, treatment of HGGs is a palliative therapy, with local failure being the near universal mode of recurrence and progression. Further investigation is needed to refine the role that radiation plays in the treatment of these patients as understanding of the molecular and genetic mechanisms of gliomas evolves.

REFERENCES

1. CBTRUS Statistical Report: primary brain and central nervous system tumors diagnosed in the

United States in 2004-2007. Available at: http://www.cbtrus.org. CBTRUS; 2011. Accessed January 1, 2012.

2. Anderson E, Grant R, Lewis SC, et al. Randomized Phase III controlled trials of therapy in malignant glioma: where are we after 40 years? Br J Neurosurg 2008;22(3):339–49.

3. Laperriere N, Zuraw L, Cairncross G. Radiotherapy for newly diagnosed malignant glioma in adults: a systematic review. Radiother Oncol 2002;64(3):259–73.

4. Walker MD, Alexander E Jr, Hunt WE, et al. Evaluation of BCNU and/or radiotherapy in the treatment of anaplastic gliomas. A cooperative clinical trial. J Neurosurg 1978;49(3):333–43.

5. Bao S, Wu Q, McLendon RE, et al. Glioma stem cells promote radioresistance by preferential activation of the DNA damage response. Nature 2006;444(7120):756–60.

6. Begg AC. Radiobiology: state of the present art. A conference report. Int J Radiat Biol 2010;86(1):71–8.

7. Firat E, Heinemann F, Grosu AL, et al. Molecular radiobiology meets clinical radiation oncology. Int J Radiat Biol 2010;86(3):252–9.

8. Albesiano E, Han JE, Lim M. Mechanisms of local immunoresistance in glioma. Neurosurg Clin N Am 2010;21(1):17–29.

9. Noda SE, El-Jawahri A, Patel D, et al. Molecular advances of brain tumors in radiation oncology. Semin Radiat Oncol 2009;19(3):171–8.

10. Milas L, Hittelman WN. Cancer stem cells and tumor response to therapy: current problems and future prospects. Semin Radiat Oncol 2009;19(2):96–105.

11. Blazek ER, Foutch JL, Maki G. Daoy medulloblastoma cells that express CD133 are radioresistant relative to CD133- cells, and the CD133+ sector is enlarged by hypoxia. Int J Radiat Oncol Biol Phys 2007;67(1):1–5.

12. Zagzag D, Lukyanov Y, Lan L, et al. Hypoxia-inducible factor 1 and VEGF upregulate CXCR4 in glioblastoma: implications for angiogenesis and glioma cell invasion. Lab Invest 2006;86(12):1221–32.

13. Rademakers SE, Span PN, Kaanders JH, et al. Molecular aspects of tumour hypoxia. Mol Oncol 2008;2(1):41–53.

14. Barcellos-Hoff MH, Park C, Wright EG. Radiation and the microenvironment–tumorigenesis and therapy. Nat Rev Cancer 2005;5(11):867–75.

15. Eyler CE, Rich JN. Survival of the fittest: cancer stem cells in therapeutic resistance and angiogenesis. J Clin Oncol 2008;26(17):2839–45.

16. Charles N, Holland EC. The perivascular niche microenvironment in brain tumor progression. Cell Cycle 2010;9(15):3012–21.

17. Aigner L, Bogdahn U. TGF-beta in neural stem cells and in tumors of the central nervous system. Cell Tissue Res 2008;331(1):225–41.

18. Barani IJ, Cuttino LW, Benedict SH, et al. Neural stem cell-preserving external-beam radiotherapy of central nervous system malignancies. Int J Radiat Oncol Biol Phys 2007;68(4):978–85.

19. Reya T, Morrison SJ, Clarke MF, et al. Stem cells, cancer, and cancer stem cells. Nature 2001;414(6859):105–11.

20. Sanai N, Alvarez-Buylla A, Berger MS. Neural stem cells and the origin of gliomas. N Engl J Med 2005;353(8):811–22.

21. Singh SK, Hawkins C, Clarke ID, et al. Identification of human brain tumour initiating cells. Nature 2004;432(7015):396–401.

22. Qi XS, Schultz CJ, Li XA. An estimation of radiobiologic parameters from clinical outcomes for radiation treatment planning of brain tumor. Int J Radiat Oncol Biol Phys 2006;64(5):1570–80.

23. Jones B, Sanghera P. Estimation of radiobiologic parameters and equivalent radiation dose of cytotoxic chemotherapy in malignant glioma. Int J Radiat Oncol Biol Phys 2007;68(2):441–8.

24. Jelsma R, Bucy PC. The treatment of glioblastoma multiforme of the brain. J Neurosurg 1967;27(5):388–400.

25. Shapiro WR, Young DF. Treatment of malignant glioma. A controlled study of chemotherapy and irradiation. Arch Neurol 1976;33(7):494, 450.

26. Andersen AP. Postoperative irradiation of glioblastomas. Results in a randomized series. Acta Radiol Oncol Radiat Phys Biol 1978;17(6):475–84.

27. Walker MD, Green SB, Byar DP, et al. Randomized comparisons of radiotherapy and nitrosoureas for the treatment of malignant glioma after surgery. N Engl J Med 1980;303(23):1323–9.

28. Kristiansen K, Hagen S, Kollevold T, et al. Combined modality therapy of operated astrocytomas grade III and IV. Confirmation of the value of postoperative irradiation and lack of potentiation of bleomycin on survival time: a prospective multicenter trial of the Scandinavian Glioblastoma Study Group. Cancer 1981;47(4):649–52.

29. Sandberg-Wollheim M, Malmstrom P, Stromblad LG, et al. A randomized study of chemotherapy with procarbazine, vincristine, and lomustine with and without radiation therapy for astrocytoma grades 3 and/or 4. Cancer 1991;68(1):22–9.

30. Bleehen NM, Stenning SP. A Medical Research Council trial of two radiotherapy doses in the treatment of grades 3 and 4 astrocytoma. The Medical Research Council Brain Tumour Working Party. Br J Cancer 1991;64(4):769–74.

31. Khan MK, Hunter GK, Vogelbaum M, et al. Evidence-based adjuvant therapy for gliomas: current concepts and newer developments. Indian J Cancer 2009;46(2):96–107.

32. Nelson DF, Diener-West M, Horton J, et al. Combined modality approach to treatment of

malignant gliomas–re-evaluation of RTOG 7401/ECOG 1374 with long-term follow-up: a joint study of the Radiation Therapy Oncology Group and the Eastern Cooperative Oncology Group. NCI Monogr 1988;(6):279–84.

33. Chan JL, Lee SW, Fraass BA, et al. Survival and failure patterns of high-grade gliomas after three-dimensional conformal radiotherapy. J Clin Oncol 2002;20(6):1635–42.

34. Shin KH, Urtasun RC, Fulton D, et al. Multiple daily fractionated radiation therapy and misonidazole in the management of malignant astrocytoma. A preliminary report. Cancer 1985;56(4):758–60.

35. Genc M, Zorlu AF, Atahan IL. Accelerated hyperfractionated radiotherapy in supratentorial malignant astrocytomas. Radiother Oncol 2000;56(2):233–8.

36. Payne DG, Simpson WJ, Keen C, et al. Malignant astrocytoma: hyperfractionated and standard radiotherapy with chemotherapy in a randomized prospective clinical trial. Cancer 1982;50(11):2301–6.

37. Shin KH, Muller PJ, Geggie PH. Superfractionation radiation therapy in the treatment of malignant astrocytoma. Cancer 1983;52(11):2040–3.

38. Deutsch M, Green SB, Strike TA, et al. Results of a randomized trial comparing BCNU plus radiotherapy, streptozotocin plus radiotherapy, BCNU plus hyperfractionated radiotherapy, and BCNU following misonidazole plus radiotherapy in the postoperative treatment of malignant glioma. Int J Radiat Oncol Biol Phys 1989;16(6):1389–96.

39. Lustig RA, Seiferheld W, Berkey B, et al. Imaging response in malignant glioma, RTOG 90-06. Am J Clin Oncol 2007;30(1):32–7.

40. Curran WJ Jr, Scott CB , Yung WK, et al. No survival benefit of hyperfractionated (HFX) radiotherapy (RT) to 72.0 Gy and carmustine versus standard RT and carmustine for malignant glioma patients: preliminary results of RTOG 90-06 [meeting abstract]. Paper presented at: American Society of Clinical Oncology (ASCO) 1996. Philadelphia, May 18-21, 1996.

41. Wallner KE, Galicich JH, Krol G, et al. Patterns of failure following treatment for glioblastoma multiforme and anaplastic astrocytoma. Int J Radiat Oncol Biol Phys 1989;16(6):1405–9.

42. Hochberg FH, Pruitt A. Assumptions in the radiotherapy of glioblastoma. Neurology 1980;30(9):907–11.

43. Shapiro WR, Green SB, Burger PC, et al. Randomized trial of three chemotherapy regimens and two radiotherapy regimens and two radiotherapy regimens in postoperative treatment of malignant glioma. Brain Tumor Cooperative Group Trial 8001. J Neurosurg 1989;71(1):1–9.

44. Tsien C, Moughan J, Michalski JM, et al. Phase I three-dimensional conformal radiation dose escalation study in newly diagnosed glioblastoma: Radiation Therapy Oncology Group Trial 98-03. Int J Radiat Oncol Biol Phys 2009;73(3):699–708.

45. Kil WJ, Cerna D, Burgan WE, et al. In vitro and in vivo radiosensitization induced by the DNA methylating agent temozolomide. Clin Cancer Res 2008;14(3):931–8.

46. van Rijn J, Heimans JJ, van den Berg J, et al. Survival of human glioma cells treated with various combination of temozolomide and X-rays. Int J Radiat Oncol Biol Phys 2000;47(3):779–84.

47. Wedge SR, Porteous JK, Glaser MG, et al. In vitro evaluation of temozolomide combined with X-irradiation. Anticancer Drugs 1997;8(1):92–7.

48. Wick W, Wick A, Schulz JB, et al. Prevention of irradiation-induced glioma cell invasion by temozolomide involves caspase 3 activity and cleavage of focal adhesion kinase. Cancer Res 2002;62(6):1915–9.

49. Stupp R, Mason WP, van den Bent MJ, et al. Radiotherapy plus concomitant and adjuvant temozolomide for glioblastoma. N Engl J Med 2005;352(10):987–96.

50. Friedman HS, McLendon RE, Kerby T, et al. DNA mismatch repair and O6-alkylguanine-DNA alkyltransferase analysis and response to Temodal in newly diagnosed malignant glioma. J Clin Oncol 1998;16(12):3851–7.

51. Athanassiou H, Synodinou M, Maragoudakis E, et al. Randomized phase II study of temozolomide and radiotherapy compared with radiotherapy alone in newly diagnosed glioblastoma multiforme. J Clin Oncol 2005;23(10):2372–7.

52. Hart MG, Grant R, Garside R, et al. Temozolomide for high grade glioma. Cochrane Database Syst Rev 2008;4:CD007415.

53. Prados MD, Seiferheld W, Sandler HM, et al. Phase III randomized study of radiotherapy plus procarbazine, lomustine, and vincristine with or without BUdR for treatment of anaplastic astrocytoma: final report of RTOG 9404. Int J Radiat Oncol Biol Phys 2004;58(4):1147–52.

54. Prados MD, Scott C, Sandler H, et al. A phase 3 randomized study of radiotherapy plus procarbazine, CCNU, and vincristine (PCV) with or without BUdR for the treatment of anaplastic astrocytoma: a preliminary report of RTOG 9404. Int J Radiat Oncol Biol Phys 1999;45(5):1109–15.

55. Rong Y, Durden DL, Van Meir EG, et al. 'Pseudopalisading' necrosis in glioblastoma: a familiar morphologic feature that links vascular pathology, hypoxia, and angiogenesis. J Neuropathol Exp Neurol 2006;65(6):529–39.

56. Gray LH, Conger AD, Ebert M, et al. The concentration of oxygen dissolved in tissues at the time of irradiation as a factor in radiotherapy. Br J Radiol 1953;26(312):638–48.

57. Bennett M, Feldmeier J, Smee R, et al. Hyperbaric oxygenation for tumour sensitisation to radiotherapy: a systematic review of randomised controlled trials. Cancer Treat Rev 2008;34(7): 577–91.

58. Bennett M, Feldmeier J, Smee R, et al. Hyperbaric oxygenation for tumour sensitisation to radiotherapy. Cochrane Database Syst Rev 2005;4:CD005007.

59. Kohshi K, Kinoshita Y, Terashima H, et al. Radiotherapy after hyperbaric oxygenation for malignant gliomas: a pilot study. J Cancer Res Clin Oncol 1996;122(11):676–8.

60. Kohshi K, Kinoshita Y, Imada H, et al. Effects of radiotherapy after hyperbaric oxygenation on malignant gliomas. Br J Cancer 1999;80(1-2): 236–41.

61. Ogawa K, Ishiuchi S, Inoue O, et al. Phase II trial of radiotherapy after hyperbaric oxygenation with multiagent chemotherapy (procarbazine, nimustine, and vincristine) for high-grade gliomas: long-term results. Int J Radiat Oncol Biol Phys 2011; 82(2):732–8.

62. Ogawa K, Yoshii Y, Inoue O, et al. Phase II trial of radiotherapy after hyperbaric oxygenation with chemotherapy for high-grade gliomas. Br J Cancer 2006;95(7):862–8.

63. Ogawa K, Yoshii Y, Inoue O, et al. Prospective trial of radiotherapy after hyperbaric oxygenation with chemotherapy for high-grade gliomas. Radiother Oncol 2003;67(1):63–7.

64. Kohshi K, Yamamoto H, Nakahara A, et al. Fractionated stereotactic radiotherapy using gamma unit after hyperbaric oxygenation on recurrent high-grade gliomas. J Neurooncol 2007;82(3):297–303.

65. Coleman CN, Noll L, Howes AE, et al. Initial results of a phase I trial of continuous infusion SR 2508 (etanidazole): a radiation therapy oncology group study. Int J Radiat Oncol Biol Phys 1989;16(4):1085–7.

66. Urtasun R, Band P, Chapman JD, et al. Radiation and high-dose metronidazole in supratentorial glioblastomas. N Engl J Med 1976;294(25):1364–7.

67. Overgaard J. Clinical evaluation of nitroimidazoles as modifiers of hypoxia in solid tumors. Oncol Res 1994;6(10–11):509–18.

68. Huncharek M. Meta-analytic re-evaluation of misonidazole in the treatment of high grade astrocytoma. Anticancer Res 1998;18(3B):1935–9.

69. Sheehan J, Sherman J, Cifarelli C, et al. Effect of trans sodium crocetinate on brain tumor oxygenation. Laboratory investigation. J Neurosurg 2009; 111(2):226–9.

70. Sheehan JP, Popp B, Monteith S, et al. Trans sodium crocetinate: functional neuroimaging studies in a hypoxic brain tumor. J Neurosurg 2011;115(4): 749–53.

71. Sheehan J, Ionescu A, Pouratian N, et al. Use of trans sodium crocetinate for sensitizing glioblastoma multiforme to radiation: laboratory investigation. J Neurosurg 2008;108(5):972–8.

72. Sheehan J, Cifarelli CP, Dassoulas K, et al. Trans-sodium crocetinate enhancing survival and glioma response on magnetic resonance imaging to radiation and temozolomide. J Neurosurg 2010; 113(2):234–9.

73. Moskowitz SI, Jin T, Prayson RA. Role of MIB1 in predicting survival in patients with glioblastomas. J Neurooncol 2006;76(2):193–200.

74. Chakravarti A, Seiferheld W, Tu X, et al. Immunohistochemically determined total epidermal growth factor receptor levels not of prognostic value in newly diagnosed glioblastoma multiforme: report from the Radiation Therapy Oncology Group. Int J Radiat Oncol Biol Phys 2005;62(2):318–27.

75. Bredel M, Scholtens DM, Yadav AK, et al. NFKBIA deletion in glioblastomas. N Engl J Med 2011; 364(7):627–37.

76. Esteller M, Garcia-Foncillas J, Andion E, et al. Inactivation of the DNA-repair gene MGMT and the clinical response of gliomas to alkylating agents. N Engl J Med 2000;343(19):1350–4.

77. Hegi ME, Diserens AC, Gorlia T, et al. MGMT gene silencing and benefit from temozolomide in glioblastoma. N Engl J Med 2005;352(10): 997–1003.

78. Chakravarti A, Chakladar A, Delaney MA, et al. The epidermal growth factor receptor pathway mediates resistance to sequential administration of radiation and chemotherapy in primary human glioblastoma cells in a RAS-dependent manner. Cancer Res 2002;62(15):4307–15.

79. Rivera AL, Pelloski CE, Gilbert MR, et al. MGMT promoter methylation is predictive of response to radiotherapy and prognostic in the absence of adjuvant alkylating chemotherapy for glioblastoma. Neuro Oncol 2010;12(2):116–21.

80. Curran WJ Jr, Scott CB, Horton J, et al. Recursive partitioning analysis of prognostic factors in three Radiation Therapy Oncology Group malignant glioma trials. J Natl Cancer Inst 1993;85(9):704–10.

81. Li J, Wang M, Won M, et al. Validation and simplification of the Radiation Therapy Oncology Group recursive partitioning analysis classification for glioblastoma. Int J Radiat Oncol Biol Phys 2011; 81(3):623–30.

82. Sharma RR, Singh DP, Pathak A, et al. Local control of high-grade gliomas with limited volume irradiation versus whole brain irradiation. Neurol India 2003;51(4):512–7.

83. Hermanto U, Frija EK, Lii MJ, et al. Intensity-modulated radiotherapy (IMRT) and conventional three-dimensional conformal radiotherapy for high-grade gliomas: does IMRT increase the integral dose to normal brain? Int J Radiat Oncol Biol Phys 2007; 67(4):1135–44.

84. Narayana A, Yamada J, Berry S, et al. Intensity-modulated radiotherapy in high-grade gliomas: clinical and dosimetric results. Int J Radiat Oncol Biol Phys 2006;64(3):892–7.

85. Barnett GH, Linskey ME, Adler JR, et al. Stereotactic radiosurgery–an organized neurosurgery-sanctioned definition. J Neurosurg 2007;106(1):1–5.

86. Cardinale R, Won M, Choucair A, et al. A phase II trial of accelerated radiotherapy using weekly stereotactic conformal boost for supratentorial glioblastoma multiforme: RTOG 0023. Int J Radiat Oncol Biol Phys 2006;65(5):1422–8.

87. Pouratian N, Crowley RW, Sherman JH, et al. Gamma knife radiosurgery after radiation therapy as an adjunctive treatment for glioblastoma. J Neurooncol 2009;94(3):409–18.

88. Sarkaria JN, Mehta MP, Loeffler JS, et al. Radiosurgery in the initial management of malignant gliomas: survival comparison with the RTOG recursive partitioning analysis. Radiation Therapy Oncology Group. Int J Radiat Oncol Biol Phys 1995;32(4):931–41.

89. Hall WA, Djalilian HR, Sperduto PW, et al. Stereotactic radiosurgery for recurrent malignant gliomas. J Clin Oncol 1995;13(7):1642–8.

90. Kondziolka D, Flickinger JC, Bissonette DJ, et al. Survival benefit of stereotactic radiosurgery for patients with malignant glial neoplasms. Neurosurgery 1997;41(4):776–83 [discussion: 783–5].

91. Loeffler JS, Alexander E 3rd, Shea WM, et al. Radiosurgery as part of the initial management of patients with malignant gliomas. J Clin Oncol 1992;10(9):1379–85.

92. Shrieve DC, Alexander E 3rd, Black PM, et al. Treatment of patients with primary glioblastoma multiforme with standard postoperative radiotherapy and radiosurgical boost: prognostic factors and long-term outcome. J Neurosurg 1999;90(1):72–7.

93. Nwokedi EC, DiBiase SJ, Jabbour S, et al. Gamma knife stereotactic radiosurgery for patients with glioblastoma multiforme. Neurosurgery 2002;50(1):41–6 [discussion: 46–7].

94. Hsieh PC, Chandler JP, Bhangoo S, et al. Adjuvant gamma knife stereotactic radiosurgery at the time of tumor progression potentially improves survival for patients with glioblastoma multiforme. Neurosurgery 2005;57(4):684–92 [discussion: 684–92].

95. Combs SE, Thilmann C, Edler L, et al. Efficacy of fractionated stereotactic reirradiation in recurrent gliomas: long-term results in 172 patients treated in a single institution. J Clin Oncol 2005;23(34):8863–9.

96. Combs SE, Widmer V, Thilmann C, et al. Stereotactic radiosurgery (SRS): treatment option for recurrent glioblastoma multiforme (GBM). Cancer 2005;104(10):2168–73.

97. Maranzano E, Anselmo P, Casale M, et al. Treatment of recurrent glioblastoma with stereotactic radiotherapy: long-term results of a mono-institutional trial. Tumori 2011;97(1):56–61.

98. Villavicencio AT, Burneikiene S, Romanelli P, et al. Survival following stereotactic radiosurgery for newly diagnosed and recurrent glioblastoma multiforme: a multicenter experience. Neurosurg Rev 2009;32(4):417–24.

99. Souhami L, Seiferheld W, Brachman D, et al. Randomized comparison of stereotactic radiosurgery followed by conventional radiotherapy with carmustine to conventional radiotherapy with carmustine for patients with glioblastoma multiforme: report of Radiation Therapy Oncology Group 93-05 protocol. Int J Radiat Oncol Biol Phys 2004;60(3):853–60.

100. Tsao MN, Mehta MP, Whelan TJ, et al. The American Society for Therapeutic Radiology and Oncology (ASTRO) evidence-based review of the role of radiosurgery for malignant glioma. Int J Radiat Oncol Biol Phys 2005;63(1):47–55.

101. Tatsuzaki H, Urie MM, Linggood R. Comparative treatment planning: proton vs. x-ray beams against glioblastoma multiforme. Int J Radiat Oncol Biol Phys 1992;22(2):265–73.

102. Park JK, Hodges T, Arko L, et al. Scale to predict survival after surgery for recurrent glioblastoma multiforme. J Clin Oncol 2010;28(24):3838–43.

103. Mandl ES, Dirven CM, Buis DR, et al. Repeated surgery for glioblastoma multiforme: only in combination with other salvage therapy. Surg Neurol 2008;69(5):506–9 [discussion: 509].

104. Mayer R, Sminia P. Reirradiation tolerance of the human brain. Int J Radiat Oncol Biol Phys 2008;70(5):1350–60.

105. Kong DS, Lee JI, Park K, et al. Efficacy of stereotactic radiosurgery as a salvage treatment for recurrent malignant gliomas. Cancer 2008;112(9):2046–51.

106. Shaw E, Scott C, Souhami L, et al. Single dose radiosurgical treatment of recurrent previously irradiated primary brain tumors and brain metastases: final report of RTOG protocol 90-05. Int J Radiat Oncol Biol Phys 2000;47(2):291–8.

107. Fokas E, Wacker U, Gross MW, et al. Hypofractionated stereotactic reirradiation of recurrent glioblastomas: a beneficial treatment option after high-dose radiotherapy? Strahlenther Onkol 2009;185(4):235–40.

108. Srividya MR, Thota B, Arivazhagan A, et al. Age-dependent prognostic effects of EGFR/p53 alterations in glioblastoma: study on a prospective cohort of 140 uniformly treated adult patients. J Clin Pathol 2010;63(8):687–91.

109. Chaichana K, Parker S, Olivi A, et al. A proposed classification system that projects outcomes based on preoperative variables for adult patients with glioblastoma multiforme. J Neurosurg 2010;112(5):997–1004.

110. Laws ER, Parney IF, Huang W, et al. Survival following surgery and prognostic factors for recently diagnosed malignant glioma: data from the Glioma Outcomes Project. J Neurosurg 2003;99(3):467–73.

111. Sijben AE, McIntyre JB, Roldan GB, et al. Toxicity from chemoradiotherapy in older patients with glioblastoma multiforme. J Neurooncol 2008;89(1): 97–103.

112. Keime-Guibert F, Chinot O, Taillandier L, et al. Radiotherapy for glioblastoma in the elderly. N Engl J Med 2007;356(15):1527–35.

113. Roa W, Brasher PM, Bauman G, et al. Abbreviated course of radiation therapy in older patients with glioblastoma multiforme: a prospective randomized clinical trial. J Clin Oncol 2004;22(9): 1583–8.

Radiation Options for High-Grade Gliomas

Benedict Beng Teck Taw, MBBS, FRCSEd(SN), FCSHK[a],
Alessandra A. Gorgulho, MD, MSc[b], Michael T. Selch, MD[c],
Antonio A.F. De Salles, MD, PhD[d,e],*

KEYWORDS

- High-grade glioma • Radiosurgery • Radiotherapy
- Stereotaxy • Fractionation

High-grade gliomas (HGGs) include World Health Organization (WHO) grade 3 anaplastic astrocytoma and grade 4 glioblastoma multiforme (GBM). Although HGG rarely results in distant metastasis, the condition's seemingly relentless local microproliferation renders its cure impossible (at least in the current technology). Even with the latest imaging and surgical technologies, the exact demarcation of the tumor and its proliferation cannot be determined. This makes the localization of the target an unachievable task. Another unique nature of brain tumor is that the brain is an unforgiving organ that contains many vital structures that many a time HGG involves. The outcome for HGG remains grim despite advancing multimodality treatments, including surgery, chemotherapy, and radiotherapy.

The exact mechanism of radiotherapy is still uncertain. However, the majority supports the notion that double-stranded breaks of the nuclear DNA are the most important cellular effect of radiation. This breakage causes an irreversible loss of reproductive integrity of the cell and eventual cell death. Radiotherapy also uses ionizing radiation to interact with water molecules within the cell, which releases free radicals, whereby causing additional DNA damage.[1]

Soon after the discovery of x-rays by Roentgen in 1895,[2] there were reports that patients with cancers were being successfully treated with radiotherapy.[3]

Frankel and German[4] published one of the earliest reports on radiotherapy for glioblastoma in 1958. The investigators reviewed 219 cases of GBM. Forty-seven patients received radiation doses varying between 2700 and 5900 rads (cGy), and 21 of these patients completed radiotherapy within 60 days after operation. When compared with 62 patients who underwent surgery alone and were alive 60 days after operation, the investigators found that there was a significantly greater percentage of survivors in the irradiated group during the first 12 months. This difference disappeared after the first year. The investigators concluded that routine postoperative radiation effectively prolonged the palliative effects of surgery and proposed a more general usage of radiotherapy. In terms of surgery, they found that a more radical removal offered the best prognosis with regard to operative mortality and survival time.

Radiotherapy is now routinely used as part of the treatment regimen for HGG. Its efficacy and

a Division of Neurosurgery, Department of Surgery, University of Hong Kong, Hong Kong, SAR, China
b Department of Neurosurgery, David Geffen School of Medicine, University of California, Los Angeles, 300 UCLA Medical Plaza, Suite B212, Los Angeles, CA 90095, USA
c Department of Radiation Oncology, David Geffen School of Medicine, University of California, Los Angeles, 200 UCLA Medical Plaza, Suite B265, Los Angeles, CA 90095, USA
d Department of Neurosurgery, David Geffen School of Medicine, University of California, Los Angeles, 10495 Le Conte Avenue, Suite 2120, Los Angeles, CA 90095, USA
e Department of Radiation Oncology, David Geffen School of Medicine, University of California, Los Angeles, 10495 Le Conte Avenue, Suite 2120, Los Angeles, CA 90095, USA
* Corresponding author. Department of Neurosurgery, David Geffen School of Medicine, 10495 Le Conte Avenue, Los Angeles, CA 90095.
E-mail address: afdesalles@yahoo.com

Neurosurg Clin N Am 23 (2012) 259–267
doi:10.1016/j.nec.2012.01.003
1042-3680/12/$ - see front matter Published by Elsevier Inc.

accuracy is continuing to be studied. Problems such as target accuracy and treatment-related complications remain the major evaluation issues. However, with advancing imaging and treatment delivery methods, conclusions and treatment protocols are improving safety and efficacy.

This article reviews the history as well as the recent advances in radiation treatments of HGG.

DEFINITION OF THE EXTENT OF RADIATION

Ionizing radiations are electromagnetic species that are capable of producing ions as they pass through matter. Photon, out of many types of radiation, is most commonly used for patient treatment. Photons may come in the form of x-rays or gamma rays. These rays are widely available in the hospital setting, produced by affordable linear accelerators (LINACs) or cobalt units. Ionizing heavy particles are also used for radiotherapy. They are generated by larger and expensive cyclotrons and are therefore less available than photons in health care. The most commonly used heavy particle is the proton; however, there is also a large experience with alpha particles generated from helium. More recently, the interest on carbon-generated beam is increasing. The advantage of these expensive particle beams is that they can be sharply stopped as they cross the tumor, therefore depositing the maximum ionizing radiation energy in the tumor itself, without exit dose to normal tissue, as occurring with photons.

ESTABLISHMENT OF RADIATION AS PART OF THE MULTIMODALITY TREATMENT OF HGGs

Although radiation therapy has been used in treating primary brain tumors since the early 1900s, there was no scientific evidence that it was efficacious and safe. In 1979, Walker and colleagues[5] published their report on the analysis of dose-effect relationship for malignant gliomas based on the experience of the Brain Tumor Study Group. They compared the median survival in patients who did not undergo radiotherapy (18 weeks) with that in those who were irradiated using radiation doses of 45 Gy or less (13.5 weeks), 50 Gy (28 weeks), and 60 Gy (42 weeks). The investigators found an increase of 1.3 times in median life span associated with the higher dose between 5000- and 6000-rads (cGy) groups. They concluded that radiotherapy had a significant influence on the survival of patients with malignant glioma, and a clear-cut dose-effect relationship was found. At around the same time, the Scandinavian Glioblastoma Study Group also published the results of a multicenter randomized trial on adjuvant

irradiation for operated HGGs,[6] disclosing that 45-Gy whole-brain irradiation increased median survival from 5.2 to 10.0 months. To investigate the relationship between radiation dosage and survival, Salazar and colleagues[7] compared groups of postoperative patients with GBM who were given radiation doses of 50, 60, and 75 Gy. The investigators found patients' survival to be 30, 42, and 56 weeks among the groups given 50, 60, and 75 Gy, respectively. The increase in median survival was only significant between the extremes and not between the intermediate dose, leading to the conclusion that higher radiation doses (75 Gy) did not significantly alter overall survival and could increase risk of radiation necrosis. Still in the 1990s, a randomized trial by the Medical Research Council also demonstrated an improvement in median survival from 9 to 12 months when 60 Gy was compared with 45 Gy.[8] Both this and the Brain Tumor Cooperative Group trials led to the conclusion that 60 Gy is the ideal dose for adjuvant postoperative radiotherapy for HGGs.

In a systematic review of radiotherapy for newly diagnosed malignant glioma, 6 randomized trials detected a significant survival benefit favoring postoperative radiotherapy compared with no radiotherapy.[9] Another randomized trial detected a small improvement in survival with 60 Gy in 30 fractions over 45 Gy in 20 fractions. It was concluded that postoperative external beam radiotherapy (EBRT) is recommended as standard therapy for patients with malignant glioma. The high dose volume should incorporate the enhancing tumor plus a limited margin (eg, 2 cm) for planning target volume (PTV), and the total dose delivered should be in the range of 50 to 60 Gy in fraction sizes of 1.8 to 2.0 Gy.

In 2005, a joint European Organization for Research and Treatment of Cancer (EORTC) and National Cancer Institute of Canada (NCIC) randomized trial found that concomitant and adjuvant temozolomide significantly increased the median survival of patients with GBM from 12.1 to 14.6 months and more than doubled the 2-year survival (26.5% vs 10.4%).[10] The current standard treatment after resection or biopsy of GBM is fractionated focal radiotherapy (60 Gy, 30–33 fractions of 1.8–2 Gy, or equivalent doses per fractionations) with concomitant chemotherapy with temozolomide (dose of 75 mg/m^2) daily (7 days per week) followed by 5-day cycles every 4 weeks to complete. The result of the 5-year analysis of this trial was published in 2009.[11] The investigators found that benefits of adjuvant temozolomide with radiotherapy lasted throughout 5 years of follow-up in all clinical prognostic subgroups, including patients aged 60 to 70 years.

Other chemotherapeutic agents have also been tried along with radiation for the treatment of HGGs. In a retrospective study examining the effect of reirradiation with bevacizumab for recurrent HGGs, patients who were previously treated with standard radiotherapy received bevacizumab (10 mg/kg intravenous) on day 1 and day 15 during administration of 36 Gy in 18 fractions.[12] It was noted that the overall survival was significantly better in patients receiving bevacizumab than in those receiving no additional substance or temozolomide. The conclusion was that reirradiation with bevacizumab is feasible and effective for recurrent HGGs.

IMPORTANCE OF SURGERY FOR RADIATION TREATMENT

Surgery is usually performed for either tissue diagnosis or tumor debulking purposes. In a review of the literature of both HGGs and low-grade gliomas, Sanai and Berger[13] showed that more extensive tumor resection is associated with longer life expectancy. Increasing the extent of resection was also found to be associated with improved survival independent of age, degree of disability and WHO grade, or subsequent treatment modalities used in both primary and repeat resection of malignant gliomas.[14] However, for tumors that are located in eloquent areas of the brain or for patients with poor premorbid status, a biopsy of the tumor may be more appropriate.

MODERN TECHNIQUES OF RADIATION FOR HGGs BASED ON MODERN IMAGING

Gliomas have no capsule and infiltrate the brain, particularly along the white matter tracts diffusely.[15] This makes definition of the tumor extent extremely difficult with the conventional radiologic technology. Without a definite margin, it is virtually impossible to plan a radiation treatment targeting only the tumor and sparing normal tissue. The current practice is to irradiate the tumor-involved tissue based on T2-weighted MRI along with an additional 2-cm margin. This practice is based on studies showing that most tumors recur within a 2-cm margin.[16]

However, modern MRI sequences promise to shed light on this difficult issue. Diffusion tensor imaging (DTI) is a modification of diffusion-weighted imaging that is sensitive to the preferential diffusion of brain water along axonal fibers and hence is useful in demonstrating white matter tract anatomy and can detect subtle changes in diseased white matter tracts (**Fig. 1**). Thus, many studies have been performed to investigate the usefulness of DTI in demonstrating the extent of HGGs. One of these studies compared DTI with T2-weighted 3-T MRI. The investigators found that subtle white matter disruption is identified using DTI beyond what was seen on T2-weighted images of patients with HGGs.[17] This DTI white matter disruption was not apparent in metastatic lesions or low-grade gliomas. Correlative studies of DTI abnormalities and histologic confirmation have been conducted to determine the accuracy of DTI in detecting tumor infiltration by HGG. One study found a sensitivity of 96% and a specificity of 85%.[18]

In an attempt to put DTI planning to test, Jena and colleagues[19] compared standard planning with individualized planning based on DTI findings. Standard plans were generated using a clinical target volume (CTV) margin of 2.5-cm added to the gross tumor volume (GTV) and were compared with DTI-based plans in which the CTV was generated by adding a 1-cm margin to the tumor-involved margin. The investigators found that DTI could reduce the size of the PTV by a mean of 35% and resulted in an escalated dose (mean, 67 Gy; range, 64–74 Gy), with normal tissue complication probability (NTCP) matching that of conventional treatment plans. Findings from studies that showed most tumors recurred in the high-dose treatment volume rather than at the margin seem to suggest that local tumor recurrence may not be caused by inadequate treatment volume or margin but rather insufficient dose to the central tumor.[20] Thus the investigators conclude that DTI can be used to individualize radiotherapy target volume with reduction of CTV, yielding modest dose escalation without increasing the NTCP.

L-(methyl-11C) methionine–labeled positron emission tomography (MET-PET) has been shown to have higher specificity and sensitivity in tumor delineation than MRI.[21] L-(methyl-11C) methionine (MET) is a natural amino acid avidly taken up by glioma cells, with only a low uptake in normal brain tissue. Comparative analysis between computed tomography (CT), MRI, MET-PET, and stereotactic biopsies has shown that MET-PET has greater accuracy in defining the extent of gliomas than CT and MRI. In a study comparing MET-PET and MRI for GTV definition for radiotherapy planning of HGG,[22] it was found that the size and location of residual MET uptake differ considerably from that found on postoperative MRI. Given the known high accuracy of MET-PET for detection of tumor tissue, these findings suggest that MET-PET may significantly improve the definition of target volumes in patients with HGGs. It was also proposed that using MET-PET/MRI fusion imaging

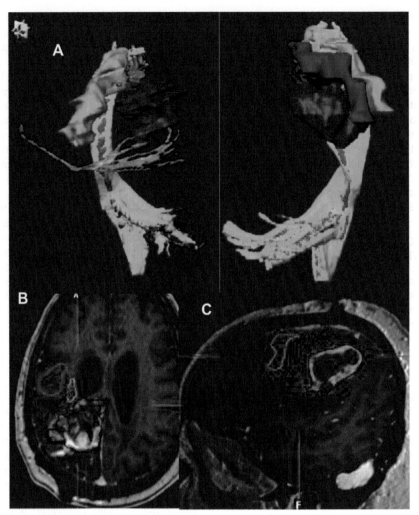

Fig. 1. Fiber tracking superimposed to gadolinium-enhanced MRI to disclose the relationship of the tumor to the eloquent cortical and white matter areas. These areas are to be avoided in surgery and in radiosurgery planning. (*A*) Visualization of the relationship of the tumor with the cortex (*magenta* and *green*), with the projection of the cortical tracts also in green. It has disclosed 2 angles of visualization. (*B*) Axial view of the tumor in the right parietal area. (*C*) Sagittal view of the relationship of the tumor with the motor area. (*B*) and (*C*) are gadolinium-enhanced T1-weighted magnetic resonance images.

and combining the biological characterization of the tissue with accurate presentation of the anatomy, a more precise delineation of the target volume for radiotherapy planning could be achieved. An important disadvantage of MET includes the low physical half-life of about 20 minutes, requiring an on-site cyclotron.

As further evidence to support the usage of MET-PET in radiotherapy planning for HGG, one study looked at the usage of MET-PET/CT/MRI fusion to determine the GTV for stereotactic fractionated radiotherapy for reirradiation of recurrent HGGs.[23] In this prospective nonrandomized single-institution trial using stereotactic fractionated radiotherapy (SFRT) reirradiation plus temozolomide, MET-PET or iodine I 123 α-methyl

tyrosine single-photon computed emission tomography (SPECT)/CT/MRI fusion and CT/T1 plus gadolinium-enhanced MRI integrated radiation treatment plans were compared. Six fractions of 5 Gy were administered in 6 days. Temozolomide, 200 mg/m² body surface per day, was administered in 1 to 2 cycles before SFRT and 4 to 5 cycles after SFRT. The median survival time for patients with treatment planning based on PET(SPECT)/CT/MRI was significantly longer than those having radiation planning using anatomic imaging (CT/MRI) alone, 9 months versus 5 months, respectively. It was concluded that biological imaging–optimized SFRT plus temozolomide in recurrent HGGs was feasible and safe and led to a significantly longer survival.

HGGs are generally considered to be radioresistant because of the hypoxic nature of the cells. Molecular oxygen is known to be a powerful modifier of cell sensitivity to radiation. The biological effect of ionizing radiation has been reported to be increased by about 3-fold when irradiation is performed under well-oxygenated conditions.[24] Hyperbaric oxygenation (HBO) is used to assist in the repair of radiation-induced damage, because it is thought that high oxygen tension promotes neovascularization in tissues of irradiated patients. A recent phase 2 trial investigating the long-term results of radiotherapy administered immediately after HBO with multiagent chemotherapy in adults with HGGs was published.[25] Patients with histologically confirmed malignant gliomas were irradiated daily with 2-Gy fractions for 5 consecutive days per week up to a total dose of 60 Gy. Each fraction was administered immediately after HBO. The chemotherapeutic agents used were procarbazine, nimustine, and vincristine; these were given during and after radiotherapy. The median overall survivals in patients with GBM and grade 3 glioma were 17.2 and 113.4 months, respectively. No patient developed neutropenic fever, intracranial hemorrhage, or serious nonhematologic or late toxicities. It was concluded that the use of radiotherapy immediately after HBO with chemotherapy for HGGs was safe, with virtually no late toxicities, and seemed effective.

High linear energy transfer–charged particle therapy with carbon ions has been investigated in the treatment of HGGs because of its better dose localization in the tumor volume and greater biological effectiveness. Because carbon ions have inverted dose profile and high local dose deposition within the Bragg peak, precise dose application and sparing of normal tissue are possible. A phase 1/2 clinical trial for patients with malignant gliomas treated with combined radiotherapy, chemotherapy, and carbon ion radiotherapy was published in 2007.[26] Patients with confirmed HGGs were treated with 50 Gy in 25 fractions for 5 weeks of radiotherapy followed by carbon ion radiotherapy in 8 fractions for 2 weeks. Nimustine hydrochloride at a dose of 100 mg/m^2 was given with radiotherapy. Carbon ion dose was increased from 16.8 to 24.8 Gy equivalent in 10% incremental steps. The median survival times for grade 3 gliomas and GBM were 35 months and 17 months, respectively. The median progression-free survival and median survival time showed 4 and 7 months for the low-dose group, 7 and 19 months for middle-dose group, and 14 and 26 months for high-dose group. It was thus concluded that carbon ion radiation seems to be effective in the treatment of HGGs

and that dose escalation of carbon ions has a statistical significance in the overall survival and progression-free survival of HGGs. This and other studies have led to a randomized phase 1/2 trial evaluating the effects of carbon ion radiotherapy versus fractionated stereotactic radiotherapy (FSRT) in recurrent or progressive gliomas.[27] In phase 1 of the carbon ion radiotherapy versus fractionated steretotactic radiotherapy in patients with recurrent or progressive gliomas (CINDERELLA) trial, the recommended dose of carbon ion radiotherapy was determined in a dose escalation scheme. In phase 2, the recommended dose was evaluated in the experimental arm compared with the standard arm, FSRT with a total dose of 36 Gy in single doses of 2 Gy. The primary end point of phase 1 was toxicity. For the randomized phase 2, the primary end point was survival after reirradiation at 12 months and the secondary end point was progression-free survival.

ROLE OF STEREOTACTIC RADIOSURGERY AND STEREOTACTIC RADIOTHERAPY FOR MANAGEMENT OF HGGs

Stereotactic radiosurgery (SRS) is a technique in which high doses of radiation can be delivered accurately in a single session to small intracranial targets in such a way that the dose falloff outside the target volume is very sharp (**Fig. 2**). One of the first reports on the usage of LINAC-based radiosurgery using noncoplanar arcs for the treatment of brain tumors was published in 1985.[28] Of the 6 patients with adequate follow-up, 1 had a grade III astrocytoma, but the patient's condition worsened within 2 months and required reoperation. Several studies were published on patients treated with SRS boost in the primary treatment of HGGs. Median survival of patients quoted showed no benefit in survival when compared with results of historical controls. The authors' data showed no benefit of SRS for primary and recurrent malignant gliomas.[29] Selection bias with these studies was raised, including small tumor size, more complete resection, good response to initial therapy, and premorbid good performance status. Shrieve and colleagues[30] published the results of a study investigating the usage of 6-megavolt LINAC radiosurgery as an adjunctive therapy for patients with confirmed GBM after EBRT. The investigators reported a median survival of 19.9 months; patients with Radiation Therapy Oncology Group (RTOG) class 3 had a significantly longer survival than class 4 and 5, and younger patients with better functional status fared better. It was concluded that

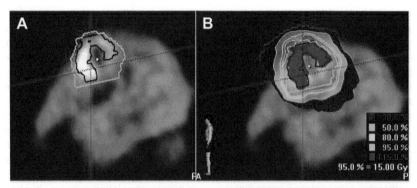

Fig. 2. Positron emission tomography with fludeoxyglucose F 18 aiding in the planning for radiosurgery. Notice that intensity modulation was used to increase the dose concentration to the glucose-avid portion of the GBM. (*A*) Delineation of the area of GTV. (*B*) Dose distribution with higher isodose coverage over the specifically chosen area of the tumor.

radiosurgery boost had a survival advantage in selected patients. In another retrospective study that reviewed Gamma Knife radiosurgery (GKR) as an adjuvant therapy for postoperative patients with GBM, a group of patients that was treated with EBRT alone was compared with patients who were treated with EBRT plus a GKR boost within 6 weeks after EBRT.[31] Median EBRT dose was 59.7 Gy and median GKR dose was 17.1 Gy. The median survival of the EBRT-only group versus the EBRT plus GKR group was 13 months and 25 months, respectively (*P* = .034). Thus it was concluded that GKR boost in conjunction with surgery and EBRT significantly improved the overall survival time. Contrary to this finding, Buatti and colleagues[32] reported the findings of LINAC SRS boost for patients with GBM with a tumor size of up to 4 cm and found that all 11 patients had disease progression within 1 year and only 3 of the 11 patients were alive at the 13-month follow-up. The efficacy of SRS boost was challenged. In 2004, the RTOG group reported the findings on a multi-institutional randomized prospective phase 3 trial evaluating SRS boost in patients treated for GBM (protocol 9305).[33] The use of SRS boost followed immediately by EBRT (60 Gy) was compared with EBRT (60 Gy) only in patients with GBM. The dose of radiosurgery was tumor size dependent and ranged from 15 to 24 Gy. Both groups received carmustine (BCNU) (80 mg/m^2) chemotherapy. Median survival was 13.5 months for the SRS plus EBRT group compared with 13.6 months in the EBRT-only group. The 2- and 3-year survival ranges also had no significant differences. Therefore, SRS boost before EBRT and BCNU showed no improvement in survival. This contradicted several earlier reports that indicated an improved survival for SRS-treated patients and could be attributed

to a selection bias. However, there was a difference in the temporal sequencing of the SRS; this may have affected the results of the studies.

SRS therapy has also been used as a salvage treatment in patients with recurrent malignant gliomas. Patients with a confirmed history of HGGs and who underwent previous resection or biopsies followed by fractionated brain irradiation with recurrence were treated with SRS.[34] The size of recurrence was limited to less than 3 cm, and LINAC was used in the first few patients, but most patients received GKR. This study found a significantly prolonged survival as a salvage treatment of GBM but not of grade 3 gliomas when compared with the historical control group: 23 months versus 12 months, *P*≤.0001. It was thus concluded that SRS was a safe and effective modality in selected patients with recurrent small-sized GBM.

GBM has been found to undergo molecular changes during radiotherapy, leading to accelerated proliferation with diminished effectiveness of prolonged fractionated irradiation.[35] To shorten the overall treatment time to decrease the opportunity for accelerated repopulation while delivering a total dose near or greater than standard treatment courses, accelerated radiotherapy schedules have been developed. This may be achieved by multiple treatments daily with a lower fraction size or using concomitant boost with higher doses on selected days during a treatment course.

FSRT is a method of delivering localized radiation and uses noninvasive immobilization techniques that allow fractionation. The usage of FSRT for boost delivery on a weekly basis combines the advantage of delivering a higher dose to the tumor with the potential benefit of fractionation. A phase 2 multi-institutional trial was performed to assess the feasibility, toxicity, and efficacy of dose-intense accelerated radiation therapy using weekly FSRT boost for patients with GBM.[36] Patients with GBM and postoperative enhancing tumor plus a tumor cavity diameter less than 60 mm were included. A standard radiation dose of 50 Gy was given in daily 2-Gy fractions. Patients also received 4 FSRT treatments once weekly during weeks 3 to 6. The dosage of FSRT was either 5 or 7 Gy per fraction and was given for a cumulative dose of 70 or 78 Gy in 29 (25 standard radiation therapy + 4 FSRT) treatments over 6 weeks. After radiation therapy, BCNU at 80 mg/m^2 was given for 3 days, every 8 weeks, for 6 cycles. Median survival time was 12.5 months. There was no survival difference compared with the RTOG historical database. However, patients who underwent gross total resection had a significantly longer median survival time than the historical controls with gross total resection. It was concluded that FSRT boost for GBM was feasible and well tolerated, but there was no significant survival benefit in using this dose-intense radiation therapy regimen. It was also found that gross total resection with minimal disease burden may benefit from this form of accelerated radiation therapy.

Another study evaluated the effect of FSRT for recurrent low-grade glioma and HGGs.[37] FSRT was given with a median dose of 36 Gy in median fractionation of 5 × 2 Gy/wk. The median overall survival after primary diagnosis was 21 months for patients with GBM and 50 months for patients with grade 3 gliomas. Median survival after reradiation was 8 months for GBM and 16 months for grade 3 gliomas. Progression-free survival after FSRT was 5 months for GBM and 8 months for grade 3 gliomas; it was concluded that FSRT was well tolerated and may be effective with recurrent gliomas.

Hypofractionated stereotactic radiotherapy (H-SRT) is a form of FSRT that is able to deliver treatment over 2 weeks versus 3 to 4 weeks with standard fractionation. This is particularly important when considering the grim prognosis for patients with HGGs for whom short treatment will definitely enhance the quality of life. Fogh and colleagues[38] reported the effect of H-SRT for recurrent HGGs. The aim of this study was to determine the efficacy and toxicity profile of H-SRT alone or in addition to repeated craniotomy or concomitant craniotomy. Patients with recurrent HGGs were treated with H-SRT (median dose, 35 Gy in 3.5-Gy fractions). Significant improvement in survival from H-SRT was found with factors such as younger age, smaller GTV, and shorter time between diagnosis and recurrence. No significant benefit of surgical resection or chemotherapy in this population was found

when analysis was controlled for other prognostic factors. The investigators concluded that H-SRT was well tolerated with minimal adverse effects and results in favorable survival benefit independent of reoperation or concomitant chemotherapy.

Cho and colleagues[39] published a study comparing SRS and FSRT in the treatment of recurrent HGGs. Of the 71 patients in the pool, 65% received SRS and 35% underwent FSRT. Median SRS dose was 17 Gy delivered to 50% isodose surface. In the FSRT group, the median dose of 37.5 Gy was given in 15 fractions to the median of 85% isodose surface. Actuarial median survival time was 11 months for the SRS group and 12 months for the FSRT group. Patients in the SRS group was noted to have more favorable prognostic factors, with a median age of 48 years, Karnofsky Performance Scale (KPS) of 70, and tumor volume of 10 mL versus median age of 53 years, KPS of 60, and tumor volume of 25 mL in the FSRT group. Late complications developed in 14 patients in the SRS group and 2 patients in the FSRT group ($P<.05$). It was deduced that patients who underwent FSRT had survival comparable to those with SRS but with poorer pretreatment prognostic factors and a lower risk of late complications. Thus, FSRT may be a better option for patients with larger tumors or tumors in eloquent structures.

In 2005, a systematic review of the evidence for the use of SRS or FSRT in patients with malignant glioma found that there was level 1 to 3 evidence that the use of SRS boost followed by EBRT and BCNU did not confer benefit in terms of overall survival, local tumor control, or quality of life compared with EBRT and BCNU. The use of SRS boost was also associated with increased toxicity. There was insufficient evidence regarding the benefits/harms of using SRS at the time of progression or recurrence. There was also insufficient evidence regarding the benefits/harms in the use of FSRT for newly diagnosed or progressive/recurrent malignant glioma.[40]

Some studies have found that daily repeated irradiation of malignant glioma cells with low doses compared with irradiation with a single biologically equivalent dose resulted in significantly higher cell killing. Hyperradiosensitivity defines the phenomenon that some human cell lines (including malignant glioma cells) are sensitive to killing by low radiation doses (<1 Gy).[41] Ultrafractionation radiation therapy is a novel regimen consisting of irradiating tumors several times daily, delivering low doses (<0.75 Gy) at which hyperradiosensitivity occurs. A phase 2 clinical trial has been performed to determine the safety, tolerability, and efficacy of an ultrafractionation regime in patients with newly diagnosed and inoperable GBM.[42] Three daily doses of 0.75 Gy were delivered at least 4 hours apart, 5 days per week over 6 to 7 consecutive weeks (90 fractions for a total of 67.5 Gy). Conformal irradiation included the tumor bulk with a margin of 2.5 cm. The ultrafractionation radiation regimen was safe and well tolerated with no acute grade III and/or IV central nervous system toxicity observed. Median progression-free survival and overall survival from initial diagnosis were 5.1 and 9.5 months, respectively. When compared with EORTC/NCIC trial in both progression-free survival and overall survival multivariate analysis, ultrafractionation showed superiority over radiotherapy alone but not over radiotherapy and temozolomide. Thus ultrafractionation regimen is safe and may prolong the survival of patients with GBM.

SUMMARY

There is evidence that dose escalation improves survival in patients with HGG. However, there is a turning point where the complications secondary to radiation necrosis compromise quality of life and survival of patients with primary or recurrent HGGs. The results of studies showing increased survival for patients undergoing radiosurgery were not confirmed when randomized and multi-institutional trials were performed. Stereotactic radiotherapy combined with the appropriate chemotherapeutic agent may have the merit to decrease side effects of boost using the stereotactic technique. Although highly popularized, a focal treatment such as stereotactic radiation has failed to show remarkable benefit for treatment of HGGs. It is plausible that in very special circumstances stereotactic radiation will become the standard of care in patients with HGGs. This will occur when imaging techniques, mostly molecular based, provide a better definition of the target to be irradiated.

REFERENCES

1. Hall EJ. Radiobiology for radiologist. 4th edition. Philadelphia: JB Lippincott; 1994. p. 1–13.
2. Roentgen WC. "On a new kind of rays." Translated by Arthur Stanton from the Sitzungsberichte der Würzburger Physik-medic. Gesellschaft, 1895. Nature 1896;1369(53):274–6.
3. Perez CA, Brady LW. Overview. In: Perez CA, Brady LW, editors. Principles and practice of radiation oncology. 2nd edition. Philadelphia: JB Lippincott; 1992. p. 1–63.
4. Frankel SA, German WJ. Glioblastoma multiforme review of 219 cases with regard to natural history, pathology, diagnostic methods, and treatment. J Neurosurg 1958;15:498–503.
5. Walker MD, Strike TA, Sheline GE. An analysis of dose-effect relationship in the radiotherapy of malignant gliomas. Int J Radiat Oncol Biol Phys 1979;5: 1725–31.
6. Kristiansen K, Hagen S, Kollevold T, et al. Combined modality therapy of operated astrocytomas grade III and IV. Confirmation of the value of postoperative irradiation and lack of potentiation of bleomycin on survival time: a prospective multicenter trial of the Scandinavian Glioblastoma Study Group. Cancer 1981;47:649–52.
7. Salazar OM, Rubin P, Feldstein ML, et al. High dose radiation therapy in the treatment of malignant gliomas: final report. Int J Radiat Oncol Biol Phys 1979;5:1733–40.
8. Bleethen NM, Stenning SP. A Medical Research Council trial of two radiotherapy doses in the treatment of grades 3 and 4 astrocytoma. The Medical Research Council Brain Tumor Working Party. Br J Cancer 1991;64:769–74.
9. Laperriere N, Zuraw L, Cairncross G, et al. Radiotherapy for newly diagnosed malignant glioma in adults: a systematic review. Radiother Oncol 2002; 64:259–73.
10. Stupp R, Mason WP, van den Bent MJ, et al. Radiotherapy plus concomitant and adjuvant temozolomide for glioblastoma. N Engl J Med 2005;352: 987–96.
11. Stupp R, Hegi ME, Mason WP, et al. Effects of radiotherapy with concomitant and adjuvant temozolomide versus radiotherapy alone on survival in glioblastoma in a randomized phase III study: 5-year analysis of the EORTC-NCIC trial. Lancet Oncol 2009;10:459–66.
12. Niyazi M, Ganswindt U, Schwarz SB, et al. Irradiation and bevacizumab in high-grade glioma retreatment settings. Int J Radiat Oncol Biol Phys 2012; 82(1):67–76.
13. Sanai N, Berger MS. Glioma extent of resection and its impact on patient outcome. Neurosurgery 2008; 62:753–66.
14. McGirt MJ, Chaichana KL, Gathinji M, et al. Independent association of extent of resection with survival in patients with malignant brain astrocytoma. J Neurosurg 2009;110:156–62.
15. Scherer HJ. Structural development in gliomas. Am J Cancer 1938;34:333–51.
16. Hochberg FH, Pruitt A. Assumptions in the radiotherapy of glioblastoma. Neurology 1980;30:907–11.
17. Price SJ, Burnet NG, Donovan T, et al. Diffusion tensor imaging of brain tumors at 3 T: a potential tool for assessing white matter tract invasion? Clin Radiol 2003;58:455–62.
18. Price SJ, Dean AF, Jena R. Identifying glioma infiltration of white matter using diffusion tensor imaging: an

MR image-guided biopsy study. Proc Intl Soc Mag Reson Med 2005;13:364.

19. Jena R, Price SJ, Baker C, et al. Diffusion tensor imaging: possible implications for radiotherapy treatment planning of patients with high-grade glioma. Clin Oncol 2005;17:581–90.

20. Oppitz U, Maessen D, Zunterer H, et al. 3D-recurrence-patterns of glioblastomas after CT-planned postoperative irradiation. Radiother Oncol 1999;53:53–7.

21. Mosskin M, Ericson K, Hindmarsh T, et al. Positron emission tomography compared with magnetic resonance imaging and computed tomography in supratentorial gliomas using multiple stereotactic biopsies as reference. Acta Radiol 1989;30:225–32.

22. Grosu AL, Weber WA, Riedel E, et al. L-(Methyl-11C) methionine positron emission tomography for target delineation in resected high-grade gliomas before radiotherapy. Int J Radiat Oncol Biol Phys 2005;63(1):64–74.

23. Grosu AL, Weber WA, Franz M, et al. Reirradiation of recurrent high-grade gliomas using amino acid PET (SPECT)/CT/MRI image fusion to determine gross tumor volume for stereotactic fractionated radiotherapy. Int J Radiat Oncol Biol Phys 2005;63(2):511–9.

24. Gray LH, Conger AD, Ebert M, et al. The concentration of oxygen dissolved in tissues at the time of irradiation as a factor in radiotherapy. Br J Radiol 1953;26:638–48.

25. Ogawa K, Ishiuchi S, Inoue O, et al. Phase II trial of radiotherapy after hyperbaric oxygenation with multiagent chemotherapy (procarbazine, nimustine, and vincristine) for high-grade gliomas: long-term results. Int J Radiat Oncol Biol Phys 2012;82(2):732–8.

26. Mizoe JE, Tsujii H, Hasegawa A, et al. Phase I/II clinical trial of carbon ion radiotherapy for malignant gliomas: combined X-ray radiotherapy, chemotherapy, and carbon ion radiotherapy. Int J Radiat Oncol Biol Phys 2007;69(2):390–6.

27. Combs SE, Burkholder I, Edler L, et al. Randomized phase I/II study to evaluate carbon ion radiotherapy versus fractionated stereotactic radiotherapy in patients with recurrent or progressive gliomas: the CINDERELLA trial. BMC Cancer 2010;10:533.

28. Colombo F, Benedetti A, Pozza F, et al. External stereotactic irradiation by linear accelerator. Neurosurgery 1985;16:154–60.

29. Selch MT, De Salles AA, Goetsch SJ, et al. Single-fraction radiosurgery for primary and recurrent malignant gliomas. J Radiosurg 1998;1:155–68.

30. Shrieve DC, Alexander E 3rd, Black PM, et al. Treatment of patients with primary glioblastoma multiforme with standard post-operative radiotherapy and radiosurgical boost: prognostic factors and long-term outcome. J Neurosurg 1999;90:72–7.

31. Nwokedi EC, DiBiase SJ, Jabbour S, et al. Gamma knife stereotactic radiosurgery for patients with glioblastoma multiforme. Neurosurgery 2002;50:41–6 [discussion: 46–7].

32. Buatti JM, Friedman WA, Bova FJ, et al. Linac radiosurgery for high-grade gliomas: the University of Florida experience. Int J Radiat Oncol Biol Phys 1995;32(1):205–10.

33. Souhami L, Seiferheld W, Brachman D, et al. Randomized comparison of stereotactic radiosurgery followed by conventional radiotherapy with carmustine to conventional radiotherapy with carmustine for patient with glioblastoma multiforme: report of Radiation Therapy Oncology Group 93-05 protocol. Int J Radiat Oncol Biol Phys 2004;60(3):853–60.

34. Kong DS, Lee JI, Park K, et al. Efficacy of stereotactic radiosurgery as a salvage treatment for recurrent malignant gliomas. Cancer 2008;112:2046–51.

35. Budach W, Gioioso D, Taghian A, et al. Repopulation capacity during fractionated irradiation of squamous cell carcinomas and glioblastomas in vitro. Int J Radiat Oncol Biol Phys 1997;39:743–50.

36. Cardinale R, Won M, Choucair A, et al. A phase II trial of accelerated radiotherapy using weekly stereotactic conformal boost for supratentorial glioblastoma multiforme: RTOG 0023. Int J Radiat Oncol Biol Phys 2006;65(5):1422–8.

37. Combs SE, Thilmann C, Edler L, et al. Efficacy of fractionated stereotactic reirradiation in recurrent gliomas: long-term results in 172 patients treated in a single institution. J Clin Oncol 2005;23:8863–9.

38. Fogh SE, Andrews DW, Glass J, et al. Hypofractionated stereotactic radiation therapy: an effective therapy for recurrent high-grade gliomas. J Clin Oncol 2010;28:3048–53.

39. Cho KH, Hall WA, Gerbi BJ, et al. Single dose versus fractionated stereotactic radiotherapy for recurrent high-grade gliomas. Int J Radiat Oncol Biol Phys 1999;45(5):1133–41.

40. Tsao MN, Mehta MP, Whelan TJ, et al. The American Society for Therapeutic Radiology and Oncology (ASTRO) evidence-based review of the role of radiosurgery for malignant glioma. Int J Radiat Oncol Biol Phys 2005;63(1):47–55.

41. Joiner MC, Denekamp J, Maughan RL. The use of "top-up" experiments to investigate the effect of very small doses per fraction in mouse skin. Int J Radiat Biol Relat Stud Phys Chem Med 1986;49:565–80.

42. Beauchesne P, Bernier V, Carnin C, et al. Prolonged survival for patients with newly diagnosed, inoperable glioblastoma with 3-times daily ultrafractionated radiation therapy. Neuro Oncol 2010;12(6):595–602.

Radiology: Criteria for Determining Response to Treatment and Recurrence of High-Grade Gliomas

Joshua Lucas, MD*, Gabriel Zada, MD

KEYWORDS

- High-grade gliomas • Response criteria • Neuroimaging

High-grade glioma (HGG) is the most common form of primary brain tumor in adults. The World Health Organization (WHO) classification for central nervous system gliomas includes 2 grades that constitute HGG: anaplastic astrocytoma (WHO grade 3) and glioblastoma multiforme (WHO grade 4). The evaluation of response to treatment for patients with these tumors is of high clinical value in several respects. First, a patient's response to a particular treatment must be able to be analyzed objectively and easily communicated among practitioners. If one particular treatment fails to produce favorable results, an alternative treatment strategy can be pursued. Also, an objective scale must be available for clinical trials of new treatments. Traditional end points for the assessment of efficacy in clinical trials are progression-free survival (PFS), radiographic response rate (RRR), and overall survival (OS). Unlike OS, PFS and RRR depend on reproducible and accurate imaging measurements to analyze tumor progression.[1]

The development and refinement of specific radiographic response criteria have spanned several decades and several imaging modalities, and have evolved considerably over the past 3 decades. Contrast-enhanced computed tomography (CT) scans were initially used to analyze tumor progression. Criteria that had been developed for CT imaging were expanded to include T1-weighted magnetic resonance imaging (MRI) with gadolinium contrast.[2] Both methods detect disruption of the blood-brain barrier by evaluating areas of tumor enhancement. Newer response criteria, including the recently published Response Assessment in Neuro-Oncology (RANO) criteria, attempt to address limitations of prior response criteria and use fluid-attenuated inversion recovery (FLAIR) and T2-weighted MRI combined with T1-weighted MRI with gadolinium contrast to evaluate tumor size. Further study of advanced MR techniques, such as perfusion/permeability imaging and diffusion-weighted imaging, and functional assessment of tumors with MR spectroscopy (MRS) and positron emission tomography (PET) scanning, will likely allow for more accurate response criteria to be developed in the future. In this review, various schemes that have been developed and implemented to determine response to treatment and recurrence of HGG, and the status of current and emerging neuroimaging modalities used to make these assessments, are reviewed.

DEVELOPMENT OF CRITERIA FOR DETERMINING RESPONSE

Starting in the 1970s, several investigators have attempted to create practical criteria for assessing tumor response to treatment based on

Disclosures: Funding Sources: Dr Lucas: None. Dr Zada: None.
Conflicts of Interest: Dr Lucas: None. Dr Zada: None.
Department of Neurosurgery, University of Southern California, 1200 North State Street, Suite 3300, Los Angeles, CA 90033, USA
* Corresponding author.
E-mail address: joshuawlucas@gmail.com

Neurosurg Clin N Am 23 (2012) 269–276
doi:10.1016/j.nec.2012.01.006
1042-3680/12/$ – see front matter Published by Elsevier Inc.

combinations of neuroimaging studies, patient clinical status, and relative interventions, such as corticosteroid administration. Although the basic principles of each of these schemes have remained more or less consistent with regard to determining treatment response versus tumor progression, the neuroimaging modalities used to make these determinations and specific criteria have evolved considerably. Starting with the Levin criteria in the late 1970s to the most recent implementation of the RANO criteria in 2010, the various criteria for assessing tumor response to multimodality treatment regimens are discussed in the following sections.

Levin Criteria (1977)

An early attempt to classify response to treatment of HGGs was published by Levin and colleagues[3] in 1977. The grading scheme they developed incorporated 4 separate modalities, including the neurologic examination, a radionuclide brain scan, an electroencephalogram, and a CT scan. Each was individually analyzed and any change from baseline was graded on a scale from +3 ("markedly better") to –3 ("markedly worse"). The CT scan was analyzed specifically for interval changes in tumor size, central lucency, degree of edema, degree of contrast enhancement, and size of the ventricular system. The corticosteroid dosages required by the patient at the time of grading were also accounted for as part of the assessment. This system represents one of the earliest published attempts at characterizing response to treatment of HGGs with the use of CT imaging.

WHO Oncology Response Criteria (1979)

In 1979, WHO developed criteria for grading response to therapy that was not specific for HGG, but applicable to all types of cancer.[4,5] Assessment of tumor size was based on 2-dimensional analysis of the tumor. The product of the 2 largest cross-sectional diameters of a specific enhancing lesion seen on CT scan was used as the primary measure of tumor size.

The criteria proposed by WHO identified 4 response categories. Complete response (CR) was characterized by complete disappearance of the lesion on subsequent CT scans. Partial response (PR) was characterized by a greater than 50% reduction in tumor size. Progressive disease (PD) indicated that tumor size had increased by more than 25% on repeat imaging. Stable disease (SD) was characterized by a reduction in size of less than 50% or an increase in size of less than 25%. Macdonald and colleagues[2]

would be the first group to apply these categories of progression to brain tumors specifically.

Macdonald Criteria (1990)

In 1990, Macdonald and colleagues[2] published a new set of criteria demonstrating that the WHO criteria of 1979 could be applied directly to brain tumors, specifically HGGs. Like the WHO criteria, the Macdonald criteria used the maximal cross-sectional enhancing diameters of a specific lesion on CT scan as the primary tumor measure. In addition to radiographic response, Macdonald and colleagues[2] incorporated the clinical assessment of the patient and the current corticosteroid dose into the response grading scheme.

The categories of response in the Macdonald criteria are similar to the WHO Oncology Response criteria with regard to changes in tumor size. CR was defined as complete disappearance of tumor, with the additional requirements of no corticosteroids and stable or improved neurologic examination. PR was characterized by greater than 50% reduction in tumor size along with no new lesions, stable or reduced corticosteroid requirements, and stable or improved neurologic examination. PD was defined as any of the following: greater than 25% enlargement of tumor size, a new lesion, or clinical deterioration. SD was defined as a stable clinical examination that did not qualify as CR, PD, or PR.

Over the next several years, the Macdonald criteria would be met with some criticism.[6,7] Because of reliance on 2-dimensional assessment of tumor size, irregularly shaped tumors are difficult to assess and may therefore result in a high degree of interobserver variability. The criteria also provide little guidance for measuring tumors within or adjacent to cystic cavities or surgical cavities, and for multifocal tumors. Another limitation of the Macdonald criteria is that the primary tumor measurement relies only on enhancing portions of the tumor, so nonenhancing portions are not taken into consideration. Furthermore, the degree of contrast enhancement can be very nonspecific. Factors that may influence enhancement include corticosteroid dosages, the amount of contrast used during the scan, postsurgical changes, treatment-related inflammation, seizure activity, ischemia, subacute radiation effects and radiation necrosis, and antiangiogenic agents.[8–13]

The Macdonald criteria have since been adapted to include MRI with gadolinium contrast, under the same assumption that breakdown of the blood-brain barrier and disrupted vascular architecture will also manifest as contrast enhancement. Because corticosteroids can influence the amount of contrast enhancement, Macdonald and colleagues[2] proposed that patients be kept on stable doses of corticosteroids when assessing for response. When new doses of corticosteroids were required, Macdonald and colleagues[2] originally proposed waiting 2 weeks for reassessment; however, new evidence suggests that 5 days are likely sufficient. The Macdonald criteria were the most widely used method of assessing response until the RANO criteria were published in 2010.

Response Evaluation Criteria in Solid Tumors (2000, 2009)

The Response Evaluation Criteria in Solid Tumors (RECIST) were introduced in 2000,[14] and then revised in 2009[15] for the evaluation of systemic cancers. In contrast to the WHO Oncology Response criteria, the RECIST criteria are based on the longest unidirectional single diameter in the axial plane. When multiple lesions are present, the diameters are summed to provide the primary tumor size measurement. As part of the RECIST criteria, the categories of response also differed from WHO criteria in that PR was defined as a greater than 30% decrease in the sums of maximal diameters of tumors, PD was characterized by a greater than 20% increase in the sums of diameters of tumors, and SD was defined as a lesion not classified as PD or PR.

The revised RECIST guidelines defined a minimum of 2 and a maximum of 5 lesions to be counted in cases of multiple lesions. Also, pathologic lymph nodes were incorporated into the assessment. To prevent overcalling progression, the revised RECIST guidelines also suggest a 5-mm absolute minimum increase requirement to diagnose PD. Several studies have suggested that the RECIST criteria have good concordance with both 2-dimensional measurements (Macdonald criteria) and volumetric measurements when determining response in both adult and pediatric high-grade gliomas.[16–18]

DEVELOPMENT OF THE CURRENT STANDARD CRITERIA (RANO CRITERIA)
Limitations of the Macdonald Criteria

Multimodality therapy for HGGs has evolved dramatically since the publication of the Macdonald criteria. Standard first-line therapy for high-grade gliomas currently involves maximal tumor resection followed by radiotherapy and concurrent and adjuvant temozolomide.[19] Therapy with antiangiogenic agents, such as bevacizumab and cediranib, or additional chemotherapy regimens, is reserved for patients demonstrating recurrence or tumor progression following first-line therapy.

Recently observed effects of these current treatment modalities, namely pseudoprogression and pseudoresponse, have presented new challenges to the practicality of the Macdonald criteria in determining response to treatment.

Pseudoprogression

Pseudoprogression refers to the phenomenon whereby an increase in contrast enhancement does not accurately reflect actual tumor progression, and is thought to occur as a result of increased vascular permeability in tumors primarily following treatment with radiation and temozolomide.[20,21] Several studies have reported that 20% to 30% of patients treated with radiation and temozolomide develop pseudoprogression on the first postradiation MRI,[22,23] and that pseudoprogression is most likely to occur 4 to 12 weeks after completion of radiation therapy. Pseudoprogression will eventually resolve on subsequent MRI. To be considered pseudoprogression, the new region of enhancement must be within the radiation field.[21] Of note, this phenomenon occurs more often in patients with methylated MGMT-promoter tumors.[22]

The clinical significance of pseudoprogression may be profound. Nontumoral enhancement mistaken for PD may result in premature discontinuation of adjuvant therapy that is actually effective. Also, pseudoprogression may have implications for response reporting in clinical trials, especially in trails using PFS and RRR as primary end points.[24]

To evaluate tumor progression in these patients, FLAIR and T2-weighted sequences can be obtained on MRI. Progressive increases in nonenhancing FLAIR and T2-weighted signals reflect actual tumor progression.[25–27] An increase in these signals must be differentiated from other potential causes, including the effects of radiation, decreased corticosteroids, demyelination, ischemia, infection, seizures, and postoperative changes. Changes in FLAIR and T2-weighted imaging that suggest infiltrating tumor include mass effect, infiltration of the cortical ribbon, and an involvement of an area outside the radiation field.[28] In addition, newer imaging modalities, such as MR perfusion and permeability imaging, can more easily distinguish between real progression and pseudoprogression.

Pseudoresponse

Pseudoresponse refers to a decrease in contrast uptake that does not reflect actual tumor regression. This phenomenon occurs most commonly in patients treated with antiangiogenic therapies, such as bevacizumab (an anti–vascular endothelial growth factor [VEGF] monoclonal antibody) and cedirinib (an anti-VEGF receptor monoclonal antibody), and can be seen as early as 1 to 2 days after initiation of antiangiogenic therapy.[28] Pseudoresponse is thought to be the result of normalization of vessel permeability and not a true antitumor response.[29,30] Also, increasing evidence suggests that anti-VEGF therapies increase blood vessel co-option by tumor cells. Co-opted vessels are believed to be less permeable and therefore less visible on contrast-enhanced MRI.[31–33]

RANO Group Criteria

The RANO group was an international effort to develop new standardized response criteria for clinical trials in brain tumors and response to therapy in individual patients with brain tumors.[28] In 2010, the RANO group published response criteria based on the Macdonald criteria but expanded these to define more-specific methods of measurement. The RANO criteria set more-specific guidelines for exact measurement of tumor size, and made significant changes to address the limitations of the Macdonald criteria (**Tables 1** and **2**).

For instance, the RANO group concluded that the use of maximum cross-sectional enhancing diameters on T1-weighted contrast-enhanced MRI was supported most by published evidence and should continue to be the primary tumor measure. The group also extended the Macdonald criteria to include both CT and MRI. For the least amount of variability, the group recommended that lesions be measured with the same scanner or at least one with the same magnetic strength. Strict guidelines were set for tumor measurements in cases of multiple lesions. The RANO criteria specify that a minimum of 2 lesions and a maximum of 5 lesions should be selected. Ideally, the largest lesions are selected, but favor should be given to those lesions that can be most reliably measured. The sum of the products of the cross-sectional diameters is used as the primary tumor measure. The group also set guidelines for measurement of small lesions. They determined that lesions must be visible on 2 consecutive 5-mm axial slices on CT or MRI. If larger slices are used, the size of the lesion at baseline should be at least double the slice thickness. Guidelines were also set for measurement of lesions with cystic components and those associated with surgical cavities. The RANO criteria state that the cyst or surgical cavity should not be measured, and lesions with cysts or surgical cavities must have a nodular component more than 10 mm in diameter to be included.

To address the phenomenon of pseudoprogression in patients treated with radiation and temozolomide, the RANO criteria specify that PD cannot be confirmed within the first 12 weeks following treatment unless new enhancement is found outside of the 80% isodose radiation field or tumor is unequivocally confirmed pathohistologically. Also, clinical decline alone without evidence of radiologic progression within the first 12 weeks was determined not to be sufficient for the classification of PD.

For patients receiving antiangiogenic therapies, specific additions were made to the RANO criteria to address pseudoresponse. According to the new criteria, FLAIR and T2-weighted MRI were included in all classifications of response. Lesions must have stable or decreased FLAIR and T2-weighted signals to be classified as CR, PR, or SD. A significant increase in FLAIR and T2-weighted signals was considered enough evidence to classify the tumor as PD, provided that other potential causes were excluded.

Aside from the addition of FLAIR/T2-imaging sequences and more strict requirements for defining PD, classifications within the RANO criteria remained largely the same as with the Macdonald criteria. CR was again classified as complete disappearance of tumor, no new lesions, absence of corticosteroids, and a stable or improved clinical examination. PR was defined as a greater than 50% decrease in tumor size, no new lesions, stable or decreased corticosteroid doses, and stable or improved clinical examination. PD was characterized by a greater than 25% increase in tumor size, new lesions, increased dosages of corticosteroids, or worsening clinical examination. SD comprised anything that did not belong to another category.

Of note, the RANO criteria defined a new category of nonmeasurable lesions as predominantly cystic lesions, lesions measureable in 1 dimension only, lesions having no clearly defined margins, or lesions with a maximum perpendicular diameter smaller than 1 mm. According to the RANO criteria, patients with nonmeasurable disease can achieve a "stable" classification as their best radiologic outcome.

EMERGING NEUROIMAGING MODALITIES TO ASSESS TUMOR RESPONSE

Authors of the RANO criteria and the RECIST criteria, the 2 most recent guidelines to be published, analyzed whether other forms of measurement, such as advanced MRI techniques, volumetric measurement, or functional assessment, would be more accurate as primary tumor

Table 1
RANO classifications of tumor response

Response	Criteria
Complete response	Requires all of the following: complete disappearance of all enhancing measurable and nonmeasurable disease sustained for at least 4 weeks; no new lesions; stable or improved nonenhancing (T2/FLAIR) lesions; patients must be off corticosteroids (or on physiologic replacement doses only); and stable or improved clinically. Note: Patients with nonmeasurable disease only cannot have a complete response; the best response possible is stable disease
Partial response	Requires all of the following: ≥50% decrease compared with baseline in the sum of products of perpendicular diameters of all measurable enhancing lesions sustained for at least 4 weeks; no progression of nonmeasurable disease; no new lesions; stable or improved nonenhancing (T2/FLAIR) lesions on same or lower dose of corticosteroids compared with baseline scan; the corticosteroid dose at the time of the scan evaluation should be no greater than the dose at time of baseline scan; and stable or improved clinically. Note: Patients with nonmeasurable disease only cannot have a partial response; the best response possible is stable disease
Stable disease	Requires all of the following: does not qualify for complete response, partial response, or progression; stable nonenhancing (T2/FLAIR) lesions on same or lower dose of corticosteroids compared with baseline scan. In the event that the corticosteroid dose was increased for new symptoms and signs without confirmation of disease progression on neuroimaging, and subsequent follow-up imaging shows that this increase in corticosteroids was required because of disease progression, the last scan considered to show stable disease will be the scan obtained when the corticosteroid dose was equivalent to the baseline dose
Progression	Defined by any of the following: ≥25% increase in sum of the products of perpendicular diameters of enhancing lesions compared with the smallest tumor measurement obtained either at baseline (if no decrease) or best response, on stable or increasing doses of corticosteroids[a]; significant increase in T2/FLAIR nonenhancing lesion on stable or increasing doses of corticosteroids compared with baseline scan or best response after initiation of therapy[a] not caused by comorbid events (eg, radiation therapy, demyelination, ischemic injury, infection, seizures, postoperative changes, or other treatment effects); any new lesion; clear clinical deterioration not attributable to other causes apart from the tumor (eg, seizures, medication adverse effects, complications of therapy, cerebrovascular events, infection, and so on) or changes in corticosteroid dose; failure to return for evaluation as a result of death or deteriorating condition; or clear progression of nonmeasurable disease

All measurable and nonmeasurable lesions must be assessed using the same techniques as at baseline.
Abbreviations: FLAIR, fluid-attenuated inversion recovery; MRI, magnetic resonance imaging.
[a] Stable doses of corticosteroids include patients not on corticosteroids.
Data from Wen PY, Macdonald DR, Reardon DA, et al. Updated response assessment criteria for high-grade gliomas: Response Assessment in Neuro-Oncology working group. J Clin Oncol 2010;28(11):1963–72.

measures for response criteria. The 2 studies concluded that current lack of published evidence, availability, and standardization prohibits the use of these advanced measurements in current response criteria. As more data become available regarding the ability for emerging advanced neuro-imaging techniques to accurately predict tumor response to therapy and differentiate this from pseudoprogression and pseudoresponse, various response criteria schemes will require periodic re-assessment and are likely to remain in flux. As

expected, future studies will undoubtedly incorporate these imaging modalities into updated response criteria for HGGs.

MR Perfusion and Permeability

MR perfusion

HGGs are characterized by an increase in neovascularization on both a macrovascular and microvascular scale. MR perfusion scanning yields an estimated relative cerebral blood volume that

Table 2
Summary of the proposed RANO response criteria

Criterion	CR	PR	SD	PD
T1 gadolinium-enhancing disease	None	≥50% ↓	< 50% ↓ but <25% ↑	≥25% ↑[a]
T2/FLAIR	Stable or ↓	Stable or ↓	Stable or↓	↑[a]
New lesion	None	None	None	Present[a]
Corticosteroids	None	Stable or ↓	Stable or ↓	NA[b]
Clinical status	Stable or ↑	Stable or ↑	Stable or ↑	↓[a]
Requirement for response	All	All	All	Any[a]

Abbreviations: CR, complete response; FLAIR, fluid-attenuated inversion recovery; NA, not applicable; PD, progressive disease; PR, partial response; RANO, Response Assessment in Neuro-Oncology; SD, stable disease; ↓, decreased; ↑, increased.
[a] Progression occurs when this criterion is present.
[b] Increase in corticosteroids alone will not be taken into account in determining progression in the absence of persistent clinical deterioration.
Data from Wen PY, Macdonald DR, Reardon DA, et al. Updated response assessment criteria for high-grade gliomas: Response Assessment in Neuro-Oncology working group. J Clin Oncol 2010;28(11):1963–72.

reflects the amount of capillaries with a given space on imaging.[30] The amount of hyperperfusion in a tumor is a marker for tumor aggressiveness and behavior. Only solid, non-necrotic, noncystic areas of tumors can be assessed. Parametric response mapping, created with perfusion scan postprocessing, has been reported to be useful in distinguishing real progression from pseudoprogression.[34]

MR permeability

Another characteristic of HGGs is increased vascular leakiness, caused by abnormal permeability of immature capillaries. Increasing amounts of vascular leakage have been shown to correlate with increasing grade in HGGs.[35] T1-weighted dynamic contrast-enhanced MRI is used to produce a variable called the transport constant (Ktrans), which corresponds to the quantity of contrast extravasation and, in turn, vascular permeability.[36,37] Corrected perfusion maps that account for extravascular extravasation of contrast have been shown to correlate more accurately with tumor grade.[38,39]

MR Diffusion-Weighted Imaging

Diffusion-weighted MRI studies the movement of water molecules within tissue, and can be used to analyze response to therapy within tumor cells. Effective therapies can potentially change the cellular density of HGGs, the architecture of individual tumor cells, and the state of water within tumor cells. In many cases, these changes are visible on diffusion-weighted imaging (DWI) before morphologic changes in the tumor are able to be

visualized.[40] The apparent diffusion coefficient (ADC) is the standard of measurement with DWI, as it provides a measure of the diffusion properties of water in brain tissue at the voxel level. Multiple voxels can be analyzed to create an ADC map.[30]

ADC maps have been shown to be effective in differentiating radiation-induced necrosis from recurrent lesions.[41–43] Contrast enhancement can be seen in the walls of the surgical cavity 48 to 72 hours postoperatively.[44,45] Baseline MRI should therefore be obtained within 24 to 48 hours, and no later than 72 hours.[28] The addition of DWI to this MRI can identify areas of ischemia that will become contrast enhancing several weeks postoperatively.[12] Without DWI, these areas of ischemia are often confused with enhancing tumor.

MR Spectroscopy

MRS provides information about the biochemical composition of tumors. Markers used for analysis include glucose (tumor metabolism), choline (membrane turnover and proliferation), creatine (energy homeostasis), N-acetyl-aspartate (intact glioneural structures), and lactate or lipids (necrosis).[30] Current limitations of MRS include signal-to-noise ratios that require large voxel sizes, which eliminate the ability to image small tumors.

PET Scanning

PET scanning assesses the metabolic state of HGGs.[30] To localize areas of tumor with increased anaerobic metabolism, 18F-fluorodeoxyglucose (18F-FDG) is commonly used. Localized hypoxia within HGGs forces cells to convert to anaerobic metabolism.[46] Also, anaerobic glycolysis occurs in spite of adequate oxygen levels in advanced cancers.[47] Tumor cells therefore have increased uptake of 18F-FDG, which can be seen on PET imaging.

Also used as markers are 11C-methionine, 18F-fluoroethyltyrosine (18F-FET), and 18F-fluorothymidine. Upregulation of DNA and protein synthesis in cancer cells creates an increased turnover of nucleosides and amino acids, and these markers are subsequently incorporated into new genetic and protein products. The 11C-methionine and 18F-FET are more specific than 18F-FDG because they are more selectively taken up by tumor cells than by healthy brain tissue. Disadvantages of PET include scarce availability, cost, and mild exposure to radioactive material.[30]

SUMMARY

The development of radiologic criteria for the assessment of response to treatment in HGGs has evolved considerably over the past decades. Currently, T1-weighted MR imaging with gadolinium contrast combined with FLAIR and T2-weighted sequences is the standard imaging modality used to assess tumors. Considerable evolution in the criteria of various tumor response grading schemes have been observed since the widespread implementation of CT imaging in the 1970s. The 2010 RANO criteria, the most recent attempt to provide comprehensive guidelines for the measurement and analyses of HGGs, have incorporated methods by which to exclude the phenomena of pseudoprogression and pseudoresponse. The RANO criteria can be implemented in both direct patient care and clinical trials. Future studies assessing emerging advanced neuroimaging techniques, combined with more widespread availability, will facilitate the development of future evidence-based radiologic response criteria with more accuracy in differentiating tumor response versus progression.

REFERENCES

1. Wen PY, Norden AD, Drappatz J, et al. Response assessment challenges in clinical trials of gliomas. Curr Oncol Rep 2010;12(1):68–75.
2. Macdonald DR, Cascino TL, Schold SC, et al. Response criteria for phase II studies of supratentorial malignant glioma. J Clin Oncol 1990;8:1277–80.
3. Levin VA, Crafts DC, Norman DM, et al. Criteria for evaluating patients undergoing chemotherapy for malignant brain tumors. J Neurosurg 1977;47(3):329–35.
4. World Health Organization. WHO handbook for reporting results of cancer treatment. Offset Publication

No. 48. Geneva (Switzerland): World Health Organization; 1979.
5. Miller A, Hoogstraten B, Staquet M, et al. Reporting results of cancer treatment. Cancer 1981;47:207–14.
6. Sorensen AG, Batchelor TT, Wen PY, et al. Response criteria for glioma. Nat Clin Pract Oncol 2008;5: 634–44.
7. van den Bent MJ, Vogelbaum MA, Wen PY, et al. End point assessment in gliomas: novel treatments limit usefulness of classical Macdonald's criteria. J Clin Oncol 2009;27:2905–8.
8. Cairncross JG, Macdonald DR, Pexman JH, et al. Steroid induced changes in patients with recurrent malignant glioma. Neurology 1988;38:724–6.
9. Watling CJ, Lee DH, Macdonald DR, et al. Corticosteroid induced magnetic resonance imaging changes in patients with recurrent malignant glioma. J Clin Oncol 1994;12:1886–9.
10. Henegar MM, Moran CJ, Silbergeld DL. Early postoperative magnetic resonance imaging following nonneoplastic cortical resection. J Neurosurg 1996;84:174–9.
11. Finn MA, Blumenthal DT, Salzman KL, et al. Transient postictal MRI changes in patients with brain tumors may mimic disease progression. Surg Neurol 2007; 67:246–50.
12. Ulmer S, Braga TA, Barker FG, et al. Clinical and radiographic features of peritumoral infarction following resection of glioblastoma. Neurology 2006;67:1668–70.
13. Kumar AJ, Leeds NE, Fuller GN, et al. Malignant gliomas: MR imaging spectrum of radiation therapy- and chemotherapy-induced necrosis of the brain after treatment. Radiology 2000;217:377–84.
14. Therasse P, Arbuck S, Eisenhauer E, et al. New guidelines to evaluate the response to treatment in solid tumors. European Organization for Research and Treatment of Cancer, National Cancer Institute of the United States, National Cancer Institute of Canada. J Natl Cancer Inst 2000;92:205–16.
15. Eisenhauer EA, Therasse P, Bogaerts J, et al. New response evaluation criteria in solid tumours: revised RECIST guideline (version 1.1). Eur J Cancer 2009; 45:228–47.
16. Warren KE, Patronas N, Aikin AA, et al. Comparison of one-, two-, and three-dimensional measurements of childhood brain tumors. J Natl Cancer Inst 2001; 93:1401–5.
17. Shah GD, Kesari S, Xu R, et al. Comparison of linear and volumetric criteria in assessing tumor response in adult high-grade gliomas. Neuro Oncol 2006;8:38–46.
18. Galanis E, Buckner JC, Maurer MJ, et al. Validation of neuroradiologic response assessment in gliomas: measurement by RECIST, two-dimensional, computer-assisted tumor area, and computer-assisted tumor volume methods. Neuro Oncol 2006;8:156–65.
19. Stupp R, Mason WP, van den Bent MJ, et al. Radiotherapy plus concomitant and adjuvant

temozolomide for glioblastoma. N Engl J Med 2005; 352:987–96.

20. de Wit MC, de Bruin HG, Eijkenboom WM, et al. Immediate post-radiotherapy changes in malignant glioma can mimic tumour progression. Neurology 2004;63:535–7.

21. Brandsma D, Stalpers L, Taal W, et al. Clinical features, mechanisms, and management of pseudo-progression in malignant gliomas. Lancet Oncol 2008;9:453–61.

22. Brandes AA, Franceschi E, Tosoni A, et al. MGMT promoter methylation status can predict the incidence and outcome of pseudoprogression after concomitant radiochemotherapy in newly diagnosed glioblastoma patients. J Clin Oncol 2008;26: 2192–7.

23. Brandes AA, Tosoni A, Spagnolli F, et al. Disease progression or pseudoprogression after concomitant radiochemotherapy treatment: pitfalls in neuro-oncology. Neuro Oncol 2008;10:361–7.

24. Lutz K, Radbruch A, Wiestler B, et al. Neuroradiological response criteria for high-grade gliomas. Clin Neuroradiol 2011;21(4):199–205.

25. Norden AD, Young GS, Setayesh K, et al. Bevacizumab for recurrent malignant gliomas: efficacy, toxicity, and patterns of recurrence. Neurology 2008;70:779–87.

26. Narayana A, Raza S, Golfinos JG, et al. Bevacizumab therapy in recurrent high grade glioma: impact on local control and survival. J Clin Oncol 2008;26:691s.

27. Norden AD, Drappatz J, Wen PY. Novel antiangiogenic therapies for malignant gliomas. Lancet Neurol 2008;7:1152–60.

28. Wen PY, Macdonald DR, Reardon DA, et al. Updated response assessment criteria for high-grade gliomas: Response Assessment in Neuro-Oncology working group. J Clin Oncol 2010;28(11):1963–72.

29. Quant EC, Wen PY. Response assessment in neuro-oncology. Curr Oncol Rep 2011;13:50–6.

30. Dhermain FG, Hau P, Lanfermann H, et al. Advanced MRI and PET imaging for assessment of treatment response in patients with gliomas. Lancet Neurol 2010;9:906–20.

31. Rubenstein J, Kim J, Ozawa T, et al. Anti-VEGF antibody treatment of glioblastoma prolongs survival but results in increased vascular cooption. Neoplasia 2000;2:306–14.

32. Paez-Ribes M, Allen E, Hudock J, et al. Antiangiogenic therapy elicits malignant progression of tumors to increased local invasion and distant metastasis. Cancer Cell 2009;15:220–31.

33. Bergers G, Hanahan D. Modes of resistance to anti-angiogenic therapy. Nat Rev Cancer 2008;8:592–603.

34. Tsien C, Galban CJ, Chenevert TL, et al. Parametric response map as an imaging biomarker to distinguish progression from pseudoprogression in high-grade glioma. J Clin Oncol 2010;28:2293–9.

35. Roberts HC, Roberts TP, Brasch RC, et al. Quantitative measurement of microvascular permeability in human brain tumours achieved using dynamic contrast-enhanced MR imaging: correlation with histologic grade. AJNR Am J Neuroradiol 2000;21: 891–9.

36. Tofts PS, Brix G, Buckley DL, et al. Estimating kinetic parameters from dynamic contrast-enhanced T(1)-weighted MRI of a diffusable tracer: standardized quantities and symbols. J Magn Reson Imaging 1999;10:223–32.

37. Haroon HA, Buckley DL, Patankar TA, et al. A comparison of Ktrans measurements obtained with conventional and first pass pharmacokinetic models in human gliomas. J Magn Reson Imaging 2004;19:527–36.

38. Cao Y, Shen Z, Chenevert TL, et al. Estimate of vascular permeability and cerebral blood volume using Gd-DTPA contrast enhancement and dynamic T2*-weighted MRI. J Magn Reson Imaging 2006;24: 288–96.

39. Boxerman JL, Schmainda KM, Weisskoff RM. Relative cerebral blood volume maps corrected for contrast agent extravasation significantly correlate with glioma tumor grade, whereas uncorrected maps do not. AJNR Am J Neuroradiol 2006;27:859–67.

40. Chenevert TL, Sundgren PC, Ross BD. Diffusion imaging: insight to cell status and cytoarchitecture. Neuroimaging Clin N Am 2006;16:619–32.

41. Barajas RF Jr, Chang JS, Segal MR, et al. Differentiation of recurrent glioblastoma multiforme from radiation necrosis after external beam radiotherapy with dynamic susceptibility-weighted contrast enhanced perfusion MR imaging. Radiology 2009;253:486–96.

42. Hu LS, Baxter LC, Smith KA, et al. Relative cerebral blood volume values to diffrentiate high-grade glioma recurrence from posttreatment radiation effect: direct correlation between image-guided tissue histopathology and localized dynamic susceptibility-weighted contrast-enhanced perfusion MR imaging measurements. AJNR Am J Neuroradiol 2009;30: 552–8.

43. Hein PA, Eskey CJ, Dunn JF, et al. Diffusion-weighted imaging in the follow-up of treated high-grade gliomas: tumor recurrence versus radiation injury. AJNR Am J Neuroradiol 2004;25:201–9.

44. Sato N, Bronen RA, Sze G, et al. Postoperative changes in the brain: MR imaging findings in patients without neoplasms. Radiology 1997;204: 839–46.

45. Cairncross JG, Pexman JH, Rathbone MP. Postsurgical contrast enhancement mimicking residual brain tumour. Can J Neurol Sci 1985;12:75.

46. Dang CV, Semenza GL. Oncogenic alterations of metabolism. Trends Biochem Sci 1999;24:68–72.

47. Warburg O. On the origin of cancer cells. Science 1956;123:309–14.

Pseudoprogression and Treatment Effect

Arman Jahangiri, BS, Manish K. Aghi, MD, PhD*

KEYWORDS

- Glioblastoma • Recurrence • Angiogenesis • Imaging
- Progression

The median survival from the time patients are diagnosed with glioblastoma, the most common malignant primary tumor, was improved to 15 months with the introduction of the Stupp protocol in 2005 and has been improved to 23 months[1] in small retrospective series with the aggressive use of more advanced therapeutic modalities at the time of recurrence, like antiangiogenic therapy with vascular endothelial growth factor (VEGF) neutralizing antibody bevacizumab.[2]

The Stupp protocol was established in a phase II, randomized clinical trial by Stupp and colleagues[3] and involves administering a total of 60 Gy of radiation during 30 sessions spanning a 6-week period while treating simultaneously with 75 mg/m^2 of temozolomide on a daily basis. Adjuvant temozolomide chemotherapy is then administered in six 28-day cycles with a dose of 150 mg/m^2 for the initial cycle followed by 200 mg/m^2 for the remaining 5 cycles. Despite the improved survival rate established by the Stupp protocol, most patients continue to experience tumor recurrence, which necessitates close follow-up with magnetic resonance imaging (MRI).[3,4] Although many have reported that there is no difference in the percentage of recurrence in distal locations[5–7] after the Stupp protocol treatment, others have suggested an increased proportion of distal recurrence in patients being treated with temozolomide as compared with radiotherapy alone.[4]

Antiangiogenic therapy became a mainstay in the treatment of recurrent glioblastoma since a pair of phase II clinical trials showed efficacy of bevacizumab and irinotecan in treating recurrent glioblastoma,[8,9] leading to the 2009 accelerated Food and Drug Administration approval of bevacizumab for recurrent glioblastoma, with a pair of large, randomized, phase III clinical trials underway evaluating the efficacy of bevacizumab in treating newly diagnosed glioblastoma.

Clinicians have long noted common transient impacts of radiation on MRI contrast enhancement. When occurring in the first 3 months after radiation, this effect imitates early tumor progression and has earned the term pseudoprogression. Another effect witnessed after therapy is lesion enhancement in patients undergoing cranial radiation, which takes place in 3% to 24% of patients 3 to 12 months after treatment and is referred to as radiation necrosis.[10–12] Additionally, the identification of nonenhancing fluid-attenuated inversion recovery (FLAIR) bright infiltrative growth representing glioblastoma recurrence after antiangiogenic therapy has cofounded the ability of clinicians to recognize glioblastoma recurrence using conventional MRI and the Macdonald criteria,[13] which are based on gadolinium enhancement. The goal of this article is to review the most recent advancements made in radiology and cancer biology that can be used to improve the ability of physicians to distinguish true recurrence from pseudoprogression or radiation-induced necrosis in patients with glioblastoma receiving radiation, temozolomide, or antiangiogenic therapy.

PSEUDOPROGRESSION: EARLY TRANSIENT ENHANCING LESIONS

Pseudoprogression is defined as enhancing changes seen on MRI within the first 3 months after treatment of glioblastoma with fractionated

Department of Neurological Surgery, University of California at San Francisco (UCSF), 505 Parnassus Avenue, Room M779, San Francisco, CA, USA
* Corresponding author.
E-mail address: aghim@neurosurg.ucsf.edu

Neurosurg Clin N Am 23 (2012) 277–287
doi:10.1016/j.nec.2012.01.002
1042-3680/12/$ – see front matter © 2012 Published by Elsevier Inc.

radiotherapy. Pseudoprogression represents treatment effects rather than treatment failure, which, with time, either successively recovers or stabilizes without being linked to subordinate outcomes.[14] Since postoperative radiotherapy and concomitant temozolomide were established as the standard treatment of glioblastoma, there has been an increase in pseudoprogression from 10% in patients with glioblastoma treated with radiotherapy alone up to nearly 30% in patients treated with radiotherapy and concomitant chemotherapy.[3,12,14–16]

Pseudoprogression is a transient process that results from increased permeability and leakage of gadolinium through both the dysfunctional blood-brain barrier in the irradiated region as well as the capillary bed of the tumor.[17] Pseudoprogression reflects response to treatment rather than treatment failure and with time it improves or stabilizes and has not shown to have any correlation with poorer outcomes[18] and in some studies has been shown to be associated with improved outcomes.[19] Based on postoperative MRI studies, pseudoprogression occurs within the first 2 months following treatment as opposed to radiation necrosis, which can take an average of 3 to 12 months before it is witnessed on imaging.[12,20] The increase in incidence of pseudoprogression since the advent of simultaneous administration of chemotherapy and radiotherapy has been suggested to be a marker for improved response to treatment, a hypothesis supported by a study in which patients with glioblastoma with pseudoprogression had greater overall survival than those without pseudoprogression.[19]

Three factors have been proposed in the literature to increase the incidence of pseudoprogression in patients with glioblastoma: methylated O6—methyl guanine-DNA methyl transferase (MGMT) status, higher doses of radiation, and concomitant administration of chemotherapy and radiation.[16]

Temozolomide is an alkylating cytostatic prodrug that undergoes rapid conversion and is hydrolyzed to its active metabolite, 3-methyl-(triazen-1-yl)imidazole-4-carboximide (MTIC). MTIC functions to methylate DNA at several positions, the most important of which is the O6 position of guanine, which leads to cell death.[21] MGMT is an enzyme that removes this methylation to prevent the lethal DNA damage the cell would otherwise sustain. Cells that have epigenetic silencing of the MGMT gene, achieved through promoter methylation, are unable to produce the enzyme and are, therefore, more sensitive and responsive to the temozolomide-induced cell death.[22,23] One study was able to demonstrate that 66% of their patients with pseudoprogression had methylated MGMT promoters, whereas 89% of patients who

had true progression while on temozolomide showed unmethylated MGMT promoters. This study was able to establish pseudoprogression to be more common with a ratio of 2:1 in patients whose tumors exhibited methylated MGMT promoters, whereas disease progression is more likely with a ratio of 3:1 in patients whose tumors exhibited unmethylated MGMT promoters.[19]

Since MGMT promoter methylation status has been proven to serve as a marker for pseudoprogression, there has been a wide search for a highly sensitive and specific screening assay. Currently, methylation-specific polymerase chain reaction (MSP) is the standard method used to test for MGMT promoter methylation status. The biggest drawback for this method is its inability to provide quantitative results, which leads to some inaccuracy predicting prognosis, and the likelihood of pseudoporgression.[24] Methylation-specific multiplex ligation probe amplification (MS-MLPA) has been recently introduced as a semiquantitative method for testing methylation status of multiples genes in a simultaneous fashion while also proving to be a consistent method for determining the methylation status of MGMT promoter in tumor tissue.[25,26] One recent study found that the combination of MSP and MS-MLPA can further augment the diagnostic accuracy of pseudoprogression to 93%, which could have a significant impact on clinical decisions.[24]

RADIATION NECROSIS: DELAYED ENHANCING LESIONS

Since the randomized clinical trials in the 1970s demonstrating an improvement in overall survival, postoperative whole-brain radiotherapy at a daily dose of 2 Gy per fraction given over a 6-week period for a total dose of 60 Gy has become part of the standard treatment of glioblastoma.[3,27] Patients treated with radiation therapy in this manner often exhibit enhancement in radiation within 3 to 12 months of completing radiation. This phenomenon is called radiation necrosis and is now a common manifestation of radiotherapy seen in 3% to 24% of cases,[10–12] with an even higher incidence noted in patients receiving temozolomide treatment concurrent to radiotherapy.[12,14] The enhancement seen on conventional MRI may be secondary to the radiation-induced damage of the blood-brain barrier, which causes gadolinium leakage into the interstitium and produces a ring-enhancing lesion that can be easily misread as tumor recurrence.[28,29]

Radiation necrosis can be witnessed as early as 3 months and its presence has been reported as late as 5 years after the original treatment, although most cases typically occur within the first 2 years after radiation.[30] One study reports the incidence of radiation necrosis in patients with glioblastoma treated at 60 Gy with conventional fractionated external beam radiotherapy to be just at 1%,[31] but as mentioned previously, there has been an increase in its incidence since the introduction of adjuvant chemotherapeutic agents, such as temozolomide.[12,14] Radiation-induced necrosis most commonly occurs at the location that has received the maximum dose of radiation, which usually falls in the purlieu of the tumor site and close to the margins of the surgical cavity of the resected tumor.[14,32] The periventricular white matter is known to be a common location for the occurrence of radionecrosis and is highly vulnerable to ischemic effects of postradiation vasculopathy, a phenomenon which may be explained by the poor blood supply this location receives from long medullary arteries lacking collateral vessels.[10,14,32]

The clinical presentation of radiation necrosis often mimics that of tumor recurrence. Patients can present with a broad set of symptoms, such as headache, seizures, behavioral changes, focal neurologic deficits, wheras some may be asymptomatic.[14,33] It is imperative to distinguish between the recurrence and radiation necrosis because the approach to treatment is fairly specific to each and can lead to unnecessary morbidity and even mortality if the incorrect treatment modality is pursued. A common finding using conventional MRI of radiation necrosis may be a mass of enhancing lesions seen on T1-weighted imaging with gadolinium contrast administration, but there is no imaging correlation that can differentiate radiation necrosis from true progression or pseudoprogression, especially on the initial post-radiotherapy temozolomide scan.[17] The main shortcoming of conventional MRI, which limits its ability to distinguish viable tumor mass from radiation necrosis, is that it only recognizes disruptions made to the blood-brain barrier and edema.[33–36] In a previous study looking for specific markers of radiation necrosis on conventional MRI, individual signs were not found to be valuable markers of tumor recurrence, whereas the combination of 2 signs in addition to the involvement of the corpus callosum and numerous enhancing lesions was a statistically significant marker for recurrence.[37] A more recent study that used a larger sample size was able to recognize subependymal enhancement as an individual marker for the early progression of tumor on conventional MRI. Even though this marker was statistically significant, the investigators from the study recognize that radiation necrosis at higher doses may lead to radiographic

findings that can mimic subependymal enhancement, hence, its less than perfect ability to serve as a definitive marker for recurrence.[18]

Several clinical factors have been associated with an increase in the risk of radiation necrosis in patients with glioma, which include the following: older age, high fraction doses (<2.5 Gy/d), hyperfractionation, lower conformity index, shorter overall treatment time, stereotactic radiosurgery, interstitial brachytherapy, reirradiation, and radiation combined with adjuvant chemotherapy.[10,16,38–44] Radiation necrosis is directly related to the volume of irradiated brain in addition to the dose of radiation that is delivered, with a precipitous increase with doses exceeding 65 Gy in fractions of 1.8 to 2.0 Gy.[14,38,39,45] One study found the administration of chemotherapy alongside radiation increases the risk of cerebral necrosis fourfold.[39] Furthermore, the brain parenchyma surrounding a glioma has been shown to be particularly sensitive to chemotherapy and radiation. Such risks must be taken into account when making a distinction between treatment effects versus tumor recurrence.

Tumor cells have been shown to be interspersed in many histologic specimens of radiated necrotic tissue, with one study showing that 55% of pathologically examined cases of radiation necrosis demonstrated viable tumor coexistence within areas of necrosis.[39] To determine whether chemotherapy should be continued or switched, the percentage of viable tumor cells versus necrotic tissue in the specimen is taken into account, with the threshold for switching chemotherapy being met typically if the specimen contains greater than 50% viable tumor cells.[16]

Pathophysiology of Radiation Necrosis

The histopathologic features observed in radiation necrosis are demonstrated in **Fig. 1**. Vascular endothelial cells and oligodendrocytes have been shown to serve as the direct targets of radiation in the central nervous system.[46] These 2 targets are directly injured and independently lead to necrosis (see **Fig. 1**A) and demyelination both within the normal tissue and the tumor. The development of acute and subacute radiation injury is secondary to the clonogenic death of endothelial cells, and vascular lesions also play a key role in late radiation injury.[47] The direct consequence of endothelial cell death from radiation is thought to induce the breakdown of the blood-brain barrier leading to ischemia, vasogenic edema, and hypoxia.[15] The hypoxic tissue then upregulates VEGF, which plays a major role in increasing vascular permeability and is shortly followed by tissue necrosis and demyelination (see **Fig. 1**B).

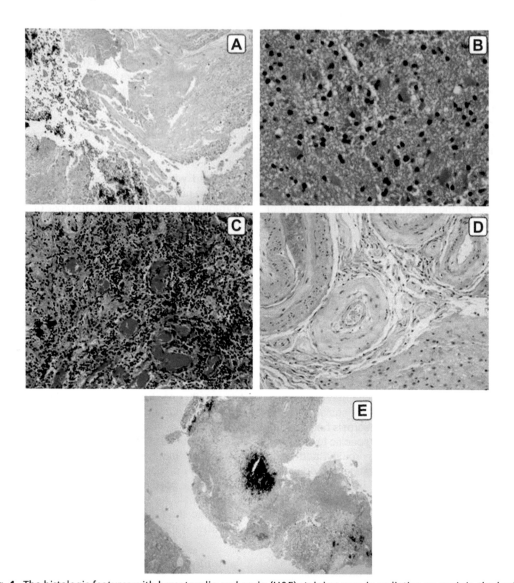

Fig. 1. The histologic features with hematoxylin and eosin (H&E) staining seen in radiation necrosis in the brain. (*A*) Necrosis is a defining feature and on occasion has dystrophic calcifications, shown here in blue. (*B*) Gliosis is also a defining feature. (*C*) Inflammation is typically seen. (*D*) Vascular hyalinization is seen from time to time. (*E*) Dystrophic calcification, shown here in blue, is occasionally present. (original magnification ×20). (*Courtesy of* T. Tihan, University of California at San Francisco, Department of Neuropathology.)

Unfortunately, radiotherapy has also been shown to stimulate glioma cells to secrete an increased amount of VEGF, causing a decrease in apoptosis in both endothelial cells and tumor cells while increasing angiogenesis in the tumor environment (see **Fig. 1**C), which is a mechanism that may account for the radiation-resistance that develops in gliomas.[48] The increase in VEGF production can be counteracted by the addition of bevacizumab, an antibody to VEGF that is now used frequently in cases of glioblastoma recurrence. Therefore, bevacizumab can function to decrease enhancement and edema while substantially improving the radiographic appearance of radiation necrosis, which mimics tumor progression.[18,49]

The mechanism by which radiation induces endothelial cell apoptosis is largely caused by damage to the cell membrane, although DNA damage still plays a role. The incited damage to the cellular membrane activates acid sphingomyelinase, which is an enzyme involved in sphingolipid metabolism and produces ceramide, a bioactive lipid well known for its physiologic role in apoptosis.[50,51] Radiation-induced DNA damage activates ceramide synthase, which serves as an additional source of ceramide, which causes additional endothelial cell apoptosis through the P53-dependent stimulation of the mitochondrial and death-receptor pathways.[52]

The current understanding of the pathophysiology of radiation-induced necrosis may be further used for treatment and molecular prevention of the radiologic and clinical effects of radiation necrosis. In one study, protein kinase C (PKC) was shown to prevent radiation damage because the downregulation of acid sphingomyelinase is a PKC-dependent mechanism, whereas PKC also functions to inhibit ceramide-dependent apoptosis.[53,54] In a study conducted by Fuks and colleagues, basic fibroblast growth factor was used to stimulate PKC activity, allowing for the inhibition of radiation-induced endothelial cells in both in vivo and in vitro experiments.

ANTIANGIOGENIC THERAPY FOR GLIOBLASTOMA: RADIOLOGIC AND NONRADIOLOGIC BIOMARKERS OF EFFICACY

Bevacizumab, a monoclonal anti-VEGF antibody, has been studied in phase II trials of patients with recurrent glioblastoma and demonstrated a 23-week medial progression-free survival when administered in combination with irinotecan.[8,9] A study of patients with glioblastoma treated with bevacizumab revealed decreased tumor hypoxia and increased tumoral VEGF expression, which were directly associated with radiographic response and prolonged survival following treatment.[55]

VEGF levels have been evaluated in the plasma and tumor fluid samples from patients with glioblastoma, which showed a relative elevation, whereas levels within the tumor cavity were elevated even higher in patients experiencing recurrence of the disease as compared with those with stable disease after resection.[56,57] Furthermore, a direct correlation has been established

between VEGF overexpression and poor prognosis based on glioblastoma tumor histology.[58] Antiangiogenic therapy has been proposed to normalize the vasculature within the tumor, allowing for thinning of the superfluous perivascular and endothelial cells and lessening the tortuosity of blood vessels while reducing the interstitial pressure. This decrease in pressure is suggested to enhance the transport of chemotherapy to the tumor cells while improving oxygenation.[59] Using bevacizumab as the agent for VEGF blockade, another study demonstrated a reduction of the microvascular density while improving the function of intratumoral vessels, which enables the penetration of chemotherapy.[60]

Unfortunately, anti-VEGF treatment in animal models has shown to increase the infiltrative growth capability of the tumor,[61] which allows for bright recurrent lesions on FLAIR MRI sequencing but is nonenhancing because of their decreased vascular permeability.[62–64]

Impact of Antiangiogenic Therapy on Imaging

Typically, the abnormal vasculature along with the highly permeable blood-brain barrier of glioblastoma permits leakage of contrast material from the tumor capillaries, which leads to an amplified enhancement of T1-weighted imaging (**Fig. 2**).[65] Antiangiogenic agents, such as bevacizumab, decrease the leak of contrast agent into the interstitium, which markedly decreases contrast enhancement. Therefore, a decrease in contrast enhancement of the tumor does not reflect a true cytostatic or cytotoxic tumor, and the dependence on contrast enhancement alone can cause an overestimation of the response to treatment, which has earned the term pseudoresponse,[66–68] representing in effect the converse of the pseudoprogression described earlier. The occurrence of radiation necrosis further takes away from

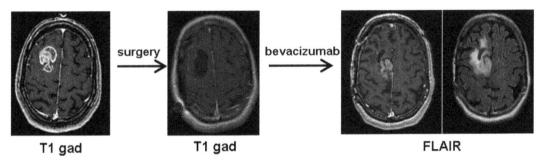

T1 gad   T1 gad   FLAIR

Fig. 2. Radiographic changes associated with bevacizumab treatment following surgical resection. Following complete resection of an enhancing right frontal glioblastoma in this 63-year-old woman, treatment with bevacizumab and irinotecan for 6 months led to increased FLAIR-bright nonenhancing infiltrative signal abnormality close to the location of the original tumor, with resection of the FLAIR-bright nonenhancing tissue seen at the right above, revealing infiltrating recurrent glioblastoma.

determining the true response of glioblastoma to antiangiogenic therapy because it is speculated that at least part of the radiologic response witnessed following bevacizumab therapy is caused by the palliation of radiation necrosis as opposed to a true tumor response.[69] These barriers have necessitated new imaging modalities that can better assess tumor response in patients receiving antiangiogenic therapy. To make this task a reality, such techniques will need the ability to distinguish true tumor progression from pseudoprogression while unraveling nonenhancing tumor from gliosis. Some of these novel techniques will be introduced and discussed later.

RESPONSE ASSESSMENT IN NEURO-ONCOLOGY CRITERIA FOR HIGH-GRADE GLIOMAS

Until recently, the MacDonald Criteria,[13] first published in 1990, served as the standard for determining response assessment in high-grade gliomas. It provided an objective radiologic assessment of the tumor response based primarily on 2-dimensional enhancing tumor area deriving from contrast-enhanced computed tomography.[70] The use of corticosteroids and fluctuations in patients' neurologic status were also taken into consideration. The Macdonald criteria were also further applied to MRI, which is now the standard modality used for assessing treatment response in glioblastoma. These criteria had several limitations, some of which include the difficult task of measuring unevenly shaped tumors, the lack of evaluating the nonenhancing tumor parts, and interobserver variability, among many others.

The response assessment in neuro-oncology criteria[71] were established in 2010 by an international working group in recognition of the intrinsic drawbacks of conventional criteria for enhancing tumors. These drawbacks include radiochemotherapy-induced pseudoprogression, nonenhancing tumor following antiangiogenic treatment, and the absence of steroid factoring into the response.[71,72] The criteria for response assessment incorporating MRI and clinical factors were divided into categories: complete response, partial response, stable disease, and progression.[71]

To be placed into the complete response category all of the following conditions must be met: disappearance of all enhancing and nonmeasurable disease for no less than 4 weeks, absence of new lesions, stable or improved nonenhancing lesions on T2/FLAIR, steroid therapy must be stopped or maintained at physiologic replacement doses, and patients must be stable or improved clinically.[71]

The partial response category requires a 50% or greater decrease of enhancing tumor in diameter as compared with baseline for no less than 4 weeks, absence of new lesions, stable or improved nonenhancing lesions on T2/FLAIR with the cessation of steroid therapy, or maintenance at physiologic replacement doses.[71]

If patients do not meet the criteria for complete response, partial response, or progression but have stable or improved nonenhancing lesions on T2/FLAIR with the cessation of steroid therapy or maintenance at physiologic replacement doses, they fall in the stable disease category.[71]

Lastly, patients who meet any of the following are considered to be in the progression category: an increase of 25% or greater in the sum of diameters of enhancing lesions at replacement physiologic steroid doses or less, a substantial increase in T2/FLAIR nonenhancing lesions, presence of any new lesions, or any neurologic deterioration.

DISTINGUISHING TREATMENT EFFECT OR PSEUDOPROGRESSION FROM TRUE PROGRESSION

Conventional MRI with gadolinium contrast enhancement fails to differentiate between true tumor recurrence, pseudoprogression, or radiation necrosis.[14,29,37,73] This form of imaging is also unable to distinguish true treatment response from the anti-VEGF treatment's impact at palliating radiation necrosis, a distinction that is important because anti-VEGF is used more commonly with drugs, such as bevacizumab.[69] Although new studies have suggested findings on conventional MRI, such as subependymal enhancement to distinguish early tumor progression from pseudoprogression with a high specificity, its low sensitivity along with a low negative predictive value demonstrate limited usage in most patients suspected of pseudoprogression.[18]

Several clinical concerns have increased the demand for novel imaging techniques to distinguish recurrence from radiation necrosis or pseudoprogression. Unfortunately, the morbidity associated with surgical resection of radiation necrosis, otherwise indistinguishable from tumor recurrence is quite high,[74] as is the administration of ineffective treatment for these enhancing pseudoprogression lesions which otherwise would resolve over time. Novel radiographic modalities, such as diffusion-weighted imaging (DWI) sequencing on MRI, positron emission tomography (PET), and magnetic resonance spectroscopy (MRS), have demonstrated encouraging results for differentiating treatment effects from tumor recurrence, although large prospective trials are needed to prove their sensitivity and specificity.

Radiographic Modalities

DWI MRI sequences detect the displacement of water molecules and can report the quantitative values in the form of apparent diffusion coefficient (ADC). The extent of restriction to water diffusion in brain tissue is inversely related to the integrity of cell membranes and cellularity of tissue.[75–77] Highly cellular areas with restricted diffusion will display low ADC value as compared with areas with less cellularity that will have high ADC levels.[78] DWI has been used to help determine if enhancing lesions in treated glioblastoma represent true progression, with the hypothesis being that recurrent tumor would have a lower ADC values (caused by increased cellularity), which has now been confirmed by several studies.[79–82] In a retrospective study by Hein and colleagues,[79] DWI MRI obtained 1 month after radiation therapy with or without chemotherapy were reviewed, and 18 patients having areas with atypical enhancement were selected. ADC values and ratios were averaged for patients with recurrent disease compared with those with treatment effect. The mean ADC ratio in those with recurrence was calculated at 1.43, which was significantly lower than the 1.82 in those without recurrence ($P<.001$). The mean of the ADC values was also significantly lower in patients with tumor recurrence, calculated at 1.18×10^{-3} mm/s^2 versus 1.40×10^{-3} mm/s^2 in the nonrecurrent group ($P<.006$).[79] Larger studies will need to be conducted to determine the sensitivity and specificity of DWI MRI for distinguishing recurrent glioblastoma from treatment effect.

Diffusion tensor imaging (DTI) is a more complete and intricate version of DWI. DTI applies diffusion-sensitization gradients in multiple directions determining the directionality of water diffusion. This information is reported within a parameter called fractional anisotropy (FA), which can detect peritumoral swelling, radiation necrosis, and infiltrating tumor cells.[83] In a recent study of 35 patients with new contrast-enhancing lesions located in areas of postoperative radiated tumor, DWI and DTI were used to examine whether a distinction between true recurrence as opposed to radiation necrosis could be made. Patients with a recurrent tumor were found to have considerably higher FA ratios with a mean of 0.45 compared with those with radiation necrosis with a value of just 0.32 ($P<.01$).[84] Based on this study, the sensitivity and specificity were calculated at 85.0% and 86.7%, respectively. This finding shows that DTI could have a promising role in differentiating postoperative radiation injury from recurrent disease, and larger studies should be conducted to validate its value and potential.

Proton MRS (^{1}H-MRS) provides information on the metabolic composition of brain tissue and can play a major role in distinguishing recurrence from radiation necrosis. Choline and choline-containing compounds (Cho) are shown to be detected at higher levels and represent radiation necrosis (**Fig. 3**).[85] In a study of 33 patients with postoperative enhancing lesions, patients with recurrent tumor had an elevation in Cho to creatine and Cho/N-acetylaspartate (NAA) ratios compared with those with radiation necrosis. The Cho/NAA had a specificity of 69% and a sensitivity of 85% in detecting true recurrence.[86] Other studies have shown that MRS can be as useful as pathologic testing in distinguishing tumor recurrence from radiation necrosis with 100.0% specificity, 94.0% sensitivity, and a 96.1% diagnostic accuracy.[12,87,88] With such promising results, further studies are needed in which pathologic samples are compared with the results of ^{1}H-MRS to compare the efficacy of each method.

Dynamic susceptibility contrast-enhanced perfusion imaging (DSC) can determine relative cerebral blood volume (rCBV), which may be useful

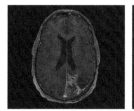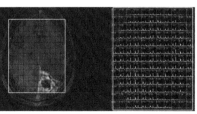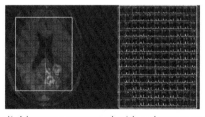

Fig. 3. Pseudoprogression on MRS imaging. A 48-year-old man with glioblastoma presented with enhancement consistent with possible recurrence, MRS showed evidence of elevated choline and depressed NAA in the area of FLAIR signal hyperintensity within the left frontal and parietal lobes thought to be consistent with recurrence; however, en bloc resection of enhancing tissue for pathologist revealed no signs of recurrent tumor. NAA, N-acetylaspartate.

because it is a reflection of the underlying angiogenesis and the microvasculature.[89,90] DSC has recently been used with reports of decreased rCBV in radiation necrosis as opposed to increased values in tumor recurrence.[89,91] A recent study of 13 patients with postoperative contrast-enhancing lesions found that those with tumor recurrence had higher rCBV compared with those with radiation necrosis.[92] These findings were correlated to the patients' histopathologic findings with 100.0% specificity and 91.7% sensitivity. One other study used ferumoxytol as the contrast agent as opposed to gadolinium, and found there to be an increase in the accuracy noted for the differentiation of pseudoprogression from true progression.[93]

PET scanning is a form of functional imaging capable of localization of anatomic regions based on the distribution of certain biochemical or metabolic products, which has shown promising results in distinguishing treatment effects from tumor recurrence.[16,94] Although initial results of fluorine-18 fluorodeoxyglucose (^{18}F-FDG) PET were encouraging, with almost 100% accuracy reported in various studies,[95,96] more recent studies have found the sensitivity and specificity for ^{18}F-FDG to be much lower, 86% and 22%, respectively.[97] A recent study used thymidine analogue 3′-deoxy-3′-18F-fluorothymidine ([18]FLT), which has longer-lived label with increased specificity for thymidine kinase 1 within the cytosol and several labeled metabolites.[98] When compared with ^{18}F-FDG, [18]FLT was shown to be much more sensitive in imaging recurrent tumors and better at predicting tumor progression and survival.[99] Further studies are demanded to establish the characteristics of this new radiotracer.

SUMMARY

The postoperative administration of adjuvant temozolomide and radiation is the new standard of care in patients with newly diagnosed glioblastoma. Pseudoprogression and radiation necrosis are common treatment effects that add much confusion in the detection of tumor recurrence using conventional MRI with gadolinium enhancement. These challenges are confounded with the recent increasing use of antiangiogenic therapy to treat newly diagnosed and recurrent glioblastoma. Until randomized trials prove the efficacy of existing advanced imaging modalities or until newer, more effective modalities are developed, advanced radiographic techniques, such as DWI, PET, MRS, and DSC, can be used in conjunction with the clinical judgment of the neurosurgeon, neuro-oncologist, and radiation oncologist

working together to make an informed estimation of the chances that an imaging finding represents true progression. Such decision making must balance the morbidity of delayed diagnosis of tumor progression with the morbidity caused by unnecessary surgical intervention or changes in chemotherapy for lack of progression.

REFERENCES

1. Clark AJ, Lamborn KR, Butowski NA, et al. Neurosurgical management and prognosis of patients with glioblastoma that progress during bevacizumab treatment. Neurosurgery 2011;70(2):361–70.
2. Stupp R, Hegi ME, Mason WP, et al. Effects of radiotherapy with concomitant and adjuvant temozolomide versus radiotherapy alone on survival in glioblastoma in a randomised phase III study: 5-year analysis of the EORTC-NCIC trial. Lancet Oncol 2009;10:459–66.
3. Stupp R, Mason WP, van den Bent MJ, et al. Radiotherapy plus concomitant and adjuvant temozolomide for glioblastoma. N Engl J Med 2005;352: 987–96.
4. Brandes AA, Tosoni A, Franceschi E, et al. Recurrence pattern after temozolomide concomitant with and adjuvant to radiotherapy in newly diagnosed patients with glioblastoma: correlation with MGMT promoter methylation status. J Clin Oncol 2009;27: 1275–9.
5. Wick W, Stupp R, Beule AC, et al. A novel tool to analyze MRI recurrence patterns in glioblastoma. Neuro Oncol 2008;10:1019–24.
6. Milano MT, Okunieff P, Donatello RS, et al. Patterns and timing of recurrence after temozolomide-based chemoradiation for glioblastoma. Int J Radiat Oncol Biol Phys 2010;78:1147–55.
7. Oh J, Sahgal A, Sanghera P, et al. Glioblastoma: patterns of recurrence and efficacy of salvage treatments. Can J Neurol Sci 2011;38:621–5.
8. Vredenburgh JJ, Desjardins A, Herndon JE 2nd, et al. Phase II trial of bevacizumab and irinotecan in recurrent malignant glioma. Clin Cancer Res 2007;13:1253–9.
9. Vredenburgh JJ, Desjardins A, Herndon JE 2nd, et al. Bevacizumab plus irinotecan in recurrent glioblastoma multiforme. J Clin Oncol 2007;25:4722–9.
10. Kumar AJ, Leeds NE, Fuller GN, et al. Malignant gliomas: MR imaging spectrum of radiation therapy- and chemotherapy-induced necrosis of the brain after treatment. Radiology 2000;217:377–84.
11. Giglio P, Gilbert MR. Cerebral radiation necrosis. Neurologist 2003;9:180–8.
12. Yaman E, Buyukberber S, Benekli M, et al. Radiation induced early necrosis in patients with malignant gliomas receiving temozolomide. Clin Neurol Neurosurg 2010;112:662–7.

13. Macdonald DR, Cascino TL, Schold SC Jr, et al. Response criteria for phase II studies of supratentorial malignant glioma. J Clin Oncol 1990;8:1277–80.

14. Brandsma D, Stalpers L, Taal W, et al. Clinical features, mechanisms, and management of pseudoprogression in malignant gliomas. Lancet Oncol 2008;9:453–61.

15. Wong CS, Van der Kogel AJ. Mechanisms of radiation injury to the central nervous system: implications for neuroprotection. Mol Interv 2004;4:273–84.

16. Yang I, Aghi MK. New advances that enable identification of glioblastoma recurrence. Nat Rev Clin Oncol 2009;6:648–57.

17. Sanghera P, Rampling R, Haylock B, et al. The concepts, diagnosis and management of early imaging changes after therapy for glioblastomas. Clin Oncol (R Coll Radiol) 2011. [Epub ahead of print].

18. Young RJ, Gupta A, Shah AD, et al. Potential utility of conventional MRI signs in diagnosing pseudoprogression in glioblastoma. Neurology 2011;76:1918–24.

19. Brandes AA, Franceschi E, Tosoni A, et al. MGMT promoter methylation status can predict the incidence and outcome of pseudoprogression after concomitant radiochemotherapy in newly diagnosed glioblastoma patients. J Clin Oncol 2008;26:2192–7.

20. Taal W, Brandsma D, de Bruin HG, et al. Incidence of early pseudo-progression in a cohort of malignant glioma patients treated with chemoirradiation with temozolomide. Cancer 2008;113:405–10.

21. Danson SJ, Middleton MR. Temozolomide: a novel oral alkylating agent. Expert Rev Anticancer Ther 2001;1:13–9.

22. Hegi ME, Diserens AC, Gorlia T, et al. MGMT gene silencing and benefit from temozolomide in glioblastoma. N Engl J Med 2005;352:997–1003.

23. Chakravarti A, Erkkinen MG, Nestler U, et al. Temozolomide-mediated radiation enhancement in glioblastoma: a report on underlying mechanisms. Clin Cancer Res 2006;12:4738–46.

24. Park CK, Kim J, Yim SY, et al. Usefulness of MS-MLPA for detection of MGMT promoter methylation in the evaluation of pseudoprogression in glioblastoma patients. Neuro Oncol 2011;13:195–202.

25. Jeuken JW, Cornelissen SJ, Vriezen M, et al. MS-MLPA: an attractive alternative laboratory assay for robust, reliable, and semiquantitative detection of MGMT promoter hypermethylation in gliomas. Lab Invest 2007;87:1055–65.

26. Nygren AO, Ameziane N, Duarte HM, et al. Methylation-specific MLPA (MS-MLPA): simultaneous detection of CpG methylation and copy number changes of up to 40 sequences. Nucleic Acids Res 2005;33: e128.

27. Walker MD, Alexander E Jr, Hunt WE, et al. Evaluation of BCNU and/or radiotherapy in the treatment of anaplastic gliomas. A cooperative clinical trial. J Neurosurg 1978;49:333–43.

28. Covarrubias DJ, Rosen BR, Lev MH. Dynamic magnetic resonance perfusion imaging of brain tumors. Oncologist 2004;9:528–37.

29. Bisdas S, Naegele T, Ritz R, et al. Distinguishing recurrent high-grade gliomas from radiation injury: a pilot study using dynamic contrast-enhanced MR imaging. Acad Radiol 2011;18:575–83.

30. Marks JE, Wong J. The risk of cerebral radionecrosis in relation to dose, time and fractionation. A follow-up study. Prog Exp Tumor Res 1985;29:210–8.

31. DeAngelis LM. Brain tumors. N Engl J Med 2001; 344:114–23.

32. Moody DM, Bell MA, Challa VR. Features of the cerebral vascular pattern that predict vulnerability to perfusion or oxygenation deficiency: an anatomic study. AJNR Am J Neuroradiol 1990;11:431–9.

33. Alexiou GA, Tsiouris S, Kyritsis AP, et al. Glioma recurrence versus radiation necrosis: accuracy of current imaging modalities. J Neurooncol 2009;95: 1–11.

34. Carvalho PA, Schwartz RB, Alexander E 3rd, et al. Detection of recurrent gliomas with quantitative thallium-201/technetium-99m HMPAO single-photon emission computerized tomography. J Neurosurg 1992;77:565–70.

35. Byrne TN. Imaging of gliomas. Semin Oncol 1994; 21:162–71.

36. Leeds NE, Jackson EF. Current imaging techniques for the evaluation of brain neoplasms. Curr Opin Oncol 1994;6:254–61.

37. Mullins ME, Barest GD, Schaefer PW, et al. Radiation necrosis versus glioma recurrence: conventional MR imaging clues to diagnosis. AJNR Am J Neuroradiol 2005;26:1967–72.

38. Marks JE, Baglan RJ, Prassad SC, et al. Cerebral radionecrosis: incidence and risk in relation to dose, time, fractionation and volume. Int J Radiat Oncol Biol Phys 1981;7:243–52.

39. Ruben JD, Dally M, Bailey M, et al. Cerebral radiation necrosis: incidence, outcomes, and risk factors with emphasis on radiation parameters and chemotherapy. Int J Radiat Oncol Biol Phys 2006;65:499–508.

40. Chamberlain MC, Glantz MJ, Chalmers L, et al. Early necrosis following concurrent Temodar and radiotherapy in patients with glioblastoma. J Neurooncol 2007;82:81–3.

41. Nieder C, Andratschke N, Wiedenmann N, et al. Radiotherapy for high-grade gliomas. Does altered fractionation improve the outcome? Strahlenther Onkol 2004;180:401–7.

42. Kong DS, Lee JI, Park K, et al. Efficacy of stereotactic radiosurgery as a salvage treatment for recurrent malignant gliomas. Cancer 2008;112:2046–51.

43. Perry A, Schmidt RE. Cancer therapy-associated CNS neuropathology: an update and review of the literature. Acta Neuropathol 2006;111:197–212.

44. Lawrence YR, Li XA, el Naqa I, et al. Radiation dose-volume effects in the brain. Int J Radiat Oncol Biol Phys 2010;76:S20–7.

45. Sheline GE, Wara WM, Smith V. Therapeutic irradiation and brain injury. Int J Radiat Oncol Biol Phys 1980;6:1215–28.

46. Tofilon PJ, Fike JR. The radioresponse of the central nervous system: a dynamic process. Radiat Res 2000;153:357–70.

47. Fajardo LF. Is the pathology of radiation injury different in small vs large blood vessels? Cardiovasc Radiat Med 1999;1:108–10.

48. Gupta VK, Jaskowiak NT, Beckett MA, et al. Vascular endothelial growth factor enhances endothelial cell survival and tumor radioresistance. Cancer J 2002; 8:47–54.

49. Kim JH, Chung YG, Kim CY, et al. Upregulation of VEGF and FGF2 in normal rat brain after experimental intraoperative radiation therapy. J Korean Med Sci 2004;19:879–86.

50. Lin T, Genestier L, Pinkoski MJ, et al. Role of acidic sphingomyelinase in Fas/CD95-mediated cell death. J Biol Chem 2000;275:8657–63.

51. Rodemann HP, Blaese MA. Responses of normal cells to ionizing radiation. Semin Radiat Oncol 2007;17:81–8.

52. Miyashita T, Krajewski S, Krajewska M, et al. Tumor suppressor p53 is a regulator of bcl-2 and bax gene expression in vitro and in vivo. Oncogene 1994;9:1799–805.

53. Fuks Z, Persaud RS, Alfieri A, et al. Basic fibroblast growth factor protects endothelial cells against radiation-induced programmed cell death in vitro and in vivo. Cancer Res 1994;54: 2582–90.

54. Haimovitz-Friedman A, Balaban N, McLoughlin M, et al. Protein kinase C mediates basic fibroblast growth factor protection of endothelial cells against radiation-induced apoptosis. Cancer Res 1994;54: 2591–7.

55. Sathornsumetee S, Cao Y, Marcello JE, et al. Tumor angiogenic and hypoxic profiles predict radiographic response and survival in malignant astrocytoma patients treated with bevacizumab and irinotecan. J Clin Oncol 2008;26:271–8.

56. Salmaggi A, Eoli M, Frigerio S, et al. Intracavitary VEGF, bFGF, IL-8, IL-12 levels in primary and recurrent malignant glioma. J Neurooncol 2003;62: 297–303.

57. Takano S, Yoshii Y, Kondo S, et al. Concentration of vascular endothelial growth factor in the serum and tumor tissue of brain tumor patients. Cancer Res 1996;56:2185–90.

58. Nam DH, Park K, Suh YL, et al. Expression of VEGF and brain specific angiogenesis inhibitor-1 in glioblastoma: prognostic significance. Oncol Rep 2004;11:863–9.

59. Jain RK. Normalizing tumor vasculature with anti-angiogenic therapy: a new paradigm for combination therapy. Nat Med 2001;7:987–9.

60. Inai T, Mancuso M, Hashizume H, et al. Inhibition of vascular endothelial growth factor (VEGF) signaling in cancer causes loss of endothelial fenestrations, regression of tumor vessels, and appearance of basement membrane ghosts. Am J Pathol 2004;165:35–52.

61. Du R, Lu KV, Petritsch C, et al. HIF1alpha induces the recruitment of bone marrow-derived vascular modulatory cells to regulate tumor angiogenesis and invasion. Cancer Cell 2008;13:206–20.

62. Kunkel P, Ulbricht U, Bohlen P, et al. Inhibition of glioma angiogenesis and growth in vivo by systemic treatment with a monoclonal antibody against vascular endothelial growth factor receptor-2. Cancer Res 2001;61:6624–8.

63. Norden AD, Young GS, Setayesh K, et al. Bevacizumab for recurrent malignant gliomas: efficacy, toxicity, and patterns of recurrence. Neurology 2008;70:779–87.

64. Rubenstein JL, Kim J, Ozawa T, et al. Anti-VEGF antibody treatment of glioblastoma prolongs survival but results in increased vascular cooption. Neoplasia 2000;2:306–14.

65. Rees JH, Smirniotopoulos JG, Jones RV, et al. Glioblastoma multiforme: radiologic-pathologic correlation. Radiographics 1996;16:1413–38 [quiz: 1462–3].

66. Pope WB, Young JR, Ellingson BM. Advances in MRI assessment of gliomas and response to anti-VEGF therapy. Curr Neurol Neurosci Rep 2011;11:336–44.

67. Brandsma D, van den Bent MJ. Pseudoprogression and pseudoresponse in the treatment of gliomas. Curr Opin Neurol 2009;22:633–8.

68. Clarke JL, Chang S. Pseudoprogression and pseudoresponse: challenges in brain tumor imaging. Curr Neurol Neurosci Rep 2009;9:241–6.

69. Gonzalez J, Kumar AJ, Conrad CA, et al. Effect of bevacizumab on radiation necrosis of the brain. Int J Radiat Oncol Biol Phys 2007;67:323–6.

70. Miller AB, Hoogstraten B, Staquet M, et al. Reporting results of cancer treatment. Cancer 1981;47:207–14.

71. Wen PY, Macdonald DR, Reardon DA, et al. Updated response assessment criteria for high-grade gliomas: response assessment in neuro-oncology working group. J Clin Oncol 2010;28:1963–72.

72. Mehta AI, Kanaly CW, Friedman AH, et al. Monitoring radiographic brain tumor progression. Toxins (Basel) 2011;3:191–200.

73. Kim YH, Oh SW, Lim YJ, et al. Differentiating radiation necrosis from tumor recurrence in high-grade gliomas: assessing the efficacy of 18F-FDG PET, 11C-methionine PET and perfusion MRI. Clin Neurol Neurosurg 2010;112:758–65.

74. McPherson CM, Warnick RE. Results of contemporary surgical management of radiation necrosis using frameless stereotaxis and intraoperative

magnetic resonance imaging. J Neurooncol 2004; 68:41–7.

75. Gauvain KM, McKinstry RC, Mukherjee P, et al. Evaluating pediatric brain tumor cellularity with diffusion-tensor imaging. AJR Am J Roentgenol 2001;177: 449–54.

76. Guo Y, Cai YQ, Cai ZL, et al. Differentiation of clinically benign and malignant breast lesions using diffusion-weighted imaging. J Magn Reson Imaging 2002;16:172–8.

77. Sugahara T, Korogi Y, Kochi M, et al. Usefulness of diffusion-weighted MRI with echo-planar technique in the evaluation of cellularity in gliomas. J Magn Reson Imaging 1999;9:53–60.

78. Koh DM, Collins DJ. Diffusion-weighted MRI in the body: applications and challenges in oncology. AJR Am J Roentgenol 2007;188:1622–35.

79. Hein PA, Eskey CJ, Dunn JF, et al. Diffusion-weighted imaging in the follow-up of treated high-grade gliomas: tumor recurrence versus radiation injury. AJNR Am J Neuroradiol 2004;25:201–9.

80. Asao C, Korogi Y, Kitajima M, et al. Diffusion-weighted imaging of radiation-induced brain injury for differentiation from tumor recurrence. AJNR Am J Neuroradiol 2005;26:1455–60.

81. Sundgren PC, Fan X, Weybright P, et al. Differentiation of recurrent brain tumor versus radiation injury using diffusion tensor imaging in patients with new contrast-enhancing lesions. Magn Reson Imaging 2006;24:1131–42.

82. Verma R, Zacharaki EI, Ou Y, et al. Multiparametric tissue characterization of brain neoplasms and their recurrence using pattern classification of MR images. Acad Radiol 2008;15:966–77.

83. Gerstner ER, Sorensen AG. Diffusion and diffusion tensor imaging in brain cancer. Semin Radiat Oncol 2011;21:141–6.

84. Xu JL, Li YL, Lian JM, et al. Distinction between postoperative recurrent glioma and radiation injury using MR diffusion tensor imaging. Neuroradiology 2010; 52:1193–9.

85. Schlemmer HP, Bachert P, Herfarth KK, et al. Proton MR spectroscopic evaluation of suspicious brain lesions after stereotactic radiotherapy. AJNR Am J Neuroradiol 2001;22:1316–24.

86. Smith EA, Carlos RC, Junck LR, et al. Developing a clinical decision model: MR spectroscopy to differentiate between recurrent tumor and radiation change in patients with new contrast-enhancing lesions. AJR Am J Roentgenol 2009;192:W45–52.

87. Zeng QS, Li CF, Liu H, et al. Distinction between recurrent glioma and radiation injury using magnetic resonance spectroscopy in combination with diffusion-weighted imaging. Int J Radiat Oncol Biol Phys 2007;68:151–8.

88. Zeng QS, Li CF, Liu H, et al. Multivoxel 3D proton MR spectroscopy in the distinction of recurrent glioma from radiation injury. J Neurooncol 2007; 84:63–9.

89. Sugahara T, Korogi Y, Tomiguchi S, et al. Post-therapeutic intraaxial brain tumor: the value of perfusion-sensitive contrast-enhanced MR imaging for differentiating tumor recurrence from nonneoplastic contrast-enhancing tissue. AJNR Am J Neuroradiol 2000;21:901–9.

90. Cha S, Knopp EA, Johnson G, et al. Dynamic contrast-enhanced T2-weighted MR imaging of recurrent malignant gliomas treated with thalidomide and carboplatin. AJNR Am J Neuroradiol 2000;21:881–90.

91. Di Costanzo A, Pollice S, Trojsi F, et al. Role of perfusion-weighted imaging at 3 Tesla in the assessment of malignancy of cerebral gliomas. Radiol Med 2008;113:134–43.

92. Hu LS, Baxter LC, Smith KA, et al. Relative cerebral blood volume values to differentiate high-grade glioma recurrence from posttreatment radiation effect: direct correlation between image-guided tissue histopathology and localized dynamic susceptibility-weighted contrast-enhanced perfusion MR imaging measurements. AJNR Am J Neuroradiol 2009;30:552–8.

93. Gahramanov S, Raslan AM, Muldoon LL, et al. Potential for differentiation of pseudoprogression from true tumor progression with dynamic susceptibility-weighted contrast-enhanced magnetic resonance imaging using ferumoxytol vs. gadoteridol: a pilot study. Int J Radiat Oncol Biol Phys 2011;79:514–23.

94. Yang I, Huh NG, Smith ZA, et al. Distinguishing glioma recurrence from treatment effect after radio-chemotherapy and immunotherapy. Neurosurg Clin N Am 2010;21:181–6.

95. Di Chiro G, Oldfield E, Wright DC, et al. Cerebral necrosis after radiotherapy and/or intraarterial chemotherapy for brain tumors: PET and neuropathologic studies. AJR Am J Roentgenol 1988;150:189–97.

96. Doyle WK, Budinger TF, Valk PE, et al. Differentiation of cerebral radiation necrosis from tumor recurrence by [18F]FDG and 82Rb positron emission tomography. J Comput Assist Tomogr 1987;11: 563–70.

97. Ricci PE, Karis JP, Heiserman JE, et al. Differentiating recurrent tumor from radiation necrosis: time for re-evaluation of positron emission tomography? AJNR Am J Neuroradiol 1998;19:407–13.

98. Jacobs AH, Thomas A, Kracht LW, et al. 18F-fluoro-L-thymidine and 11C-methylmethionine as markers of increased transport and proliferation in brain tumors. J Nucl Med 2005;46:1948–58.

99. Chen W, Cloughesy T, Kamdar N, et al. Imaging proliferation in brain tumors with 18F-FLT PET: comparison with 18F-FDG. J Nucl Med 2005;46:945–52.

The Role of BCNU Polymer Wafers (Gliadel) in the Treatment of Malignant Glioma

Seema Nagpal, MD

KEYWORDS

- Gliadel • BCNU wafers • Local chemotherapy • Glioma

After surgical removal, direct delivery of anti neoplastic agents to the tumor site is the oldest strategy of adjuvant cancer therapy. Brachytherapy, the direct delivery of radiation via an encapsulated source, was first used at the turn of the twentieth century to treat a wide variety of cancers. It was not commonly used to treat brain tumors, however. In the 1950s and 1960s systemic chemotherapies became available, but were quickly found to be ineffective against gliomas. The inability of most drugs to penetrate the blood-brain barrier and the subsequent dose-limiting systemic toxicity when attempting to reach therapeutic drug levels in brain led clinicians to revisit the concept of local drug delivery.

Clinicians used intracarotid injection,[1] direct application of drug to the cavity,[2,3] and diffusion via semipermeable silastic rubber membranes[4] with drugs, such as cyclophosphamide, vincristine, and methotrexate. These proved largely ineffective and no better than systemic administration, probably because the drugs had little activity against glioma.

In the mid-1970s, the nitrosoureas, 1,3-bis(2-chloroethyl)-1-nitrosourea (BCNU; carmustine) and 1-(2-chloroethyl)-3-cyclohexyl-1-nitrosourea (CCNU; lomustine), were introduced and had moderate efficacy against gliomas.[4,5] Unfortunately, doses that produced response rates as high as 50% caused significant leukopenia or thrombocytopenia,[6] as well as a non–dose-related pulmonary fibrosis. The half-life of BCNU is only 15 to 30 minutes, but patients may need six weeks or longer between doses to allow adequate bone marrow recovery. Attempts to deliver BCNU intra-arterially and by direct injection into the postresection surgical cavity yielded results no better than systemic therapy. Patients who received intra-arterial BCNU had an increased risk of blindness.[7]

In the late 1970s, Langer and Folkman[8] demonstrated that polymers could provide a sustained release of proteins and other macromolecules. This mechanism could theoretically deliver chemotherapy beyond the blood-brain barrier. The initial polymers were nonbiodegradable and the rate of drug release slowed with time, making them unattractive for use in brain. In the 1980s, completely degradable polymers became available and were rapidly incorporated into surgical practice, in the form of absorbable sutures. The newer polymers work by surface erosion, with the layers being resorbed one after the other, analogous to peeling layers from an onion, and allowing more constant drug delivery.[9] Ultimately, these polymers were used to create the Gliadel wafer.

ANIMAL AND PHARMACOKINETIC STUDIES

Tamargo and colleagues[10] published the first paper using BCNU-embedded wafers in 1993. Rats with intracranial 9L gliosarcomas implanted with the wafers had 2- to 3-fold longer survivals than those treated with intraperitoneal BCNU

I have no disclosures.
Division of Neuro-Oncology, Department of Neurology, Stanford Advanced Medicine Center, 875 Blake Wilbur Drive, CC2221, Stanford, CA 94305-5826, USA
E-mail address: snagpal@stanford.edu

Neurosurg Clin N Am 23 (2012) 289–295
doi:10.1016/j.nec.2012.01.004

injections. They tested 2 different polymer bases using this model, ultimately choosing polifeprosan 20 (copolymer of 1,3-bis(p-carboxyphenoxy)propane and sebacic acid in a 20:80 M ratio) because it better protects BCNU from degradation before it is released.[11]

The initial pharmacokinetic studies on BCNU wafers were performed in rabbits, using radiolabeled BCNU. Grossman and colleagues[12] demonstrated that BCNU was distributed widely in the brain ipsilateral to the implants, at distances up to 12 mm from the wafers. Follow-up studies in monkeys measured the drug concentration at the site of implantation on day 1 at 3.5 mmol/L, decreasing to approximately 1.0 mmol/L at a distance of 3 mm from implantation. Seven days postimplant, only the area within 0.5 mm had a concentration greater than 1 mmol/L.[13] The inhibitory concentration of BCNU on human glioma lines in vitro has been reported as from 15 to 300 μmol/L,[14,15] implying that the area adjacent to the implant receives well in excess of the therapeutic drug levels for at least 7 days. Further studies in monkeys demonstrated the safety of BCNU wafers with radiation therapy,[16] and allowed for human trials to begin.

HUMAN TRIALS WITH SINGLE-AGENT BCNU WAFERS

The initial trials of single-agent BCNU wafers are summarized in **Table 1**.

A phase I to II trial in patients with recurrent glioma identified the 3.85% BCNU wafer as the most effective, based on survival from the time of implantation. The higher-dose group (6.35%) did not have more side effects, but overall survival was lower, possibly because it contained 100% glioblastoma (GB) patients. In the 2 lower-dose cohorts only 60% of patients had GB. The 3.85% wafer was chosen for use in subsequent trials, although there was no apparent difference in toxicity.[17] The phase III trial enrolled 222 patients with recurrent glioma, randomizing them to active or placebo wafers. This trial demonstrated an increased overall survival of 8 weeks ($P = .061$) and led the Food and Drug Administration (FDA) to approve Gliadel (3.85% BCNU wafer) for use in recurrent malignant glioma in 1996.

A phase I safety study of the BCNU wafer in combination with radiation therapy for newly diagnosed glioma was run concurrently with the phase III trial for recurrence. The study demonstrated an increased median survival compared with historical controls, but also showed a higher rate of severe adverse events compared with earlier trials, which included seizures, intracranial hypertension, and neurologic decline in the postoperative period. The phase III trial for newly diagnosed glioma had a lower complication rate than observed in the Phase I trial, but remained concerning. Five percent of patients in the BCNU group had cerebrospinal fluid leaks and 9.1% of patients had intracranial hypertension. Although there was a statistically significant improvement in survival in both the recurrent and up-front trials, it is important to note that patients in the placebo arms did not receive treatment after radiation therapy until they had recurrent tumor Standard practice at the time would likely have followed radiation with chemotherapy. This makes the modest results somewhat difficult to interpret (see **Table 1**).

LIMITATIONS OF BCNU WAFERS IN MALIGNANT GLIOMA

Unlike bevacizumab and oral temozolomide (TMZ), the use of BCNU wafers has not been widely adopted, despite phase III data in its favor. There are several factors that have limited its broader use. A review of patients enrolled at one center in the phase III trial showed that only 25% to 30% of patients with malignant gliomas qualified for the use of BNCU wafer. These patients were younger, with more complete resections and higher performance scores,[24] making the results difficult to generalize to the overall patient population. TMZ, a well-tolerated oral alkylating agent with good penetration of the central nervous system, was being used regularly at around the time the FDA approved Gliadel for up-front therapy in 2003. The Stupp trial, demonstrating increased survival with radiation and concurrent TMZ, was published shortly thereafter, in 2005. Although there has never been a head-to-head trial, the increase in survival using BCNU wafers is similar to radiation with TMZ or PCV (procarbazine, CCNU, vincristine).[25] In a recent retrospective review of BCNU wafers, it also appeared that patients with non–methylated methylguanine methyltransferase (non-MGMT) had shorter survivals.[26] If in the future MGMT status is used to make decisions about first-line therapy, placing BCNU wafers at the time of initial surgery is likely to become less attractive.

Another limitation to the use of BCNU wafers is the complication rate noted after 2003, when use of the wafers expanded beyond controlled trial populations. Centers with early experience using BCNU wafers reported complication rates comparable to those seen in patients who do not receive wafers.[27] However, other centers report adverse events in up to 44% of patients receiving BCNU wafers.[28] Formation of a cyst at the implantation site

Table 1
Human trials using single-agent BCNU wafers

Phase	Reference	Patients	Design	Result	Conclusions
I–II	Brem et al,[17] 1991	21 recurrent malignant glioma	Single-arm, dose escalation	Wafer with 3.85% BCNU (7.7 mg) chosen for phase III; higher dose group had lower survival	Safe and well tolerated without systemic side effects
I	Brem et al,[18] 1995	22 new glioma (21 glioblastoma multiforme)	Single-arm, historical control	Median survival was 42 wk	Safe to use in combination with XRT, but 10/22 patients had an SAE
III	Brem et al,[19] 1995	222 recurrent glioma	Double-blind, placebo-controlled	6-mo survival of 56% vs 47% (P = .061) Median survival increased by 8 wk	Marginal change in survival. Placebo patients received no active treatment other than XRT
III	Westphal et al,[20,21] 2003/2006	240 new malignant glioma	Double-blind, placebo-controlled	Median survival 13.8 vs 11.6 mo (P = .017)	Effective, but the placebo arm got no treatment other than XRT. Higher rate of cerebral edema, CSF leaks
III	Valtonen et al,[22] 1997	32 new malignant glioma (planned 100)	Double-blind, placebo-controlled	Median survival 58.1 vs 39.9 wk (P = .012)	Trial stopped early because of wafer shortage; again, randomized to no active treatment after XRT
I	Olivi et al,[23] 2003	44 recurrent malignant glioma	Single-arm, dose escalation	Wafer with 20% BCNU loading was maximum tolerated dose	Can use higher concentrations of BCNU in implanted wafers

Abbreviations: CSF, cerebrospinal fluid; SAE, severe adverse event; XRT, conventional radiation therapy.

Table 2
Trials of BCNU wafers in combination with other therapy

Reference	Patients	Drug	Design	Results	Conclusions
Weingart et al,[34] 2007	38 recurrent glioma	O6-BG	Phase I	Safe dose of bolus, followed by 7-d infusion	Move to phase II
Quinn et al,[35] 2009	52 recurrent glioblastoma multiforme requiring GTR	O6-BG	Phase II single-arm	82% 6 mo survival (56% historical control); median OS 53 weeks	13.4% infection rate, 19.2% CSF leak. May increase risk of AEs
Gururangan et al,[36] 2001	10 recurrent glioma requiring GTR	Monthly TMZ	Phase I	Safe to use 200 mg/m^2 TMZ in combination	Move to phase II
Limentani et al,[37] 2005	16 new malignant glioma	XRT followed by carboplatin	Phase I	Median progression-free survival 266 days, no grade 3 or 4 AEs	Feasible
Sampath et al,[38] 2005	10 recurrent glioma	Irinotecan	Phase I	Median survival from implant 13.5 mo	Tolerable, possibly more effective than monotherapy
Smith et al,[39] 2008	25 new malignant glioma	GammaKnife within 2 wk of surgery, followed by XRT	Phase I/II	Median Survival 50 wk 2-y survival 22%	Unclear if patients received monthly TMZ; 47% rate of radiation necrosis
Affronti et al,[40] 2009	36 new malignant glioma	XRT+TMZ, then TMZ+rotational chemotherapy	Retrospective review	No statistically significant difference in survival for patients with wafers	Safe and feasible
McGirt et al,[41] 2009	33 new malignant glioma	XRT+TMZ, followed by TMZ	Retrospective review	2-y survival 39% vs 18% if no oral TMZ after Gliadel +XRT	Safe and feasible
Bock et al,[42] 2010	44 new malignant glioma	XRT+TMZ, followed by TMZ	Retrospective review	43% of patients with grade 3 or 4 AEs	Combination may produce more toxicity
Noel et al,[26] 2011	28 new malignant glioma	XRT+TMZ, followed by TMZ	Retrospective review	OS 20.6 (Gliadel) vs 20.8 mo	No improvement in survival
Salvati et al,[43] 2011	32 new malignant glioma	XRT+TMZ, followed by TMZ	Retrospective review	No postsurgical AEs Follow-up median only 6.5 mo	Feasible

Abbreviations: AE, adverse event; GTR, gross total resection; O6-BG, O6-benzylguanine; OS, overall survival; TMZ, temozolomide; XRT, conventional radiation.

may occur in up to 11% of patients and, despite high-dose steroids, may still require surgical intervention.[29] The rate of postcraniotomy infection can be as high as 15% to 28%[30,31] at some major centers. Malignant edema, although less common, can lead to severe neurologic dysfunction and death.[30,32]

COMBINATION TRIALS WITH GLIADEL

Recurrence after treatment with BCNU wafers is nearly universal. Despite local drug delivery, the pattern of recurrence is quite similar to that seen with systemic chemotherapy and radiation therapy; 73% have local recurrence while 27% present with a combination of local and distant recurrence,[33] which has led to several trials combining BCNU wafers with other systemic and local therapies (**Table 2**). O6-benzylguanine (O6-BG) is thought to potentiate the action of BCNU by blocking the activity of a DNA repair enzyme, and seems promising based on phase I/II trials. Although a phase III trial in recurrent glioma has not been opened, O6-BG is being used in trials for newly diagnosed patients (see **Table 2**).

FUTURE DIRECTIONS

Current clinical trials that include BCNU wafers are using them in combination with other agents. An actively recruiting phase II trial is using wafers at the time of surgery, followed by TMZ and bevacizumab concurrently with radiation, then TMZ and bevacizumab concurrently until recurrence. Other local delivery mechanisms are under investigation using BCNU, other chemotherapies, and biological agents. BCNU dissolved in ethanol (DTI-015) has been used in phase I/II trials for recurrent and newly diagnosed glioma.[44,45] Convection-enhanced delivery (a constant positive pressure injection), microcapsule delivery (a diffusion-controlled mechanism), and gels are also being explored in both clinical and preclinical settings.

SUMMARY

Although BCNU wafers are included in the 2011 National Comprehensive Cancer Network guidelines (level 2B), they are just one of the options available for treatment of malignant glioma. Clinical trials support its use in patients with a smaller lesion and good performance status, but whether this is a better option than radiation with concurrent TMZ remains an unanswered question. Recent studies of patients receiving combined therapy suggest there may be a role for BCNU wafers in newly diagnosed glioma, as an addition to radiation and TMZ. Other combinations also appear to be well tolerated. The complications associated with the wafers, such as malignant edema and increased frequency of wound infection, present a barrier to widespread adoption of the technology. In addition, patients who qualify for BCNU wafers are frequently candidates for clinical trials. Up-front use of BCNU wafers can disqualify patients from participating. Future work in this area, using newer delivery mechanisms and combination therapies, shows promise for better drug delivery and overcoming drug resistance.

REFERENCES

1. Owens G, Javid R, Tallon M, et al. Arterial infusion chemotherapy of primary gliomas. JAMA 1963; 186:802–3.
2. Garfield J, Dayan AD. Postoperative intracavitary chemotherapy of malignant gliomas. A preliminary study using methotrexate. J Neurosurg 1973;39(3): 315–22.
3. Heppner F, Diemath HE. Local chemotherapy of brain tumors. Acta Neurochir (Wien) 1963;11:287–93 [in German].
4. Wilkinson HA, Kornblith P, Weems S. Focal chemotherapy of brain tumours using semipermeable membranes. J Neurol Neurosurg Psychiatry 1977; 40(4):389–94.
5. Wilson CB, Gutin P, Boldrey EB, et al. Single-agent chemotherapy of brain tumors. A five-year review. Arch Neurol 1976;33(11):739–44.
6. Fewer D, Wilson CB, Boldrey EB, et al. The chemotherapy of brain tumors. Clinical experience with carmustine (BCNU) and vincristine. JAMA 1972;222(5): 549–52.
7. Johnson DW, Parkinson D, Wolpert SM, et al. Intracarotid chemotherapy with 1,3-bis-(2-chloroethyl)-1-nitrosourea (BCNU) in 5% dextrose in water in the treatment of malignant glioma. Neurosurgery 1987;20(4):577–83.
8. Langer R, Folkman J. Polymers for the sustained release of proteins and other macromolecules. Nature 1976;263(5580):797–800.
9. Wang PP, Frazier J, Brem H. Local drug delivery to the brain. Adv Drug Deliv Rev 2002;54(7): 987–1013.
10. Tamargo RJ, Myseros JS, Epstein JI, et al. Interstitial chemotherapy of the 9L gliosarcoma: controlled release polymers for drug delivery in the brain. Cancer Res 1993;53(2):329–33.
11. Fleming AB, Saltzman WM. Pharmacokinetics of the carmustine implant. Clin Pharmacokinet 2002;41(6): 403–19.
12. Grossman SA, Reinhard C, Colvin OM, et al. The intracerebral distribution of BCNU delivered by surgically implanted biodegradable polymers. J Neurosurg 1992;76(4):640–7.

13. Fung LK, Ewend MG, Sills A, et al. Pharmacokinetics of interstitial delivery of carmustine, 4-hydroperoxycyclophosphamide, and paclitaxel from a biodegradable polymer implant in the monkey brain. Cancer Res 1998;58(4):672–84.

14. Gu B, DeAngelis LM. Enhanced cytotoxicity of bioreductive antitumor agents with dimethyl fumarate in human glioblastoma cells. Anticancer Drugs 2005;16(2):167–74.

15. Hunter KJ, Deen DF, Pellarin M, et al. Effect of alpha-difluoromethylornithine on 1,3-bis(2-chloroethyl)-1-nitrosourea and cis-diamminedichloroplatinum(II) cytotoxicity, DNA interstrand cross-linking, and growth in human brain tumor cell lines in vitro. Cancer Res 1990;50(9):2769–72.

16. Brem H, Tamargo RJ, Olivi A, et al. Biodegradable polymers for controlled delivery of chemotherapy with and without radiation therapy in the monkey brain. J Neurosurg 1994;80(2):283–90.

17. Brem H, Mahaley MS Jr, Vick NA, et al. Interstitial chemotherapy with drug polymer implants for the treatment of recurrent gliomas. J Neurosurg 1991; 74(3):441–6.

18. Brem H, Ewend MG, Piantadosi S, et al. The safety of interstitial chemotherapy with BCNU-loaded polymer followed by radiation therapy in the treatment of newly diagnosed malignant gliomas: phase I trial. J Neurooncol 1995;26(2):111–23.

19. Brem H, Piantadosi S, Burger PC, et al. Placebo-controlled trial of safety and efficacy of intraoperative controlled delivery by biodegradable polymers of chemotherapy for recurrent gliomas. The Polymer-Brain Tumor Treatment Group. Lancet 1995;345(8956):1008–12.

20. Westphal M, Hilt DC, Bortey E, et al. A phase 3 trial of local chemotherapy with biodegradable carmustine (BCNU) wafers (Gliadel wafers) in patients with primary malignant glioma. Neuro Oncol 2003; 5(2):79–88.

21. Westphal M, Ram Z, Riddle V, et al. Gliadel wafer in initial surgery for malignant glioma: long-term follow-up of a multicenter controlled trial. Acta Neurochir (Wien) 2006;148(3):269–75 [discussion: 75].

22. Valtonen S, Timonen U, Toivanen P, et al. Interstitial chemotherapy with carmustine-loaded polymers for high-grade gliomas: a randomized double-blind study. Neurosurgery 1997;41(1):44–8 [discussion: 48–9].

23. Olivi A, Grossman SA, Tatter S, et al. Dose escalation of carmustine in surgically implanted polymers in patients with recurrent malignant glioma: a new approaches to brain tumor therapy CNS consortium trial. J Clin Oncol 2003;21(9):1845–9.

24. Whittle IR, Lyles S, Walker M. Gliadel therapy given for first resection of malignant glioma: a single centre study of the potential use of Gliadel. Br J Neurosurg 2003;17(4):352–4.

25. Stewart LA. Chemotherapy in adult high-grade glioma: a systematic review and meta-analysis of individual patient data from 12 randomised trials. Lancet 2002;359(9311):1011–8.

26. Noel G, Schott R, Froelich S, et al. Retrospective comparison of chemoradiotherapy followed by adjuvant chemotherapy, with or without prior Gliadel implantation (carmustine) after initial surgery in patients with newly diagnosed high-grade gliomas. Int J Radiat Oncol Biol Phys 2012;82(2):749–55.

27. Attenello FJ, Mukherjee D, Datoo G, et al. Use of Gliadel (BCNU) wafer in the surgical treatment of malignant glioma: a 10-year institutional experience. Ann Surg Oncol 2008;15(10):2887–93.

28. Menei P, Metellus P, Parot-Schinkel E, et al. Biodegradable carmustine wafers (Gliadel) alone or in combination with chemoradiotherapy: the French experience. Ann Surg Oncol 2010;17(7):1740–6.

29. Dorner L, Ulmer S, Rohr A, et al. Space-occupying cyst development in the resection cavity of malignant gliomas following Gliadel(R) implantation—incidence, therapeutic strategies, and outcome. J Clin Neurosci 2011;18(3):347–51.

30. Subach BR, Witham TF, Kondziolka D, et al. Morbidity and survival after 1,3-bis(2-chloroethyl)-1-nitrosourea wafer implantation for recurrent glioblastoma: a retrospective case-matched cohort series. Neurosurgery 1999;45(1):17–22 [discussion: 22–3].

31. McGovern PC, Lautenbach E, Brennan PJ, et al. Risk factors for postcraniotomy surgical site infection after 1,3-bis(2-chloroethyl)-1-nitrosourea (Gliadel) wafer placement. Clin Infect Dis 2003;36(6):759–65.

32. Weber EL, Goebel EA. Cerebral edema associated with Gliadel wafers: two case studies. Neuro Oncol 2005;7(1):84–9.

33. Giese A, Kucinski T, Knopp U, et al. Pattern of recurrence following local chemotherapy with biodegradable carmustine (BCNU) implants in patients with glioblastoma. J Neurooncol 2004;66(3):351–60.

34. Weingart J, Grossman SA, Carson KA, et al. Phase I trial of polifeprosan 20 with carmustine implant plus continuous infusion of intravenous O6-benzylguanine in adults with recurrent malignant glioma: new approaches to brain tumor therapy CNS consortium trial. J Clin Oncol 2007;25(4):399–404.

35. Quinn JA, Jiang SX, Carter J, et al. Phase II trial of Gliadel plus O6-benzylguanine in adults with recurrent glioblastoma multiforme. Clin Cancer Res 2009;15(3):1064–8.

36. Gururangan S, Cokgor L, Rich JN, et al. Phase I study of Gliadel wafers plus temozolomide in adults with recurrent supratentorial high-grade gliomas. Neuro Oncol 2001;3(4):246–50.

37. Limentani SA, Asher A, Heafner M, et al. A phase I trial of surgery, Gliadel wafer implantation, and

immediate postoperative carboplatin in combination with radiation therapy for primary anaplastic astrocytoma or glioblastoma multiforme. J Neurooncol 2005;72(3):241–4.

38. Sampath P, Sungarian A, Alderson L, et al. BCNU-impregnated wafers (Gliadel) plus irinotecan (Camptosar) in combination treatment for patients with recurrent glioblastoma multiforme [abstract]. Congress of Neurological Surgeons, Boston, October 8–13, 2005.

39. Smith KA, Ashby LS, Gonzalez LF, et al. Prospective trial of gross-total resection with Gliadel wafers followed by early postoperative Gamma Knife radiosurgery and conformal fractionated radiotherapy as the initial treatment for patients with radiographically suspected, newly diagnosed glioblastoma multiforme. J Neurosurg 2008;109(Suppl):106–17.

40. Affronti ML, Heery CR, Herndon JE, et al. Overall survival of newly diagnosed glioblastoma patients receiving carmustine wafers followed by radiation and concurrent temozolomide plus rotational multiagent chemotherapy. Cancer 2009;115(15):3501–11.

41. McGirt MJ, Than KD, Weingart JD, et al. Gliadel (BCNU) wafer plus concomitant temozolomide therapy after primary resection of glioblastoma multiforme. J Neurosurg 2009;110(3):583–8.

42. Bock HC, Puchner MJ, Lohmann F, et al. First-line treatment of malignant glioma with carmustine implants followed by concomitant radiochemotherapy: a multicenter experience. Neurosurg Rev 2010; 33(4):441–9.

43. Salvati M, D'Elia A, Frati A, et al. Safety and feasibility of the adjunct of local chemotherapy with biodegradable carmustine (BCNU) wafers to the standard multimodal approach to high grade gliomas at first diagnosis. J Neurosurg Sci 2011;55(1):1–6.

44. Hassenbusch SJ, Nardone EM, Levin VA, et al. Stereotactic injection of DTI-015 into recurrent malignant gliomas: phase I/II trial. Neoplasia 2003;5(1): 9–16.

45. Jenkinson MD, Smith TS, Haylock B, et al. Phase II trial of intratumoral BCNU injection and radiotherapy on untreated adult malignant glioma. J Neurooncol 2010;99(1):103–13.

Alternative Chemotherapeutic Agents: Nitrosoureas, Cisplatin, Irinotecan

Jose A. Carrillo, MD[a],*, Claudia A. Munoz, MD, MPH[b]

KEYWORDS

- Glioblastoma • Glioma • Chemotherapy • Cisplatin
- Irinotecan • Nitrosoureas • CCNU • BCNU

CHEMOTHERAPY FOR HIGH-GRADE GLIOMA

Before Food and Drug Administration (FDA) approval of temozolomide (TMZ, Temodar) for the treatment of high-grade gliomas in 2005, the mainstay of treatment focused on the use of cisplatin, irinotecan, and nitrosoureas alone and in combination. Decades of experience with these chemotherapies coupled with meta-analyses that provide evidence of significant improvement in survival when added to surgery and radiotherapy have established a position for chemotherapy in the treatment regimen of malignant gliomas.[1,2] With the establishment of TMZ concomitant with radiotherapy and adjuvant TMZ as the standard of care for the initial treatment of glioblastoma multiforme (GBM), the role for these chemotherapies has changed to that of one at the time of recurrence or progression.[3] In this article, the authors focus on the use of cisplatin, irinotecan, and the nitrosoureas in the era of TMZ and bevacizumab (Avastin). The assessment of outcomes across clinical trials is notoriously difficult. To facilitate some meaningful level of comparison, an effort was made to include like outcomes, such as overall survival (OS) and progression-free survival at 6 months (PFS-6), in addition to the radiographic response.

CISPLATIN

Cisplatin (CDDP) is a platinum-based inorganic metal complex that acts as a DNA-intercalating agent forming DNA intrastrand and interstrand cross-links, along with DNA-protein cross-links. Apoptosis and cell growth inhibition are induced as a result of the cross-links. Cisplatin has been shown to have antitumor activity against several human malignancies. The use of CDDP in brain tumors stems from its ability to cross the blood-brain barrier.[4,5] Before the advent of TMZ, researchers investigated cisplatin's use in the treatment of malignant gliomas, primarily in concert with other chemotherapeutic agents and radiotherapy.

Upfront Treatment with Cisplatin

- Cisplatin has a long history of therapeutic use in high-grade gliomas. In clinical use, cisplatin is often given in combination with other chemotherapies. In 1992 Yung and colleagues[5] conducted a single-arm study to test the efficacy of using alternating courses of 1,3-bis(2-chloroethyl)-1 nitrosourea (BCNU, carmustine) and CDDP in conjunction with radiation therapy after surgical resection to treat primary malignant

Disclosures: none to report.
[a] Department of Neurology, University of California Irvine, 101 The City Drive South, Shanbrom Hall, Suite 121, Orange, CA 92868, USA
[b] Department of Neurology, University of California Irvine, 101 The City Drive South, Orange, CA 92868, USA
* Corresponding author.
E-mail address: carrilj2@hs.uci.edu

glioma. Patients with histologic diagnosis of GBM, anaplastic astrocytoma, and anaplastic oligodendroglioma underwent surgical resection or biopsy. Radiotherapy was initiated over 6 to 7 weeks, and chemotherapy was started during the first week of radiotherapy. A total of 33 patients entered the analysis, with a median time to tumor progression of 32 weeks for patients with glioblastoma and 50 weeks for those with anaplastic glioma. Median survival time was 55 weeks for glioblastoma and 110 weeks for anaplastic glioma.[5] The 18-month survival rate was 55% overall. The results of this study suggested that BCNU alternating with CDDP in conjunction with radiotherapy is safe and also indicated that there may be benefits in OS over radiotherapy with BCNU alone.

- Lassen and colleagues[6] investigated the use of CDDP as part of a combination therapy for newly diagnosed GBM. This study was a single-arm phase II trial examining the efficacy of a combination of cisplatin, BCNU, and etoposide, followed by radiation. All patients underwent tumor resection, and then chemotherapy was started 2 to 4 weeks after surgery. The primary end point of the study was response to chemotherapy using the MacDonald criteria.[7] Radiographic partial response was achieved by 32% of patients, 39% had stable disease, and 29% had progressive disease. Complete response was not achieved in any patient. Median time to progression was 7.6 months and median survival was 11.4 months.[6] The investigators concluded that although the survival benefit fell short of historical data, a potential benefit from the regimen used in the study was the shorter total treatment time of preradiation chemotherapy making it potentially less cumbersome.

- In 2009 Silvani and colleagues[8] conducted a retrospective study examining the clinical effectiveness of using the combination of CDDP and BCNU as the first-line management of GBM. One hundred sixty patients received chemotherapy and radiotherapy in a tandem fashion. After chemotherapy, radiotherapy was administered at 1.8 to 2.0 Gy/d to a total of 60 Gy. The next cycle of chemotherapy was started after radiotherapy was completed and subsequent cycles started every 6 weeks for a total of 5 cycles. Patients in this study had a median PFS of 7.6 months and median OS of 15.6 months. Although the survival results of the study are comparable with those of Stupp and colleagues[3] with TMZ, regarding the clinical benefit of cisplatin and BCNU, the toxicities were comparably worse.[8] The results of this large trial of CDDP in GBM are compared in **Table 1**.

Cisplatin Toxicity

The main difficulty in the use of cisplatin is its toxicity profile. Hematologic side effects are the most common and tend to be the most severe. Hematologic toxicity was significant with grade 4 leukopenia and thrombocytopenia occurring in 10% and 57% respectively.[6] Ototoxicity is also frequent, making this a drug that must be used with caution. Clinically significant hearing loss and tinnitus can be seen in 13% to 19% of patients at 6 months after treatment with cisplatin, with 36% having evidence of sensorineural hearing loss on audiogram testing.[10]

IRINOTECAN

The prodrug irinotecan (CPT-11; Camptosar; 7-ethyl-10-[4-(1-piperidino)-1-piperidino]carbonyl-20-S-camptothecin) is a water soluble alkaloid derivative of camptothecin that is extracted from the Chinese tree, *Camptotheca acuminata*.[11] Irinotecan is largely metabolized in the liver by carboxylesterase enzymes to the active 7-ethyl-10-hydroxycamptothecin (SN-38), which functions

Table 1
Comparison of cisplatin-based chemotherapies in high-grade gliomas

Trial	Tumor Type	Timing of Treatment	Number of Patients	Chemotherapy	Median PFS (wk)	Median OS (wk)
Yung et al,[5] 1992	Grade III/IV	Upfront	33	BCNU + CDDP	50/32	110/55
Shinoda et al,[9] 1997	GBM	Upfront	30	CDDP	16	60
Lassen et al,[6] 1999	GBM	Upfront	27	BCNU + CDDP + Etoposide	30.4	45.6
Silvani et al,[8] 2009	GBM	Upfront	160	BCNU + CDDP	30.4	62.4

as a topoisomerase I inhibitor.[12,13] The inhibition of the enzyme produces DNA damage via interference with DNA transcription, replication, and repair.[14] Activity against central nervous system (CNS) tumors was initially demonstrated by Hare and colleagues[15] using xenografts derived from childhood and adult high-grade gliomas.

Irinotecan in Recurrent Disease

- The use of irinotecan as a single agent has had mixed results and is complicated by interactions with CYP inducers. A prospective phase II study by Chamberlain[14] of CPT-11 in 40 patients with recurrent supratentorial GBM failed to show a tumor response to treatment although the dosages used, 400 to 500 mg/m^2 every 3 weeks, were suboptimal.[14] Anticonvulsant medications with cytochrome P450–inducing features upregulate chemotherapy catabolism.[14] It was suggested that the dosages used may have been insufficient because more than 60% of patients were on anticonvulsant therapy.
- Only 48% of patients enrolled in the Friedman and colleagues'[11] phase II study of recurrent or progressive malignant gliomas received enzyme-inducing antiepileptic drugs. In this population of 80% GBM, the 60 patients enrolled experienced a median time to tumor progression of 12 weeks and a median estimated survival of 43 weeks. Confirmed partial responses on magnetic resonance imaging were seen in 15% of patients, whereas stable disease was achieved in 55% of radiographic responses.[11]

Enzyme-Inducing Antiepileptic Drugs Affect the Dosing of Irinotecan

- The effects of receiving enzyme-inducing antiepileptic drug (EIAED) therapy were taken into account in the phase II North American Brain Tumor Coalition (NABTC) study in recurrent malignant gliomas treated with irinotecan.[16] Irinotecan was administered at 350 mg/m^2 every 3 weeks in those not on EIAED therapy and 750 mg/m^2 in those on EIAED therapy until progression or a total of 12 months of treatment. Patients with GBM accounted for 75% of 51 total patients enrolled. Overall, 17.6% of the patients were PFS-6. A partial radiographic response was seen in 5.8%, stable disease in 33%, and immediate progression was seen in 58.8% of the group.[16] The predetermined PFS-6 efficacy of at least 30% was not met, leading the study

investigators to conclude that efficacy was not established in this population.[16]
- In the New Approaches to Brain Tumor Therapy (NABTT) 97-11 study, they attempted to mitigate the varied doses of prior trials and the influence of EIAED therapy by treating at the maximum tolerated dose (MTD) of irinotecan for those patients on EIAED therapy (group A) and those who were not (group B).[17] Group A was treated with an infusion of 411 mg/m^2 every week for 4 consecutive weeks out of a 6-week cycle, whereas group B received 117 mg/m^2. The primary end point was the radiographic response: 6% experienced a complete response, there were no partial responses, 28% had stable disease, and another 28% experienced disease progression during treatment. Median PFS was 7.3 months, PFS-6 was 56%, and median OS was 10.4 months.[16] Phase I of this trial was closed after 18 patients because of the failure to meet the minimum requirement of more than 2 responses.[17]

Irinotecan Toxicity

- Common toxicities seen in single-agent CPT-11 were diarrhea, nausea and vomiting, and neutropenia.[11,15,17] In CNS disease, toxicities were less frequently seen than in colorectal studies of similar doses because of the increased metabolism of CPT-11 caused by the CYP450-inducing antiepileptic drugs with subsequent increases in irinotecan clearance.[11,14] The frequency of grade 3/4 diarrhea was 33.7% and grade 3/4 neutropenia was 28% in colorectal studies.[18] In those patients treated at the MTD, grade 3/4 toxicities were encountered in 67% of patients.[17] Anticholinergic symptoms are frequently seen and commonly pretreated with atropine during infusion. The equivocal efficacy data on single-agent CPT-11 led to postulation about its role in combination therapy with newer treatments.

Irinotecan in the TMZ Era

With the statistically significant survival benefits of the alkylating agent, TMZ, along with minimal toxicity, the Stupp regimen has become the standard care for newly diagnosed GBM.[3] The role of irinotecan in addition to TMZ has been investigated in the NABTT study along with the pharmacokinetics of the combination in patients receiving EIAED therapy.[12]

- In this dose-escalation study of irinotecan combined with TMZ, the starting dose of irinotecan was 350 mg/m^2, which was escalated in 50 mg/m^2 increments to 550 mg/m^2. The MTD in the study was 500 mg/m^2.[12] Twenty-six out of 33 patients had GBMs, one was diagnosed with gliosarcoma and the remainder of the patients had anaplastic gliomas. Radiographic complete response was seen in 6%, partial response in 19%, stable disease in 36%, and progressive disease in 39%.[12]
- Quinn and colleagues[19] studied the use of TMZ plus irinotecan in 42 newly diagnosed patients with GBM before treatment with radiotherapy at the end of cycle number 3 in a phase II trial. Irinotecan was infused on days 1, 8, 22, and 29 of each cycle, with those on EIAED therapy receiving 325 mg/m^2 and 125 mg/m^2 for those not receiving EIAED therapy. The radiographic response consisted of 19% partial responses and 50% with stable disease.[19] Median PFS was 3.1 months and median OS was 13.8 months. Disappointingly, the study failed to meet the predetermined response rate of greater than or equal to 26% required to proceed with a phase III trial and had grade 3/4 adverse events of up to 36%.[19] Of interest, the level of O^6-methylguanine-DNA methyltransferase (MGMT) expression in this study failed to show a statistically significant relationship between PFS and OS as would be expected from treatment with TMZ.

Irinotecan in the Bevacizumab Era

The introduction of the humanized immunoglobulin G$_1$ monoclonal antibody that selectively inhibits vascular endothelial growth factor, bevacizumab, has changed the way chemotherapies, such as irinotecan, are used. FDA approval for bevacizumab in the recurrent setting was established in 2009 based on response data from the following study.

- The prospective phase II trial by Vrendenburgh and colleagues[20] evaluated bevacizumab plus irinotecan in 35 patients with recurrent GBM initially treated with radiotherapy and concurrent TMZ. Two dosing schedules were used, most patients received bevacizumab at 10 mg/kg and irinotecan every 2 weeks, with those on EIAEDs receiving 340 mg/m^2 and those not on EIAEDs receiving 125 mg/m^2. There was no difference between the 2 groups

statistically. A radiographic partial response was seen in 57% of patients by the Macdonald criteria.[7] The median PFS was 24 weeks and median PFS-6 was 46%, far exceeding the predetermined 20% decision rule for effectiveness. The 6-month OS was 77% and the median OS was 42 weeks.[20]
- The benefit of bevacizumab alone or in combination with CPT-11 was evaluated by Friedman and colleagues[21] in a phase II, multicenter, noncomparative trial in recurrent glioblastoma. The PFS-6 rates were 42.6% and 50.3%, and the median OS times were 9.2 months and 8.7 months, respectively, for bevacizumab alone and bevacizumab/CPT-11 groups.

NITROSOUREAS

Nitrosoureas are alkylating agents that function by cross-linking DNA. As a group, the high lipid solubility of nitrosoureas promotes crossing of the blood-brain barrier. Before TMZ, radiotherapy plus nitrosoureas was the standard of care for the treatment of GBM.[22] The most commonly used nitrosoureas in clinical practice today are 1-(2-chloroethyl)-3-cyclohexyl-1-nitrosurea (CCNU, lomustine) and BCNU. In a meta-analysis of properly randomized trials comparing radiotherapy alone with radiotherapy plus chemotherapy consisting largely of nitrosoureas in high-grade gliomas established a role for chemotherapy in the treatment regimen of gliomas after it was shown that chemotherapy significantly improved outcomes.[2] There was a statistically significant increase in PFS (overall hazard ratio [HR] of 0.83) ($P<.0001$) and a significant increase in OS (HR of 0.85) ($P<.0001$) seen with the addition of chemotherapy.[2] Nitrosoureas are commonly used as modern, standard second-line chemotherapies and are frequently relegated to the standard arm in randomized phase II trials against novel agents. Multiple nitrosourea-based polychemotherapy regimens have largely been unsuccessful in increasing efficacy as compared with single-agent nitrosourea chemotherapy.

CCNU

The chemotherapy CCNU is a derivative of 1-methyl-1-nitrosurea. CCNU is a lipid-soluble, nonionized, aqueous insoluble, oral chemotherapy that, because of high lipid solubility, is able to pass the blood-brain barrier.[23] With a wide spectrum of antitumor activity, CCNU was eventually used to treat brain tumors. CCNU is one of the few chemotherapeutic agents that are FDA approved in the treatment of GBM.

- The benefits of CCNU in place of and in addition to radiation were explored in an early randomized trial by Reagan and colleagues.[24] Sixty-three patients with high-grade gliomas at a single institution were randomized into 3 groups receiving radiotherapy alone, CCNU, or combined radiation therapy and CCNU. The group receiving chemotherapy alone experienced the lowest OS with a median 6.6 months survival. Those receiving radiotherapy consisting of whole brain irradiation had a median survival of 11.5 months. Lastly, the combined radiation and chemotherapy group demonstrated a median survival of 12.0 months.[24]
- In the phase II study by Rosenblum and colleagues,[23] patients were treated with 130 mg/m^2 every 6 weeks, and a remission rate of 37% for all patients was seen. This finding compared favorably with remission rates of 40% to 50% that were seen in earlier studies with BCNU. The results of CCNU therapy in several trials are illustrated in **Table 2**.

CCNU in the TMZ Era

- The use of CCNU plus TMZ was evaluated in the study by Herrlinger and colleagues[25] in 31 patients with newly diagnosed glioblastoma given chemotherapy concomitant with radiotherapy. The median PFS was 9 months and the PFS-6 was 61.3%, which was higher than the predefined efficacy criteria of 53.3%. The median survival time was 22.6 months, with 71% of patients surviving at 1 year and 44.7% surviving at 2 years.[25]

MGMT Methylation Status

- The association of MGMT promoter methylation with a favorable outcome in patients with glioblastoma treated with the alkylating agent TMZ has been well described.[28] MGMT methylation status was available for the determination by methylation-specific polymerase chain reaction in 19 tumors in the Herrlinger study.[25] The favorable methylation of MGMT was associated with significantly longer PFS and median survival times. The PFS was 19 months in those tumors with methylated MGMT as compared with 6 months in those with unmethylated tumors ($P = .014$).[25] The median survival time was not reached in the methylated MGMT group at 24 months as compared with 12.5 months in those unmethylated tumors.[25] These findings support the presumed similar effects on survival for nitrosoureas seen with TMZ and MGMT promoter methylation, given both agents affect the O^6-position of guanine.

CCNU Toxicity

- Early studies with CCNU in malignant brain tumors in 26 consecutive patients admitted to the Baltimore Cancer Research Center between 1970 and 1971 show that CCNU is well tolerated.[23] Immediate toxic effects, beginning 4 to 6 hours after treatment, consisted of nausea and vomiting in 70% of patients. Infrequent anorexia and rare fatigue were noted. Transient thrombocytopenia begins after the first week and reaches a nadir in the third week, before recovering to near baseline values by the fifth week. Treatment-limiting and dose-limiting delayed hematological toxicity were encountered. Nearly half of the

	Tumor Type	Timing of Treatment	Number of Patients	Chemotherapy	Median PFS (wk)	Median OS (wk)
Trial						
Reagan et al,[24] 1976	HGG	Upfront	63	CCNU	—	46
Herrlinger et al,[25] 2006	GBM	Upfront	31	CCNU + TMZ	36.0	90.4
Wick et al,[26] 2010	GBM	Recurrent	266	CCNU (vs enzastaurin)	6.4	28.4
Ballman et al,[27] 2007	GBM	Upfront	1348	CCNU + others[a]	21.2	40.8

Table 2
Results of various trials using CCNU in GBM

[a] Ballman et al is a pooled analysis of 11 North Central Cancer Treatment Group (NCCTG) trials for newly diagnosed GBM.

patients developed mild transient elevations of transaminases, alkaline phosphatase, and lactate dehydrogenase in nearly one-half of the patients.[23] The toxicity of CCNU is largely hematologic and cumulative in nature.

- When CCNU was given concomitantly with TMZ, the dose was adjusted for hematologic toxicity in 12.9% of the patients.[25] The World Health Organization grade 4 leukopenia was seen in 10% of the patients, thrombocytopenia in 16%, and anemia in 3%. One case of grade 2 pulmonary fibrosis was seen; 12.9% of the patients developed elevation of transaminases to levels consistent with drug-induced hepatitis.[25]

BCNU

BCNU is an intravenously administered nitrosourea that functions as an alkylating agent at the O^6 position of guanine, forming cross-linking between DNA strands resulting in impairment in DNA duplication and protein transcription.[13] A meta-analysis of several studies involving BCNU has demonstrated a statistically significant PFS and OS improvement in the treatment of GBM.[1,2] BCNU is one of the few chemotherapeutic agents that are FDA approved in the treatment of GBM.

BCNU Comparison with Temozolomide

- In a retrospective analysis of BCNU versus TMZ in newly diagnosed patients with GBM, Vinjamuri and colleagues[29] reported on the use of BCNU given intravenously every 8 weeks at 200 mg/m² for a maximum of 8 cycles concomitant with radiation in comparison with TMZ given concomitant with radiotherapy and adjuvantly up to 2 years. The median PFS for the 2 groups was not significant, with a median PFS of 7.7 months in the BCNU group and 5.2 months in the TMZ group (P = .8). Median OS curves were significantly different, with 11.5 months in the BCNU group and 15.9 months in the TMZ group. The BCNU and TMZ groups had a 1-year survival of 44% and 64% respectively. The 2-year survival for BCNU was 9% and 36% for TMZ.[29]

BCNU in Recurrent Disease

- Reithmeier and colleagues[30] recently investigated the use of BCNU in recurrent GBM after the initial treatment with radiotherapy and TMZ. This retrospective analysis looked at 35 patients with recurrent or progressive GBM treated with BCNU 80 mg/m² on days 1 through 3 every 8 weeks for a maximum of 6 cycles. Radiographic complete responses were not seen in any patient, 5.7% had a partial response, 54.3% were observed to have stable disease, and 31.4% developed progressive disease after the first cycle of BCNU. Median PFS was 11 weeks, PFS-6 was 13%, median OS was 22 weeks, and 6-month OS was 43%.[30]

- In a multicenter Gruppo Italiano Cooperativo di Neuro-Oncologia (GICNO) trial, the use of BCNU plus irinotecan was evaluated in recurrent or progressive GBM after first-line TMZ chemotherapy and radiotherapy.[13] BCNU 100 mg/m² was intravenously given every 6 weeks with irinotecan 175 mg/m²/wk for 4 out of 6 weeks for a maximum of 8 cycles in a total of 42 patients. There were no radiographic complete responses, 21.4% partial responses, and 50% exhibited stable disease. The median time to progression was 17 weeks and the PFS-6 was 30.3%. The median survival time was 11.7 months, with 71% of patients alive at 6 months and 44.1% alive at 12 months[13]

BCNU Toxicity

- Sclerosis of the veins is a frequent long-term sequelae of administration of intravenous BCNU.[22] Fatigue and lethargy are common and can be seen as a cause of treatment discontinuation even in the absence of tumor progression. Grade 4 pulmonary toxicities complicate treatment in 5% of cases treated with BCNU.[31] Decreased carbon monoxide diffusing capacity was seen in 14.3% of patients, with one case of acute pulmonary reaction seen in one study of 49 patients.[29]

BCNU WAFERS

BCNU wafers (poly[carboxyphenoxy-propane]sebacic acid) anhydride (Gliadel) wafers contain BCNU at 3.85% concentration. Biodegradable BCNU wafers are implanted into the tumor resection cavity at the time of surgery whereby they slowly release BCNU over a 2- to 3-week period.[32] The surgeon may implant up to 8 wafers in the resection cavity, depending on the cavity size. Based on the phase III trial by Westphal and colleagues,[32] BCNU wafers became the only interstitial chemotherapy approved for malignant glioma.

Use of BCNU Wafer Alone

- In the prospective, randomized, placebo-controlled, multicenter, multinational, double-blind trial, the effectiveness of BCNU wafers was assessed in 240 patients at the time of the first surgical resection with an intraoperative abnormality of the malignant glioma.[32] Study patients received standard radiation to the tumor site; however, systemic chemotherapy was prohibited. Median survival time was 13.9 months for the BCNU wafer group and 11.6 months for the placebo group, a statistically significant difference. The median survival within the GBM subgroup treated with BCNU wafers was 13.5 months compared with 11.4 months in the placebo wafer group, a difference that was not statistically significant. PFS was not statistically different between both treatment groups.[32]
- The long-term follow-up by Westphal and colleagues[33] followed the same group of 240 patients with malignant glioma to assess the 1-, 2-, and 3-year event rates. The proportion surviving at the 3-year point was statistically significant at 9.2% in the BCNU group versus 1.7% in the placebo wafer group. In the GBM subgroup, the median survival was 13.1 months in the BCNU wafer-treated group compared with 11.4 months in the placebo group, a non-statistically significant difference even after Cox proportional hazards model was performed to account for possible prognostic factor imbalances between the groups (**Fig. 1**).[33]

Use of BCNU Wafer with Chemotherapy

- The initial trials using BCNU wafers prohibited the use of adjuvant chemotherapy. The single-institution retrospective study by McGirt and colleagues[34] evaluated the added benefit of concomitant TMZ in addition to BCNU wafers after primary resection of GBM. All patients underwent surgical resection and adjuvant radiotherapy. Patients treated before the initiation of the Stupp protocol TMZ at the institution were evaluated and compared with those who received TMZ in addition to BCNU wafers placed at surgery. The median OS in the radiation + TMZ + BCNU wafer group was significantly improved compared with the radiation + BCNU wafer group: 21.3 months versus 12.4 months. The 2-year OS was 39% versus 18% respectively for the treatment group as compared with the

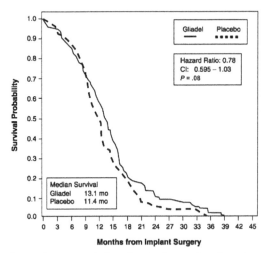

Fig. 1. GBM population. Survival curve for the subset 207 patients with GBM. The median survival time was not significantly increased among the GBM subset (P = .08). CI, confidence interval. (*Data from* Westphal M, Ram Z, Riddle V, et al. Gliadel wafer in initial surgery for malignant glioma: long-term followup of a multicenter controlled trial. Acta Neurochir 2006;148: 269–75. Used with permission Springer publishing.)

control and was independently associated with improved OS. However, when surgery was controlled for with only those patients with gross total resection receiving radiation + TMZ + BCNU wafers were compared with those receiving radiation + TMZ, the median survival was not significant.[34]

BCNU Wafer Toxicity

- BCNU wafers are generally well tolerated with adverse events profile similar to that of the placebo group in the Westphal and colleagues[32] randomized, double-blind, placebo-controlled trial. Only intracranial hypertension is seen more often in the BCNU wafer group, occurring as a late event generally greater than 6 months after implantation. Seizures, intracranial infections, and healing abnormalities were not seen more commonly in the BCNU wafer group than the placebo wafer group.[32] When added to TMZ and radiation, BCNU wafers resulted in significantly increased incidence of myelosuppression: 23% versus 0%.[34] In the era of antiangiogenic treatments, such as bevacizumab, with well-described impairments in healing, caution should be exercised in combining these 2 treatments.

FOTEMUSTINE

Fotemustine (diethyl-1-[3-(2-chloroethyl)-3-nitro-soureido]-ethylphosphonate) is a third-generation chloroethylnitrosourea, historically used less frequently than CCNU or BCNU. The agent is highly lipophilic, readily crossing the blood-brain barrier owing to the addition of the phosphoalanine carrier group.[31] Clinical studies suggest a role for fotemustine in the treatment of progressive GBM.[31] The activity of this agent has been evaluated in the TMZ era in recurrent GBM trials.[31,35,36] The activity of various chemotherapies in the recurrent GBM after the initial standard of care treatment with radiotherapy and concomitant TMZ are shown in **Table 2**.

Fotemustine Use in Recurrent GBM

- Scoccianti and colleagues[35] evaluated the fotemustine in 27 patients with recurrent glioblastoma pretreated with temozolomide. There were radiographic partial responses in 29.6% of patients, stable disease in 18.5%, and 51.8% showed disease progression. The median PFS was 5.7 months, PFS-6 was 48%, and PFS at 1 year was 18.5%. Median survival from the time of first recurrence was 9.1 months and median OS was 21.2 months. Survival from the first diagnosis at 1 year and 2 years were 92.5% and 46% respectively.[35]
- Recurrent GBM was treated with fotemustine 100 mg/m² infused on days 1, 8, and 15, followed by a 4- to 6-week rest period during induction. Maintenance fotemustine therapy was administered at 100 mg/m² every 3 weeks until progression.[36] Fifty patients were enrolled with 2% complete responses,

16% partial responses, 44% stable disease, and 38% progressive disease. A measure of efficacy control Complete Response + Partial Response + Stable Disease (CR+PR+SD) was 62%. The median PFS was 6.1 months, the PFS-6 was 51.5%, and the PFS at 1 year was 35.5%. The median survival from time of first relapse was 8.1 months, median OS was 24.5 months, and survival at 1 year and 2 years from diagnosis were 80.7% and 51.0%, respectively (**Table 3**).[36]

Fotemustine and MGMT Methylation Status

- Brandes and colleagues[31] evaluated fotemustine in recurrent or progressive glioblastoma in 43 patients. On radiographic review, 7.1% experienced partial responses, 34.9% had stable disease with a disease control rate (PR+SD) of 42.5%. The disease control rate was statistically greater in patients who were MGMT methylated (75.0%) compared with the unmethylated MGMT promoter (34.6%). The median PFS was 1.7 months, the PFS-6 was 20.9%, and median OS was 6 months.[31]

Fotemustine Toxicity

- Fotemustine was well tolerated in general, with grade 2 transaminase elevations in 4%, grade 3 thrombocytopenia in 8%, grade 3 anemia in 2%, grade 3 lymphopenia, and grade 4 neutropenia in 2%.[36] Grade 3/4 toxicities were found in 14% of cases. Toxicities increased to grade 3/4 thrombocytopenia in 20.9% and grade 3/4 neutropenia in 16.3% during the induction phase of the treatment.[31]

Table 3
Chemotherapies in GBM after initial treatment with radiotherapy and concomitant TMZ

Trial	Tumor Type	Timing of Treatment	Number of Patients	Chemotherapy	Median PFS (wk)	Median OS (wk)
Brandes et al,[13] 2004	GBM	Recurrent/ progressive	42	BCNU + CPT-11	17.0	46.8
Reithmeier et al,[30] 2010	GBM	Recurrent	35	BCNU	11	22
Brandes et al,[31] 2009	GBM	Recurrent/ progressive	43	Fotemustine	6.8	24.0
Scoccianti et al,[35] 2008	GBM	Recurrent	27	Fotemustine	22.8	36.4
Fabrini et al,[36] 2009	GBM	Recurrent	50	Fotemustine	24.4	32.4

SUMMARY

Irinotecan, cisplatin, and nitrosoureas have a long history of use in brain tumors, with demonstrated efficacy in the adjuvant treatment of malignant gliomas. In the era of TMZ with concurrent radiotherapy given as the standard of care, the use has shifted to that of treatment at progression or recurrence. Now with the widespread use of bevacizumab in the recurrent setting, irinotecan and other chemotherapies are seeing use in combination and alone in the recurrent setting. Despite future advancements in biologic and targeted agents, the activity of these chemotherapeutic agents in brain tumors will likely ensure a place in the armamentarium of neuro-oncologists for years to come.

REFERENCES

1. DeAngelis L, Burger P, Green S, et al. Malignant glioma: who benefits from adjuvant therapy? Ann Neurol 1998;44:691–5.
2. Stewart LA. Chemotherapy in adult high-grade glioma: a systematic review and meta-analysis of individual patient data from 12 randomised trials: Glioma Meta-Analysis Trialists (GMT) group. Lancet 2002;359:1011–8.
3. Stupp R, Mason W, van den Bent M, et al. Radiotherapy plus concomitant and adjuvant temozolomide for glioblastoma. N Engl J Med 2005;352: 987–96.
4. Bonnem E, Litterst C, Smith F. Platinum concentrations in human glioblastoma multiforme following the use of cisplatin. Cancer Treat Rep 1982;66:1661–3.
5. Yung WK, Janus T, Maor M, et al. Adjuvant chemotherapy with carmustine and cisplatin for patients with malignant gliomas. J Neuro Oncol 1992;12:131–5.
6. Lassen U, Kristjansen P, Wagner A, et al. Treatment of newly diagnosed glioblastoma multiforme with carmustine, cisplatin and etoposide followed by radiotherapy. A phase II study. J Neuro Oncol 1999;43:161–6.
7. Macdonald D, Cascino T, Schold S, et al. Response criteria for phase II studies of supratentorial malignant glioma. J Clin Oncol 1990;8:1277–80.
8. Silvani A, Gaviani P, Lamperti E, et al. Cisplatinum and BCNU chemotherapy in primary glioblastoma patients. J Neuro Oncol 2009;94:57–62.
9. Shinoda J, Sakai N, Hara A, et al. Clinical trial of external beam-radiotherapy combined with daily administration of low-dose cisplatin for supratentorial glioblastoma multiforme – a pilot study. J Neuro Oncol 1997;35:73–80.
10. Marshall NE, Ballman KV, Michalak JC, et al. Ototoxicity of cisplatin plus standard radiation therapy vs. accelerated radiation therapy in glioblastoma patients. J Neuro Oncol 2006;77:315–20.
11. Friedman H, Petros W, Friedman A, et al. Irinotecan therapy in adults with recurrent or progressive malignant glioma. J Clin Oncol 1999;17:1516–25.
12. Loghin M, Prados M, Wen P, et al. Phase I study of temozolomide and irinotecan for recurrent malignant gliomas in patients receiving enzyme-inducing anti-epileptic drugs: a North American brain tumor consortium study. Clin Cancer Res 2007;13:7133–8.
13. Brandes A, Tosoni A, Basso U, et al. Second-line chemotherapy with irinotecan plus carmustine in glioblastoma recurrent or progressive after first-line temozolomide chemotherapy: a phase II study of the Gruppo Italiano Cooperativo di Neuro-Oncologia (GICNO). J Clin Oncol 2004;22:4779–86.
14. Chamberlain MC. Salvage chemotherapy with CPT-11 for recurrent glioblastoma multiforme. J Neuro Oncol 2002;56:183–8.
15. Hare C, Elion G, Houghton P, et al. Therapeutic efficacy of the topoisomerase I inhibitor 7-ethyl-10-(4-[1-piperidino]-1-piperidino)-carbonyloxy-camptothecin against pediatric and adult central nervous system tumor xenografts. Cancer Chemother Pharmacol 1997;39:187–91.
16. Prados M, Lamborn K, Yung WK, et al. A phase 2 trial of irinotecan (CPT-11) in patients with recurrent malignant glioma: a North American brain tumor consortium study. J Neuro Oncol 2006;8:189–93.
17. Batchelor T, Gilbert M, Supko J, et al. Phase 2 study of weekly irinotecan in adults with recurrent malignant glioma: final report of NABTT 97-11. J Neuro Oncol 2004;6:21–7.
18. Von Hoff D, Rothenberg M, Pilot C, et al. Phase II trial of irinotecan (CPT-11) therapy for patients with previously treated metastatic colorectal cancer: overall results of FDA-reviewed pivotal US clinical trials. Proc Am Soc Clin Oncol 1997;16:228a.
19. Quinn J, Jiang S, Reardon D, et al. Phase II trial of temozolomide (TMZ) plus irinotecan (CPT-11) in adults with newly diagnosed glioblastoma multiforme before radiotherapy. J Neuro Oncol 2009;95:393–400.
20. Vrendenburgh J, Desjardins A, Herndon J, et al. Bevacizumab plus irinotecan in recurrent glioblastoma multiforme. J Clin Oncol 2007;25:4722–9.
21. Friedman H, Prados M, Wen P, et al. Bevacizumab alone and in combination with irinotecan in recurrent glioblastoma. J Clin Oncol 2009;27:4733–40.
22. Wolff J, Berrak S, Webb SE, et al. Nitrosourea efficacy in high-grade glioma: a survival gain analysis summarizing 504 cohorts with 24193 patients. J Neuro Oncol 2008;88:57–63.
23. Rosenblum M, Reynolds A, Smith K, et al. Chloroethyl-cyclohexyl-nitrosourea (CCNU) in the treatment of malignant brain tumors. J Neurosurg 1973;39: 306–14.
24. Reagan T, Bisel H, Childs D, et al. Controlled study of CCNU and radiation therapy in malignant astrocytomas. J Neurosurg 1976;44:186–90.

25. Herrlinger U, Rieger J, Koch D, et al. Phase II trial of lomustine plus temozolomide chemotherapy in addition to radiotherapy in newly diagnosed glioblastoma: UCT-03. J Clin Oncol 2006;24:4412–7.

26. Wick W, Puduvalli VK, Chamberlain MC, et al. Phase III study of enzastaurin compared with lomustine in the treatment of recurrent intracranial glioblastoma. J Clin Oncol 2010;28:1168–74.

27. Ballman KV, Buckner JC, Brown PD, et al. The relationship between six-month progression-free survival and 12-month overall survival end points for phase II trials in patients with glioblastoma multiforme. J Neuro Oncol 2007;9:29–38.

28. Hegi M, Diserens AC, Gorlia T, et al. MGMT gene silencing and benefit from temozolomide in glioblastoma. N Engl J Med 2005;352:997–1003.

29. Vinjamuri M, Adumala R, Altaha R, et al. Comparative analysis of temozolomide (TMZ) versus 1,3-bis(2-chloroethyl)-1 nitrosourea (BCNU) in newly diagnosed glioblastoma multiforme (GBM) patients. J Neuro Oncol 2009;91:221–5.

30. Reithmeier T, Graf E, Piroth T, et al. BCNU for recurrent glioblastoma multiforme: efficacy, toxicity and prognostic factors. BMC Cancer 2010;10:30–8.

31. Brandes A, Tosoni A, Franceschi E, et al. Fotemustine as second-line treatment for recurrent or progressive glioblastoma after concomitant and/or adjuvant temozolomide: a phase II trial of Gruppo Italiano Cooperativo di Neuro-Oncologia (GICNO). Cancer Chemother Pharmacol 2009;64:769–75.

32. Westphal M, Hilt D, Bortey E, et al. A phase 3 trial of local chemotherapy with biodegradable carmustine (BCNU) wafers (Gliadel wafers) in patients with primary malignant glioma. J Neuro Oncol 2003;5:79–88.

33. Westphal M, Ram Z, Riddle V, et al. Gliadel wafer in initial surgery for malignant glioma: long-term follow-up of a multicenter controlled trial. Acta Neurochir 2006;148:269–75.

34. McGirt M, Than K, Weingart J, et al. Gliadel (BCNU) wafer plus concomitant temozolomide therapy after primary resection of glioblastoma multiforme. J Neurosurg 2009;110:583–8.

35. Scoccianti S, Detti B, Sardaro A, et al. Second-line chemotherapy with fotemustine in temozolomide-pretreated patients with relapsing glioblastoma: a single institution experience. Anticancer Drugs 2008;19:613–20.

36. Fabrini M, Silvano G, Lolli I, et al. A multi-institutional phase II study on second-line fotemustine chemotherapy in recurrent glioblastoma. J Neuro Oncol 2009;92:79–86.

Temozolomide and Other Potential Agents for the Treatment of Glioblastoma Multiforme

Daniel T. Nagasawa, MD, Frances Chow, BA,
Andrew Yew, MD, Won Kim, MD, Nicole Cremer, BS,
Isaac Yang, MD*

KEYWORDS

- Temozolomide • Glioblastoma multiforme • BCNU wafers
- Bevacizumab • NovoTTF-100A

Key Points

- Glioblastoma multiforme is the most common primary central nervous system tumor, representing approximately 60% of all primary brain tumors in the United States
- Temozolomide has quickly become a part of the standard of care for the modern treatment of stage IV glioblastoma multiforme
- Despite its improvements from previous therapies, median survival remains dismal
- Epigenetic modulation of the MGMT promoter gene by hypermethylation results in decreased MGMT mRNA expression and increased response to temozolomide therapy
- Given the substantial population of patients with resistance to temozolomide treatment, the development of supplemental, combination, or alternative therapies is critical to optimize glioblastoma multiforme management
- Other Food and Drug Adminisration–approved therapies for glioblastoma include BCNU wafers, bevacizumab, and NovoTTF-100A

Glioblastoma multiforme (GBM) is the most common primary central nervous system tumor, representing approximately 60% of all primary brain tumors in the United States and characterized by aggressive invasion throughout adjacent parenchyma.[1] Although untreated patients generally do not survive beyond 3 months, even with optimal patient management median overall survival (OS) is approximately 15 months, with a 2-year survival rate of 8% to 26%.[1–5] Standard of care remains surgical resection with concomitant daily temozolomide (TMZ) and radiotherapy, followed by

---

UCLA Department of Neurosurgery, University of California Los Angeles, David Geffen School of Medicine at UCLA, 695 Charles East Young Drive South, UCLA Gonda 3357, Los Angeles, CA 90095–1761, USA
* Corresponding author.
E-mail address: iyang@mednet.ucla.edu

Neurosurg Clin N Am 23 (2012) 307–322
doi:10.1016/j.nec.2012.01.007
1042-3680/12/$ – see front matter © 2012 Elsevier Inc. All rights reserved.

adjuvant TMZ.[1] Given its tendency for rapid tumor growth, GBM is often diagnosed at a point when severe damage to eloquent structures has already occurred. Furthermore, expansion along the white matter tracts and across the corpus callosum is not uncommon, making gross total resection difficult and recurrence nearly inevitable.[2] Given that no standard of treatment has yet been established for recurrent tumors, many clinicians rely on TMZ retreatment with either standard or alternative dosing strategies. Although several studies have not reported any significant benefit from alternative dosing after GBM recurrence, numerous investigations are currently evaluating outcomes to optimize TMZ dosing in first- and second-line settings.[1]

Nevertheless, gross total resection remains the treatment goal (**Fig. 1**), with several studies demonstrating extent of removal being prognostic for OS.[3,4,6,7] It has been reported that with greater than 98% tumor resection, median survival time is 13 months, compared with 8.8 months when less is removed.[3] One recent analysis examining the role of extent of resection concluded that the added benefit of total versus subtotal resection confers at least 3 months of increased survival for patients.[4] However, if lesions are situated in eloquent areas, such as those involved in speech and language comprehension, adjuvant and less caustic therapies may be preferred in place of aggressive surgical resection.

Other prognostic factors have included patient age, apparent tumor necrosis, presence of edema, and Karnofsky Performance Status scores. Despite recent advancements in image-guided surgical resections[8] and the use of fluorescent 5-aminolevulinic acid,[9] surgery does not always translate to improved outcome, most notably in elderly patients with poor presurgical evaluation who present with necrosis, edema, and low Karnofsky Performance Status scores.[2,3,10,11] In a recent report focusing on patients with advanced age, median survival was 8.6 months with greater than 98% resection, and 7.8 months with less than 98% resection. This difference did not reach significance ($P = .13$),[3] indicating that there was no survival advantage appreciated for a gross total resection in older individuals. These patient populations with poor surgical outcomes remain in dire need of effective adjuvant therapy.

TMZ is a chemotherapeutic agent for treatment of glioblastoma,[11] considered standard of care since 2005. TMZ was first approved by the Food and Drug Administration (FDA) for use in recurrent GBM based on the phase II trial by Yung and colleagues[12,13] in which they demonstrated improved 6-month progression-free survival (PFS) and 6-month OS over procarbazine in 225 patients. In the pivotal phase III study, Stupp and colleagues[14] randomized 573 patients from 85 centers for treatment of newly diagnosed GBM with either radiation therapy alone or radiotherapy plus continuous daily TMZ. Their investigation demonstrated an improved 14.6-month median survival in the TMZ group, versus 12.1 months in the control group. Two-year survival was also increased to 26.5% compared with 10.4% for those treated with radiotherapy alone. Regarding long-term outcome, 5-year survival for groups receiving TMZ or radiation therapy alone was 9.8% and 1.9%, respectively.[14–18] Here, we discuss the advantages and limitations of TMZ as a treatment for glioblastoma, and explore possible directions for future research and therapeutic options.

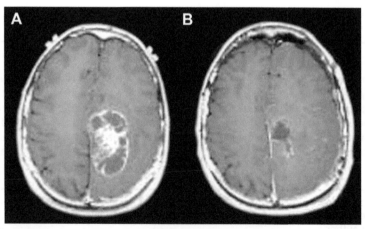

Fig. 1. Gross total resection of a glioblastoma as demonstrated by the (*A*) preoperative and (*B*) postoperative contrast-enhanced axial MRI. (*From* Hentschel SJ, Sawaya R. Optimizing outcomes with maximal surgical resection of malignant gliomas. Cancer Control 2003;10(2):109–14; with permission.)

MECHANISM OF ACTION AND PHARMACOKINETICS

TMZ is a second-generation DNA alkylating agent that disrupts malignant growth and cell cycle repair by methylating the N^7 and O^6 positions of guanine and the N^3 site on adenine 70%, 5%, and 9% of the time, respectively.[19,20] The O^6 position of guanine, although least frequently the target of TMZ, is of unique importance because its methylation results in its pairing with thymine rather than cytosine during DNA replication.[21] This pharmacologically induced injury results in crosslinking of double-stranded DNA, rendering mismatch mechanisms unable to repair the glioblastoma's damaged DNA. A series of double-stranded breaks, calcium-dependent apoptosis, and autophagy after this mismatch ultimately result in cell death.[21–23]

TMZ is an imidazotetrazine derivative prodrug that spontaneously decomposes to 5-(3-methyltriazen-1-yl)imidazole-4carboxamide (MTIC) on entering a basic environment (**Fig. 2**). Because activation of the prodrug does not require first-pass metabolism, hepatic and renal function are not a factor for its performance.[24] Because of TMZ's stability in acidic environments (pH <4), it

remains in a prodrug state while passing through the digestive system[25] and is conveniently administered orally.[26] Oral TMZ is rapidly and almost entirely (>99%) bioavailable, and physiologic conditions immediately lead to nonenzymatic decomposition of TMZ into MTIC. MTIC in turn decomposes into 4-amino-5-imidazole-carboxamide (AIC)[27,28] in acidic environments.[26,29–33]

By oral administration, mean maximum peak is at 1.2 hours and mean half-life is 1.9 hours.[29] For patients who have absorption difficulties, nausea, or are too young to swallow TMZ in pill form, intravenous TMZ is an alternative[34] that is biologically equivalent to oral TMZ, with nearly identical pharmacokinetic parameters (half-life, time of maximum peak, and clearance).[35] Because MTIC can be hydrolyzed to AIC in any tissue with subsequent clearance, TMZ does not accumulate in plasma after the standard 5-day therapy cycle. However, some AIC may remain in the body to be used as an intermediate in purine synthesis.[27–30]

Although the blood–brain barrier may be an obstacle for many therapeutic agents, TMZ is a lipophilic molecule that effectively penetrates to glioma cells.[30,36] Additionally, the blood–brain barrier surrounding these tumors is often

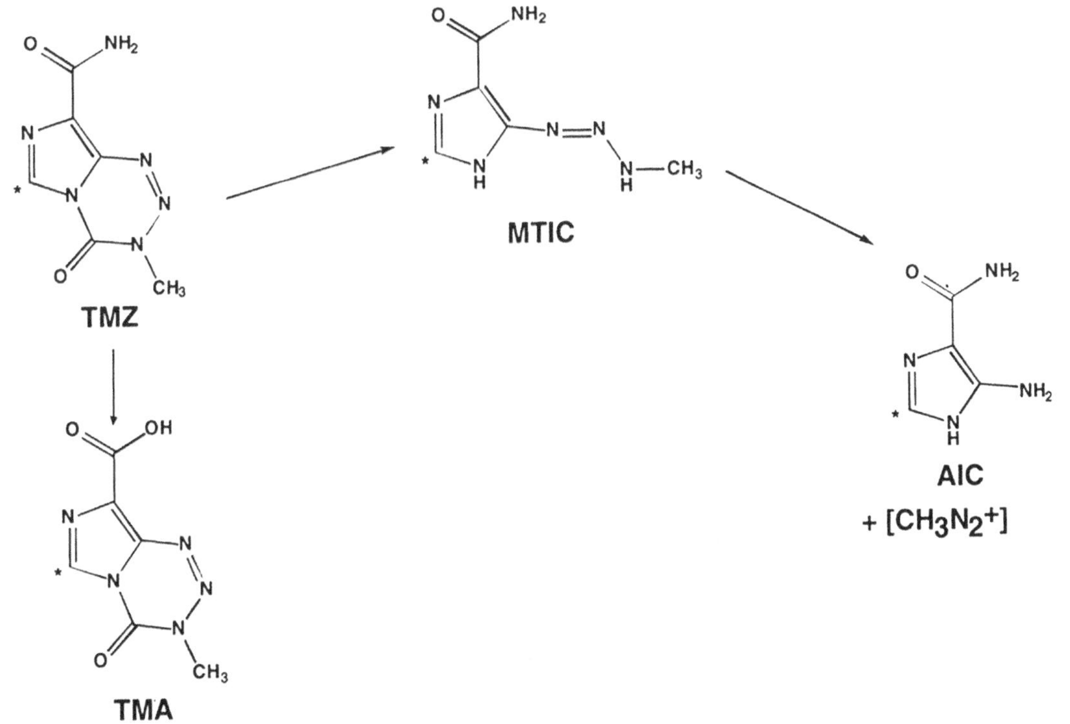

Fig. 2. Metabolic and degradation pathways of temozolomide. AIC, 4-amino-5-imidazole-carboxamide; TMA, 3-methyl-2,3-dihydro-4-oxoimidazo-[5,1-d]-tetrazine-8-carboxylic acid. (*From* Baker SD, Wirth M, Statkevich P, et al. Absorption, metabolism, and excretion of 14C-temozolomide after oral administration to patients with advanced cancer. Clin Cancer Res 1999;5(2):309–17; with permission.)

compromised, and the highly angiogenic characteristics of glioblastoma allow TMZ concentrations in malignant areas to reach higher levels than in normal surrounding tissues.[37] However, it has been suggested that GBM cells with invasion into healthy parenchyma may be exposed to decreased concentrations of TMZ compared with those in closer proximity to disruptions in the blood–brain barrier.[38]

Extensive research is currently underway to elucidate other mechanisms and cascades of TMZ toxicity on glioblastoma cells. A study into the precise changes in gene transcription and protein translation after TMZ treatment identified 1886 proteins that were expressed at greater than twofold differences.[39] Two proteins of particular interest were hypoxia-inducible factor (HIF)-1 (increased in two distinct glioblastoma cell lines between twofold and sixfold) and vascular endothelial growth factor (VEGF) (increased by twofold to fourfold). Although these specific proteins were not increased to the greatest extent compared with several others, they are implicated in control processes that are thought to promote tumorigenesis, despite the fact that TMZ has an overall antitumor effect. The stress of TMZ induces a hypoxic-like state that promotes maintenance of the regulator protein HIF-1α. In turn, HIF-1α becomes concentrated within the cell, with subsequent promotion of angiogenesis, glycolysis, cell cycle maintenance, erythropoiesis, and apoptosis.[39] Because these processes enhance tumorigenesis and autophagy,[40] authors of the study suggest the possibility of a common pathway to the activation of tumorigenesis and tumor destruction,[39] requiring further elucidation on the interplay between these seemingly opposing processes.

Furthermore, TMZ therapy may be able to activate p53 and p21$^{WAF1/Cip1}$-mediated G$_2$/M arrest with subsequent apoptosis or senescence. However, this chemotherapeutic approach in GBM cells with decreased p53 expression may have a more limited role.[38] This notion has been supported by one study demonstrating improved PFS in patients with p53 overexpression.[41]

SIDE EFFECTS AND QUALITY OF LIFE

Before the approval of TMZ, the standard of care for GBM treatment was surgical resection, followed by radiotherapy and adjuvant nitrosoureas.[14,42,43] Such agents included carmustine or the trio combination of procarbazine (an alkylating agent), lomustine (an alkylating nitrosourea), and vincristine (a mitotic inhibitor). However, these alkylating compounds, particularly lomustine, proved

highly myelosuppressive, often to the point that treatment cycles had to be halted and postponed.[11] However, studies evaluating the toxicity of TMZ demonstrated increased tolerance and improved quality of life compared with procarbazine-lomustine-vincristine therapy.[44–46]

Side effects of concomitant and adjuvant TMZ include nausea (which can be controlled by antiemetics)[47] and fatigue. Like its nitrosourea precursors, TMZ may also induce hematologic toxicity, although usually reversible and occurring in only 7% of patients.[14] Neurotoxicity may also manifest in response to TMZ, with acute events being associated with late neurotoxicity and a poorer OS.[48] However, grade III and IV adverse reactions typically present as thrombocytopenia, neutropenia,[44,49] and lymphopenia,[47] with reports of patients being at elevated risk for opportunistic infections, particularly *Pneumocystis carinii*.[14,50] In a review of TMZ-related infections, one study reported on the most frequently occurring diseases, including mucocutaneous candidiasis (28%); herpes zoster (13%); herpes simplex virus (10%); cytomegalovirus (13%); *P carinii* pneumonia (8%); hepatitis B virus (5%); and others (23%).[51] Another study suggested that higher doses of TMZ given in seven 14-day cycles led to lymphopenia in slightly more than half of their patients; however, it did not result in any infectious complications.[52] Similarly, no *P carinii* infections were reported in a children's study involving lymphopenia as a side effect of TMZ.[53] Overall, TMZ is very well-tolerated, with only 13% of patients discontinuing concomitant doses and 8% interrupting adjuvant doses because of toxicity.[14]

According to studies based on self-reported questionnaires, patients undergoing chemotherapy reported equivalent or greater quality of life (physical, emotional, social, and cognitive abilities) when under treatment with TMZ. These results were also reflective of improvement in health status because of the effectiveness of TMZ. Interestingly, quality of life status changed several weeks before disease progression, which was later measured by MRI and CT scans.[45,54]

However, a unique side effect of TMZ is pseudoprogression, the transient enhancement of diseased areas on MRI that gives the impression of tumor progression despite the overall benefit of radiotherapy and chemotherapy.[55–57] Pseudoprogression often precedes recovery and is believed to be inflammation or necrosis caused by radiation therapy and chemotherapy. TMZ cycles should be continued even if pseudoprogression occurs,[57–60] and only after three cycles should treatment be reevaluated.[61–63] Several studies report that up to 50% of progression cases are pseudoprogression,[62,63] which can be alleviated with continued TMZ administration (**Fig. 3**). As with the assessment of quality of life, the complication of pseudoprogression necessitates a more effective method of evaluating disease progression.

DOSAGE AND SCHEDULING

Because TMZ degrades within hours[29] and its effects are dose-dependent, patient adherence to dosing schedules is integral to treatment. In newly diagnosed glioblastoma, TMZ is administered concomitantly with radiation therapy at 75 mg/m^2 per day for 42 days. It is then given as an adjuvant in cycles for 5 days, each 28-day period. Dosing for the first adjuvant cycle is 150 mg/m^2 per day for 5 days, with subsequent cycles two to six at 200 mg/m^2 per day. For recurrent glioblastoma with no prior chemotherapy, dosing is 200 mg/m^2 per day for 5 days, each 28-day period. In recurrent glioblastoma with prior chemotherapy, dosing is 150 mg/m^2 per day for 5 days, each 28-day period.[64] However, alternative schedules exist and should be modified if hematologic toxicity becomes severe.

Activation of tumor cell death is an obvious goal of chemotherapy. However, several studies have suggested that TMZ may confer a cytostatic effect on a significant percentage of GBM cells, rather than a cytotoxic one. Investigations of saturating cells in 500 to 1290 μM of TMZ found 30% to 40% cell survival.[38,65,66]

One study reexamined the extensive length of dosing during concomitant treatment, claiming

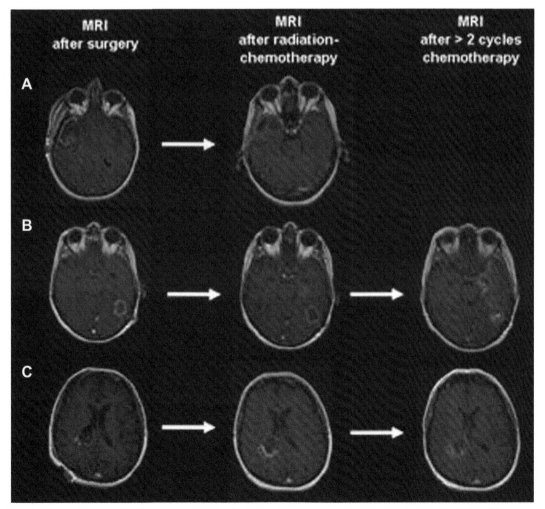

Fig. 3. T1-weighted contrast-enhanced MRI of glioblastoma demonstrating (*A*) partial response, (*B*) disease progression, and (*C*) pseudoprogression. (*From* Roldan GB, Scott JN, McIntyre JB, et al. Population-based study of pseudoprogression after chemoradiotherapy in GBM. Can J Neurol Sci 2009;36:617–22; with permission.)

that TMZ is effective even if only given during the first and last weeks of radiation therapy.[67] According to their results, median OS was reportedly 18 months, and 2-year survival rate was 34.8%. However, only 25 glioblastoma patients were included in the study, and no statistics were provided on the significance of their results compared with traditional dose scheduling. Another more extensive study compared two dose regimens of TMZ. Group A was given 50 mg/m^2 for 5 days each week on radiotherapy, whereas group B was given 75 mg/m^2 for 7 days each week on radiotherapy. Subsequently, 2-year survival rate for group A was 43%, whereas group B's 2-year survival rate was 49%, with no statistically significant difference found between groups.[68]

A study on adjuvant TMZ therapy showed that alternative dose-dense schedules (150 mg/m^2 daily for Days 1–7 and 15–28 of each 28-day cycle) confer benefits greater than standard dosing schedules, whereas metronomic adjuvant dosing (50 mg/m^2 daily, every day of 28-day cycle) did not provide any additional advantage. Two-year survival was 34.8% for dose-dense adjuvant treatment and 28% for metronomic schedules. Median OS for the dose-dense and metronomic treatments was 17.1 months and 15.1, respectively.[69] These findings reiterate the Norton-Simon model of cellular proliferation[69,70] and suggest that a dose-dense regimen may prevent glioma cells from proliferating between cycles. Although the effectiveness of alternative dosing schedules continues to be debated and requires further investigation, target dosage should minimize hematologic toxicity and avoid development of drug-resistance.[69]

Patient adherence to dosing schedules is critical in that they are designed to sufficiently overwhelm and deplete the glioma's O^6-methylguanine-DNA methyltransferase (MGMT),[14] a protein that repairs DNA by removing methyl groups from the O^6 position of guanine residues[71] and becomes permanently inactivated while reversing TMZ-induced DNA methylation. In patients with hypermethylated MGMT promoter regions, subsequent decreased protein expression leads to a reduction in DNA repair and increased tumor cell destruction.[12] General consensus throughout the literature suggests that MGMT protein expression confers an increased propensity for TMZ resistance up to 10-fold.[38,65,72]

Epigenetic modulation of the MGMT promoter gene by hypermethylation results in decreased MGMT mRNA expression and increased response to TMZ therapy (Fig. 4).[73–76] Hegi and colleagues[71] demonstrated a 21.7-month median OS in MGMT methylated patients treated with adjuvant TMZ compared with 12.7 months in patients with unmethylated promoter regions. Similarly, in MGMT-negative cells, radiotherapy with concomitant TMZ led to significant increase in survival compared with radiotherapy with adjuvant TMZ. MGMT-positive cells, however, showed no difference in survival regardless of treatment arm, supporting the significance of MGMT status in TMZ effectiveness.[19] Results remain pending from a phase III trial in which more than 1100 patients with newly diagnosed GBM received either standard-dose TMZ or dose-intensive TMZ in addition to standard therapy. This study aims to evaluate the potential of TMZ to deplete MGMT activity and improve overall patient survival.[12]

In another study involving 63 high-grade gliomas, MGMT mRNA expression was found to be a strong prognostic marker, because low levels

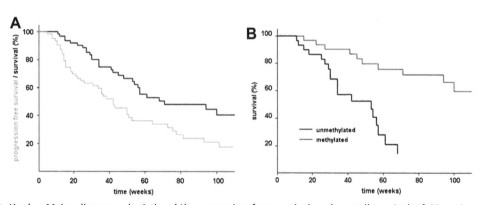

Fig. 4. Kaplan-Meier diagrams depicting (A) progression-free survival and overall survival of 63 patients with malignant gliomas, and (B) overall survival of patients according to MGMT promoter methylation status. (From Kreth S, Thon N, Eigenbrod S, et al. O6-Methylguanine-DNA methyltransferase (MGMT) mRNA expression predicts outcome in malignant glioma independent of MGMT promoter methylation. PlosOne 2011;6(2):e17156; with permission.)

was associated with prolonged time to progression, increased treatment response, and improved survival. Furthermore, mRNA expression was also correlated with MGMT promoter methylation status in most patients, and in cases of discordant findings between epigenetic and expression profiles (eg, hypermethylation with increased MGMT mRNA), MGMT mRNA was still strongly prognostic. Given evidence of incongruent findings related to methylation status and MGMT expression, methylation-independent pathways may necessitate further evaluation to elucidate the mechanisms behind MGMT mRNA expression.[75]

Sensitivity and effectiveness of TMZ treatment may be predicted by screening for epigenetic methylation of the promoter gene for MGMT. Higher methylation translates to silencing of MGMT, which is prognostic for benefit from TMZ treatment.[60,71,77–80] These patients have demonstrated a 2-year survival rate of 46%,[63] whereas only 13.8% of patients who lack such methylation survive beyond 2 years.[63,71,81–86]

TMZ AND RADIATION THERAPY

Several studies have suggested the synergistic properties of TMZ and radiotherapy.[19,65,71,87] It has been established that glioma cells under the assault of TMZ are arrested in G_2/M phase of the cell cycle, hindering them from subsequent growth and division,[40,88,89] and rendering them sensitive to radiotherapy.[89] Tsien and colleagues[90] reported findings in their study using intensity modulated radiotherapy of 75 Gy in 30 fractions, resulting in a median OS of 20.1 months. One recent evaluation of data was collected from nearly 14,000 patients throughout the United States comparing outcomes before and during the TMZ era. Before TMZ (2000–2003), patients treated with surgery and radiation therapy survived a median 12 months, whereas those within the 2005 to 2008 TMZ treatment years had a median survival of 14.2 months. However, outcomes were found to dramatically vary by age, reporting a 31.9-month survival for patients in the 20 to 29 age range, whereas those older than 80 years displayed a 5.6-month survival. Similar findings were reported by Darefsky and colleagues[91] regarding a database of nearly 20,000 patients. These findings confirm the treatment effect of TMZ in a population-based cohort.

Although the postoperative standard of care has traditionally contained fractionated irradiation doses of 60 Gy, one study evaluated the use of accelerated radiotherapy with 1.8 Gy twice daily to a total dose of 54 Gy within 3 weeks. They demonstrated that the addition of TMZ was found to prolong median OS from 11.3 to 16 months compared with those without chemotherapy. This OS was found to be similar to that of TMZ added to conventionally fractionated radiotherapy, making it a reasonable alternative. This approach has been suggested for patients with a severely limited life expectancy. However, because outpatient treatment may be quite burdensome given the frequency of treatments, considerations for quality of life should be a point of discussion.[92]

TMZ AND IMMUNOTHERAPY

Regulatory T cells may modulate the native immune system through various mechanisms. They can secrete immunosuppressive cytokines (transforming growth factor-β and interleukin-10), or may be constitutively activated and inhibit cytotoxic T lymphocytes.[93,94] In patients with melanoma, the Treg population has been shown to become decreased after prolonged exposure to low-dose TMZ.[93,95] This modulation of the GBM microenvironment may have profound effects on immunoreactivity against tumor cells. Given that radiation therapy and TMZ therapy may alter the regulatory and effector peripheral blood mononuclear cells, immunotherapeutic studies may need to consider the potential interactions of this altered immune system.[93] Furthermore, patients with GBM treated with dendritic cell vaccinations plus chemotherapy have demonstrated prolonged survival compared with those receiving the vaccination alone, with evidence suggesting that dendritic cell vaccinations may be capable of sensitizing tumor cells to the effects of TMZ.[93,96–98]

SUPPLEMENTAL, COMBINATION, AND ALTERNATIVE THERAPIES

Cancer stem cells are thought to constitute a subpopulation of tumor cells and mediate chemoresistant properties. Although the remaining tumor may undergo cell death after standard therapies, growing evidence suggests that these stem cells are responsible for GBM recurrence.[33,38] Resistance to TMZ may not only be based in genetic predisposition, but it can also be acquired, as in the case of MSH6 mutations that are found in posttreatment glioblastoma but not in pretreatment glioblastoma.[99] Given the substantial population of patients with resistance to TMZ treatment, the development of supplemental, combination, or alternative therapies is critical to optimize GBM management.

When MGMT is absent or becomes depleted, O^6-methylguanine may initiate mismatch repair (MMR) enzymes or downstream protein pathways, ultimately resulting in apoptosis and cell death. However, nearly all patients with GBM endure tumor recurrence, with most of these lesions being TMZ-resistant as a result of increased MGMT expression or decreased MMR.[100]

Although the TMZ-induced O^6-methylguanine lesion is thought to be associated with most of this chemotherapeutic's cell toxicity, the effects of N^3-methyladenine and N^7-methylguanine lesions have also been recently investigated.[100] Although N^3-methyladenine and N^7-methylguanine are thought to contribute a minimal effect on tumor destruction because of their rapid restoration by base excision repair (BER), BER inhibition may provide a potential target for applied therapeutics. The rate-limiting step in BER is thought to be DNA polymerase-β, and its inhibition has demonstrated accumulation of this pathway's substrates with increased cell sensitivity. Additionally, BER inhibition using methoxyamine hydrochloride has also been shown to increase the cytotoxic effects of N^3-methyladenine and N^7-methylguanine.[100–102]

It has been suggested that cell death after BER activation may be an energy-dependent phenomenon, because NAD^+ consumption for poly(ADP-ribose) synthesis after poly(ADP-ribose) polymerase (PARP) hyperactivation leads to ATP depletion. Alkylation sensitivity caused by failed BER may also be reversed by NAD^+ precursor supplementation, further supporting this proposed mechanism of action.[100,101] In a study by Goellner and colleagues,[100] investigators reported findings on a combined approach with inhibitors of BER (methoxyamine hydrochloride) and NAD^+ (FK866) pathways to enhance N^3-methyladenine and N^7-methylguanine tumor cell sensitivity to TMZ. They determined that TMZ resistance caused by either MMR deficiency or MGMT overexpression may be reversed by combined BER and NAD^+ biosynthetic inhibition. However, particular concern may arise from depleting NAD^+ and ATP from healthy tissue, resulting in necrotic cell death of normal parenchyma. Yet, it has been suggested that given the high energy demands of rapid tumor cell growth, the combination therapy may selectively affect GBM cells.[100,103]

In addition, PARP inhibitors may also prove beneficial in the restoration of TMZ sensitivity in MGMT unmethylated GBM, because PARP enzymes are involved in base-excision repair after TMZ N^3 and N^7 methylation. Such inhibitors have demonstrated in vitro and in vivo abilities to induce TMZ sensitivity in previously resistant glioma tumor cells.[12,104]

Another DNA repair enzyme,[45] O^6-alkylguanine-DNA alkyltransferase, plays a similar TMZ-resistant role, yet no longer remains an obstacle to treatment because its effects have been shown to be effectively inhibited by O^6-benzylguanine.[19,21,40,105,106]

Recent studies indicate that supplements, such as interferon-β, may sensitize glioma cells to TMZ treatment and can extend median OS to 19.9 months compared with TMZ-only group of 12.7 months.[107] One-year survival rates were 83.6% for the interferon-β/TMZ combination group and 67.6% for standard TMZ treatment, whereas 2-year survival rates were 34.5% and 22.1%, respectively. These effects were thought to result from the antiproliferative cascades involved with interferon-β.[107] Furthermore, other agents, such as sphingosine kinase inhibitors,[108] have also been shown to modulate and resensitize resistant gliomas to TMZ.

Current TMZ clinical trials are in pursuit of combination therapies that help to improve its effectiveness. Recent developments that target unregulated glioma growth include inhibition of tumor growth factors,[109] angiogenic agents,[110] VEGF signaling, epidermal growth factor receptors,[111] PKC/phosphatidylinositol 3-kinase (PI3K)/AKT pathways, SRC-family kinases, platelet-derived growth factor receptor, integrins, c-MET, glutamate receptors, and histone deacetylase.[1]

PI3K has been associated with cell survival, growth, and proliferation, and its regulators have been found to be mutated at a high frequency in GBM tumors. Evaluation of 209 clinical GBM samples found that 86% displayed activating mutations or genetic amplifications in the RTK/PI3K pathway.[112,113] GBM also commonly displays a mutation or loss of PTEN, a tumor suppressor that modulates the activity of PI3K and is found to be mutated or deleted in 36% of clinical GBM samples.[112,113] These PTEN alterations result in constitutively activated PI3Kinase, subsequent activation of mTOR, and resultant tumor growth and resistance to radiation.[12] Preclinical studies have suggested that inhibitors of PI3K or its downstream signaling proteins (including AKT, GSK-3, and mTOR) may confer G1 arrest of GBM cell lines in vitro and increased TMZ sensitivity in vivo.[1,114–116] In one preclinical study, a combination inhibitor of PI3K/mTOR (XL765) was used to determine the effects on intracranial, orthotopic glioma xenografts as a single agent, and as a synergistic addition to TMZ. The dual inhibition of the PI3K/mTOR pathways may be particularly important in GBM tumors, because mTOR inhibition may induce a negative feedback loop that results in increased PI3K/Akt activity. Authors of this study found that XL765 resulted in concentration-dependent cell death; inhibition of the PI3K/mTOR pathways; a decreased median tumor bioluminescence by 12-fold (indicating decreased tumor burden); and increased survival. Although TMZ alone resulted in a 30-fold decreased bioluminescence, the combination of TMZ and XL765 produced a 140-fold reduction and a trend toward improved survival compared with TMZ alone.[112] These findings indicate the potential for future phase Ib/II trials to evaluate the clinical benefit these pathway modulators may possess.

Integrins have been associated with metastasis and angiogenesis, because they play important roles in cellular adhesion, migration, and invasion. The α_v integrin inhibitor, cilengitide, has been evaluated in clinical trials reporting promising 6-month PFS rates (69%), 12-month OS (68%), 24-month OS (35%), and median OS (16 months), with particularly increased PFS and OS rates for patients with MGMT promoter methylation.[117]

Within the pediatric population, it has been discovered that malignant gliomas may be genetically distinct from those of adults, displaying a markedly decreased frequency of epidermal growth factor receptors amplification, PTEN alterations, and IDH gene mutations.[118–120] In a study evaluating 107 pediatric patients with high-grade gliomas, TMZ failed to provide any added survival benefit compared with the use of other chemotherapies during standard treatment regimens. This suggests that GBM present in pediatric patients may represent a unique entity from that of adults, necessitating age-appropriate therapeutic options.[118]

FDA-APPROVED THERAPIES

Other FDA-approved therapies for glioblastoma include BCNU wafers (approved in 1996); bevacizumab (approved in 2009); and NovoTTF-100A (approved in 2011). BCNU wafers are

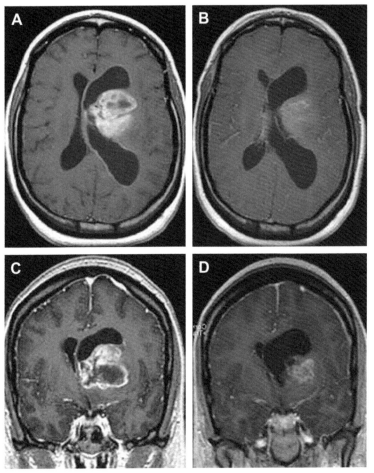

Fig. 5. Postcontrast axial and coronal T1-weighted MRIs at baseline (*A, C*) and after treatment with bevacizumab and irinotecan (*B, D*). (*From* Vredenburgh JJ, Desjardins A, Herndon JE II, et al. Bevacizumab plus irinotecan in recurrent glioblastoma multiforme. J Clin Oncol 2007;25(30):4722–9; with permission.)

a combination of carmustine chemotherapy and a polymer wafer that are administered directly into the tumor resection cavity. This therapy was approved by the FDA in 1996 for the treatment of recurrent GBM after a phase III double-blind study involving 222 patients demonstrated more than a 50% increase in 6-month survival.[121,122] After a meta-analysis of two phase III trials depicting an improved median survival of 13.1 months versus 10.9 months in the control group, FDA approval was granted in 2003 for newly diagnosed high-grade gliomas.[122–124] Thus, BCNU wafers may provide a modest treatment during the interval between surgical resection and other adjuvant therapies.[12]

Bevacizumab is a monoclonal antibody for VEGF-A that inhibits proliferation of endothelial cells and angiogenesis.[125] This therapeutic approach has been widely prescribed as treatment for other tumor types, including colorectal, breast, and lung cancers. However, its precise role for glioblastoma remains elusive. Although many studies have demonstrated improvement in radiologic response and 6-month PSF, others have failed to identify any increase in OS. However, recent findings have suggested significant benefit to patient outcomes with the administration of bevacizumab, implying the necessity for additional studies to evaluate this treatment modality (**Fig. 5**).[125–146]

NovoTTF-100A is a noninvasive external electrode system that generates "tumor treatment fields" (TTF) or alternating electric fields that arrest cell proliferation and induce apoptosis. They inhibit the proper formation of mitotic spindles, cause cells to burst when dividing,[147] and interfere with organelle assembly.[148] A phase III clinical trial showed that treatment with TTF (120 patients) had better responses and tolerance than treatment with the "best standard chemotherapy" with TMZ (117 patients). Median OS for TTF treatment was 6.6 months, compared with median OS of 6 months with chemotherapy.[148] However, the results were not statistically significant, indicating that whereas NovoTTF-100A was not a better alternative to chemotherapy, it could be considered comparable.

NovoTTF-100A offers advantages over TMZ, because the system can be used at home and lacks the side effects commonly associated with chemotherapy. Because the electric fields cannot penetrate bone, this treatment can preserve the integrity of bone marrow and other blood cells that may become injured as a result of hematologic toxicity in TMZ therapy.[147,149] NovoTTF-100A side effects include dermatitis at electrodes sites in 17% of patients[147,148,150–152] and the

theoretic risk of cardiac arrhythmia or seizures; however, these have yet to be documented in clinical trials.[6,147] NovoTTF-100A holds promise as an alternative therapy for patients who are poor surgical candidates or are unable to tolerate TMZ chemotherapy.

SUMMARY

Several advancements have been made in the treatment of glioblastoma. Benefits of TMZ include increased tolerance and improvement in OS compared with surgery alone, radiation therapy alone, or first-generation alkylating agents. Despite these advancements, myelosuppression, acquired tolerance, and dismal 2-year survival rates remain as reminders of current therapeutic limitations. Recent years have revealed novel innovations, including such therapies as BCNU wafers, bevacizumab, NovoTTF-100A, and a variety of potential adjuvants to TMZ treatment. Ultimately, it may be necessary to combine several of these approaches to best optimize the management of glioblastoma. A recent study reported that TMZ may be combined with as many as three other agents to target growth of malignant cells.[20,52] However, the potential toxicity of these multimodality treatments must be kept in mind to minimize treatment-related complications.[153] Although TMZ has provided an improvement in the management of GBM, its conferred advantage is by no means sufficient alone. Future research is necessary to augments its effects and optimize patient outcomes.

ACKNOWLEDGMENTS

Daniel Nagasawa was partially supported by an American Brain Tumor Association Medical Student Summer Fellowship in Honor of Connie Finc. Isaac Yang (senior author) was partially supported by a Visionary Fund Grant, Eli and Edythe Broad Stem Cell Research Center Scholars in Translational Medicine Program Award, and a UCLA Stein Oppenheimer grant.

REFERENCES

1. Wick W, Weller M, Weiler M, et al. Pathway inhibition: emerging molecular targets for treating glioblastoma. Neuro Oncol 2011;13(6):566–79.
2. Hentschel SJ, Lang FF. Current surgical management of glioblastoma. Cancer J 2003;9(2):113–25.
3. Lacroix M, Abi-Said D, Fourney DR, et al. A multivariate analysis of 416 patients with glioblastoma multiforme: prognosis, extent of resection, and survival. J Neurosurg 2001;95(2):190–8.

4. Sanai N, Berger MS. Glioma extent of resection and its impact on patient outcome. Neurosurgery 2008;62(4):753–64 [discussion: 264–6].

5. Galanis E, Buckner J. Chemotherapy for high-grade gliomas. Br J Cancer 2000;82(8):1371–80.

6. Sanai N, Berger MS. Operative techniques for gliomas and the value of extent of resection. Neurotherapeutics 2009;6(3):478–86.

7. Hentschel SJ, Sawaya R. Optimizing outcomes with maximal surgical resection of malignant gliomas. Cancer Control 2003;10(2):109–14.

8. Litofsky NS, Bauer AM, Kasper RS, et al. Image-guided resection of high-grade glioma: patient selection factors and outcome. Neurosurg Focus 2006;20(4):E16.

9. Stummer W, Stocker S, Wagner S, et al. Intraoperative detection of malignant gliomas by 5-aminolevulinic acid-induced porphyrin fluorescence. Neurosurgery 1998;42(3):518–25 [discussion: 525–6].

10. Kelly PJ, Hunt C. The limited value of cytoreductive surgery in elderly patients with malignant gliomas. Neurosurgery 1994;34(1):62–6 [discussion: 66–7].

11. Chinot OL, Barrie M, Frauger E, et al. Phase II study of temozolomide without radiotherapy in newly diagnosed glioblastoma multiforme in an elderly populations. Cancer 2004;100(10):2208–14.

12. Quick A, Patel D, Hadziahmetovic M, et al. Current therapeutic paradigms in glioblastoma. Rev Recent Clin Trials 2010;5(1):14–27.

13. Yung WK, Albright RE, Olson J, et al. A phase II study of temozolomide vs. procarbazine in patients with glioblastoma multiforme at first relapse. Br J Cancer 2000;83(5):588–93.

14. Stupp R, Mason WP, van den Bent MJ, et al. Radiotherapy plus concomitant and adjuvant temozolomide for glioblastoma. N Engl J Med 2005;352(10):987–96.

15. van Genugten JA, Leffers P, Baumert BG, et al. Effectiveness of temozolomide for primary glioblastoma multiforme in routine clinical practice. J Neurooncol 2010;96(2):249–57.

16. Athanassiou H, Synodinou M, Maragoudakis E, et al. Randomized phase II study of temozolomide and radiotherapy compared with radiotherapy alone in newly diagnosed glioblastoma multiforme. J Clin Oncol 2005;23(10):2372–7.

17. Combs SE, Gutwein S, Schulz-Ertner D, et al. Temozolomide combined with irradiation as postoperative treatment of primary glioblastoma multiforme. Phase I/II study. Strahlenther Onkol 2005;181(6):372–7.

18. Mirimanoff RO, Gorlia T, Mason W, et al. Radiotherapy and temozolomide for newly diagnosed glioblastoma: recursive partitioning analysis of the EORTC 26981/22981-NCIC CE3 phase III randomized trial. J Clin Oncol 2006;24(16):2563–9.

19. Chakravarti A, Erkkinen MG, Nestler U, et al. Temozolomide-mediated radiation enhancement in glioblastoma: a report on underlying mechanisms. Clin Cancer Res 2006;12(15):4738–46.

20. Zhang M, Chakravarti A. Novel radiation-enhancing agents in malignant gliomas. Semin Radiat Oncol 2006;16(1):29–37.

21. Kanzawa T, Bedwell J, Kondo Y, et al. Inhibition of DNA repair for sensitizing resistant glioma cells to temozolomide. J Neurosurg 2003;99(6):1047–52.

22. Clark AS, Deans B, Stevens MF, et al. Antitumor imidazotetrazines. 32. Synthesis of novel imidazotetrazinones and related bicyclic heterocycles to probe the mode of action of the antitumor drug temozolomide. J Med Chem 1995;38(9):1493–504.

23. Karran P, Hampson R. Genomic instability and tolerance to alkylating agents. Cancer Surv 1996;28:69–85.

24. Panetta JC, Kirstein MN, Gajjar A, et al. Population pharmacokinetics of temozolomide and metabolites in infants and children with primary central nervous system tumors. Cancer Chemother Pharmacol 2003;52(6):435–41.

25. Beale P, Judson I, Moore S, et al. Effect of gastric pH on the relative oral bioavailability and pharmacokinetics of temozolomide. Cancer Chemother Pharmacol 1999;44(5):389–94.

26. Marzolini C, Decosterd LA, Shen F, et al. Pharmacokinetics of temozolomide in association with fotemustine in malignant melanoma and malignant glioma patients: comparison of oral, intravenous, and hepatic intra-arterial administration. Cancer Chemother Pharmacol 1998;42(6):433–40.

27. Horgan CM, Tisdale MJ. Antitumour imidazotetrazines–VIII. Uptake and decomposition of a novel antitumour agent mitozolomide (CCRG 81010; M and B 39565; NSC 353451) in TLX5 mouse lymphoma in vitro. Biochem Pharmacol 1985;34(2):217–21.

28. Schulman MP, Buchanan JM. Biosynthesis of the purines. II. Metabolism of 4-amino-5-imidazolecarboxamide in pigeon liver. J Biol Chem 1952;196(2):513–26.

29. Baker SD, Wirth M, Statkevich P, et al. Absorption, metabolism, and excretion of 14C-temozolomide following oral administration to patients with advanced cancer. Clin Cancer Res 1999;5(2):309–17.

30. Reyderman L, Statkevich P, Thonoor CM, et al. Disposition and pharmacokinetics of temozolomide in rat. Xenobiotica 2004;34(5):487–500.

31. Meany HJ, Warren KE, Fox E, et al. Pharmacokinetics of temozolomide administered in combination with O6-benzylguanine in children and adolescents with refractory solid tumors. Cancer Chemother Pharmacol 2009;65(1):137–42.

32. Riccardi A, Mazzarella G, Cefalo G, et al. Pharmacokinetics of temozolomide given three times a day

in pediatric and adult patients. Cancer Chemother Pharmacol 2003;52(6):459–64.

33. Jen JF, Cutler DL, Pai SM, et al. Population pharmacokinetics of temozolomide in cancer patients. Pharm Res 2000;17(10):1284–9.

34. Motomura K, Natsume A, Fujii M, et al. Clinical experience of intravenous temozolomide therapy for gliomas. J Clin Oncol 2011;29(Suppl):[abstract: e12523].

35. Diez BD, Statkevich P, Zhu Y, et al. Evaluation of the exposure equivalence of oral versus intravenous temozolomide. Cancer Chemother Pharmacol 2010;65(4):727–34.

36. Patel M, McCully C, Godwin K, et al. Plasma and cerebrospinal fluid pharmacokinetics of intravenous temozolomide in non-human primates. J Neurooncol 2003;61(3):203–7.

37. Rosso L, Brock CS, Gallo JM, et al. A new model for prediction of drug distribution in tumor and normal tissues: pharmacokinetics of temozolomide in glioma patients. Cancer Res 2009;69(1):120–7.

38. Beier D, Schulz JB, Beier CP. Chemoresistance of glioblastoma cancer stem cells: much more complex than expected. Mol Cancer 2011;10:128.

39. Fisher T, Galanti G, Lavie G, et al. Mechanisms operative in the antitumor activity of temozolomide in glioblastoma multiforme. Cancer J 2007;13(5): 335–44.

40. Lefranc F, Facchini V, Kiss R. Proautophagic drugs: a novel means to combat apoptosis-resistant cancers, with a special emphasis on glioblastomas. Oncologist 2007;12(12):1395–403.

41. Malkoun N, Chargari C, Forest F, et al. Prolonged temozolomide for treatment of glioblastoma: preliminary clinical results and prognostic value of p53 overexpression. J Neurooncol 2012;106(1): 127–33.

42. Walker MD, Alexander E Jr, Hunt WE, et al. Evaluation of BCNU and/or radiotherapy in the treatment of anaplastic gliomas. A cooperative clinical trial. J Neurosurg 1978;49(3):333–43.

43. Walker MD, Green SB, Byar DP, et al. Randomized comparisons of radiotherapy and nitrosoureas for the treatment of malignant glioma after surgery. N Engl J Med 1980;303(23):1323–9.

44. van den Bent MJ, Taphoorn MJ, Brandes AA, et al. Phase II study of first-line chemotherapy with temozolomide in recurrent oligodendroglial tumors: the European Organization for Research and Treatment of Cancer Brain Tumor Group Study 26971. J Clin Oncol 2003;21(13):2525–8.

45. Osoba D, Brada M, Yung WK, et al. Health-related quality of life in patients with anaplastic astrocytoma during treatment with temozolomide. Eur J Cancer 2000;36(14):1788–95.

46. Perry J, Laperriere N, Zuraw L, et al. Adjuvant chemotherapy for adults with malignant glioma:

a systematic review. Can J Neurol Sci 2007;34(4): 402–10.

47. Kocher M, Kunze S, Eich HT, et al. Efficacy and toxicity of postoperative temozolomide radiochemotherapy in malignant glioma. Strahlenther Onkol 2005;181(3):157–63.

48. Lawrence YR, Wang M, Dicker AP, et al. Early toxicity predicts long-term survival in high-grade glioma. Br J Cancer 2011;104(9):1365–71.

49. Lanzetta G, Campanella C, Rozzi A, et al. Temozolomide in radio-chemotherapy combined treatment for newly-diagnosed glioblastoma multiforme: phase II clinical trial. Anticancer Res 2003;23(6D):5159–64.

50. Kovacs JA, Masur H. Prophylaxis against opportunistic infections in patients with human immunodeficiency virus infection. N Engl J Med 2000;342(19): 1416–29.

51. Kizilarslanoglu MC, Aksoy S, Yildirim NO, et al. Temozolomide-related infections: review of the literature. J BUON 2011;16(3):547–50.

52. Gilbert MR, Gonzalez J, Hunter K, et al. A phase I factorial design study of dose-dense temozolomide alone and in combination with thalidomide, isotretinoin, and/or celecoxib as postchemoradiation adjuvant therapy for newly diagnosed glioblastoma. Neuro Oncol 2010;12(11):1167–72.

53. Baruchel S, Diezi M, Hargrave D, et al. Safety and pharmacokinetics of temozolomide using a dose-escalation, metronomic schedule in recurrent paediatric brain tumours. Eur J Cancer 2006; 42(14):2335–42.

54. Taphoorn MJ, Stupp R, Coens C, et al. Health-related quality of life in patients with glioblastoma: a randomised controlled trial. Lancet Oncol 2005; 6(12):937–44.

55. Brandsma D, Stalpers L, Taal W, et al. Clinical features, mechanisms, and management of pseudoprogression in malignant gliomas. Lancet 2008; 9(5):453–61.

56. Chamberlain MC, Glantz MJ, Chalmers L, et al. Early necrosis following concurrent Temodar and radiotherapy in patients with glioblastoma. J Neurooncol 2007;82(1):81–3.

57. de Wit MC, de Bruin HG, Eijkenboom W, et al. Immediate post-radiotherapy changes in malignant glioma can mimic tumor progression. Neurology 2004;63(3):535–7.

58. Rosenthal MA, Ashley DL, Cher L. Temozolomide-induced flare in high-grade gliomas: a new clinical entity. Intern Med J 2002;32(7):346–8.

59. Taal W, Brandsma D, de Bruin HG, et al. Incidence of early pseudo-progression in a cohort of malignant glioma patients treated with chemoirradiation with temozolomide. Cancer 2008;113(2):405–10.

60. Brandes AA, Franceschi E, Tosoni A, et al. MGMT promoter methylation status can predict the incidence and outcome of pseudoprogression after

concomitant radiochemotherapy in newly diagnosed glioblastoma patients. J Clin Oncol 2008; 26(13):2192–7.

61. Easaw JC, Mason WP, Perry J, et al. Canadian recommendations for the treatment of recurrent or progressive glioblastoma multiforme. Curr Oncol 2011;18(3):e126–36.

62. Mason WP, Maestro RD, Eisenstat D, et al. Canadian recommendations for the treatment of glioblastoma multiforme. Curr Oncol 2007;14(3):110–7.

63. Roldan GB, Scott JN, McIntyre JB, et al. Population-based study of pseudoprogression after chemoradiotherapy in GBM. Can J Neurol Sci 2009; 36(5):617–22.

64. Villano J, Seery T, Bressler L. Temozolomide in malignant gliomas: current use and future targets. Cancer Chemother Pharmacol 2009;64:647–55.

65. Hermisson M, Klumpp A, Wick W, et al. O6-methylguanine DNA methyltransferase and p53 status predict temozolomide sensitivity in human malignant glioma cells. J Neurochem 2006;96(3):766–76.

66. Combs SE, Schulz-Ertner D, Roth W, et al. In vitro responsiveness of glioma cell lines to multimodality treatment with radiotherapy, temozolomide, and epidermal growth factor receptor inhibition with cetuximab. Int J Radiat Oncol Biol Phys 2007;68(3): 873–82.

67. Balducci M, D'Agostino GR, Manfrida S, et al. Radiotherapy and concomitant temozolomide during the first and last weeks in high grade gliomas: long-term analysis of a phase II study. J Neurooncol 2010;97(1):95–100.

68. Combs SE, Wagner J, Bischof M, et al. Radiochemotherapy in patients with primary glioblastoma comparing two temozolomide dose regimens. Int J Radiat Oncol Biol Phys 2008;71(4):999–1005.

69. Clarke JL, Iwamoto FM, Sul J, et al. Randomized phase II trial of chemoradiotherapy followed by either dose-dense or metronomic temozolomide for newly diagnosed glioblastoma. J Clin Oncol 2009;27(23):3861–7.

70. Simon R, Norton L. The Norton-Simon hypothesis: designing more effective and less toxic chemotherapeutic regimens. Nat Clin Pract Oncol 2006;3(8): 406–7.

71. Hegi ME, Diserens AC, Gorlia T, et al. MGMT gene silencing and benefit from temozolomide in glioblastoma. N Engl J Med 2005;352(10):997–1003.

72. Beier D, Rohrl S, Pillai DR, et al. Temozolomide preferentially depletes cancer stem cells in glioblastoma. Cancer Res 2008;68(14):5706–15.

73. Lam N, Chambers CR. Temozolomide plus radiotherapy for glioblastoma in a Canadian province: efficacy versus effectiveness and the impact of O6-methylguanine-DNA-methyltransferase promoter methylation. J Oncol Pharm Pract 2011 Nov 7. [Epub ahead of print].

74. Hegi ME, Diserens AC, Godard S, et al. Clinical trial substantiates the predictive value of O-6-methylguanine-DNA methyltransferase promoter methylation in glioblastoma patients treated with temozolomide. Clin Cancer Res 2004;10(6): 1871–4.

75. Kreth S, Thon N, Eigenbrod S, et al. O-methylguanine-DNA methyltransferase (MGMT) mRNA expression predicts outcome in malignant glioma independent of MGMT promoter methylation. PLoS One 2011;6(2):e17156.

76. Felsberg J, Rapp M, Loeser S, et al. Prognostic significance of molecular markers and extent of resection in primary glioblastoma patients. Clin Cancer Res 2009;15(21):6683–93.

77. Costa BM, Caeiro C, Guimaraes I, et al. Prognostic value of MGMT promoter methylation in glioblastoma patients treated with temozolomide-based chemoradiation: a Portuguese multicentre study. Oncol Rep 2010;23(6):1655–62.

78. Sardi I, Cetica V, Massimino M, et al. Promoter methylation and expression analysis of MGMT in advanced pediatric brain tumors. Oncol Rep 2009;22(4):773–9.

79. Weiler M, Hartmann C, Wiewrodt D, et al. Chemoradiotherapy of newly diagnosed glioblastoma with intensified temozolomide. Int J Radiat Oncol Biol Phys 2010;77(3):670–6.

80. Watanabe R, Nakasu Y, Tashiro H, et al. O6-methylguanine DNA methyltransferase expression in tumor cells predicts outcome of radiotherapy plus concomitant and adjuvant temozolomide therapy in patients with primary glioblastoma. Brain Tumor Pathol 2011;28(2):127–35.

81. Gerson SL. MGMT: its role in cancer aetiology and cancer therapeutics. Nat Rev Cancer 2004;4(4): 296–307.

82. Hotta T, Saito Y, Fujita H, et al. O6-alkylguanine-DNA alkyltransferase activity of human malignant glioma and its clinical implications. J Neurooncol 1994;21(2):135–40.

83. Belanich M, Pastor M, Randall T, et al. Retrospective study of the correlation between the DNA repair protein alkyltransferase and survival of brain tumor patients treated with carmustine. Cancer Res 1996;56(4):783–8.

84. Jaeckle KA, Eyre HJ, Townsend JJ, et al. Correlation of tumor O6 methylguanine-DNA methyltransferase levels with survival of malignant astrocytoma patients treated with bis-chloroethylnitrosourea: a Southwest Oncology Group study. J Clin Oncol 1998;16(10):3310–5.

85. Friedman HS, McLendon RE, Kerby T, et al. DNA mismatch repair and O6-alkylguanine-DNA alkyltransferase analysis and response to Temodal in newly diagnosed malignant glioma. J Clin Oncol 1998;16(12):3851–7.

86. Silber JR, Blank A, Bobola MS, et al. O6-methyl-guanine-DNA methyltransferase-deficient phenotype in human gliomas: frequency and time to tumor progression after alkylating agent-based chemotherapy. Clin Cancer Res 1999;5(4):807–14.

87. Sridhar T, Gore A, Boiangiu I, et al. Concomitant (without adjuvant) temozolomide and radiation to treat glioblastoma: a retrospective study. Clin Oncol 2009;21(1):19–22.

88. Hirose Y, Berger MS, Pieper RO. p53 effects both the duration of G2/M arrest and the fate of temozolomide-treated human glioblastoma cells. Cancer Res 2001;61(5):1957–63.

89. Stupp R, Dietrich PY, Ostermann Kraljevic S, et al. Promising survival for patients with newly diagnosed glioblastoma multiforme treated with concomitant radiation plus temozolomide followed by adjuvant temozolomide. J Clin Oncol 2002; 20(5):1375–82.

90. Tsien CI, Brown D, Normolle D, et al. Concurrent temozolomide and dose-escalated intensity-modulated radiation therapy in newly diagnosed glioblastoma. Clin Cancer Res 2012;18(1):273–9.

91. Darefsky AS, King JT Jr, Dubrow R. Adult glioblastoma multiforme survival in the temozolomide era: a population-based analysis of surveillance, epidemiology, and end results registries. Cancer 2011. DOI:10.1002/cncr.26494. [Epub ahead of print].

92. Guckenberger M, Mayer M, Buttmann M, et al. Prolonged survival when temozolomide is added to accelerated radiotherapy for glioblastoma multiforme. Strahlenther Onkol 2011;187(9):548–54.

93. Fadul CE, Fisher JL, Gui J, et al. Immune modulation effects of concomitant temozolomide and radiation therapy on peripheral blood mononuclear cells in patients with glioblastoma multiforme. Neuro Oncol 2011;13(4):393–400.

94. Wang HY, Wang RF. Antigen-specific CD4+ regulatory T cells in cancer: implications for immunotherapy. Microbes Infect 2005;7(7–8): 1056–62.

95. Su YB, Sohn S, Krown SE, et al. Selective CD4+ lymphopenia in melanoma patients treated with temozolomide: a toxicity with therapeutic implications. J Clin Oncol 2004;22(4):610–6.

96. Liau LM, Prins RM, Kiertscher SM, et al. Dendritic cell vaccination in glioblastoma patients induces systemic and intracranial T-cell responses modulated by the local central nervous system tumor microenvironment. Clin Cancer Res 2005;11(15): 5515–25.

97. Wheeler CJ, Das A, Liu G, et al. Clinical responsiveness of glioblastoma multiforme to chemotherapy after vaccination. Clin Cancer Res 2004; 10(16):5316–26.

98. Liu G, Akasaki Y, Khong HT, et al. Cytotoxic T cell targeting of TRP-2 sensitizes human malignant glioma to chemotherapy. Oncogene 2005;24(33): 5226–34.

99. Yip S, Miao J, Cahill DP, et al. MSH6 mutations arise in glioblastomas during temozolomide therapy and mediate temozolomide resistance. Clin Cancer Res 2009;15(14):4622–9.

100. Goellner EM, Grimme B, Brown AR, et al. Overcoming temozolomide resistance in glioblastoma via dual inhibition of NAD+ biosynthesis and base excision repair. Cancer Res 2011;71(6): 2308–17.

101. Tang JB, Goellner EM, Wang XH, et al. Bioenergetic metabolites regulate base excision repair-dependent cell death in response to DNA damage. Mol Cancer Res 2010;8(1):67–79.

102. Fishel ML, He Y, Smith ML, et al. Manipulation of base excision repair to sensitize ovarian cancer cells to alkylating agent temozolomide. Clin Cancer Res 2007;13(1):260–7.

103. Watson M, Roulston A, Belec L, et al. The small molecule GMX1778 is a potent inhibitor of NAD+ biosynthesis: strategy for enhanced therapy in nicotinic acid phosphoribosyltransferase 1-deficient tumors. Mol Cell Biol 2009;29(21):5872–88.

104. Russo AL, Kwon HC, Burgan WE, et al. In vitro and in vivo radiosensitization of glioblastoma cells by the poly (ADP-ribose) polymerase inhibitor E7016. Clin Cancer Res 2009;15(2):607–12.

105. Quinn JA, Jiang SX, Reardon DA, et al. Phase II trial of temozolomide plus o6-benzylguanine in adults with recurrent, temozolomide-resistant malignant glioma. J Clin Oncol 2009;27(8): 1262–7.

106. Koch D, Hundsberger T, Boor S, et al. Local intracerebral administration of O(6)-benzylguanine combined with systemic chemotherapy with temozolomide of a patient suffering from a recurrent glioblastoma. J Neurooncol 2007;82(1):85–9.

107. Motomura K, Natsume A, Kishida Y, et al. Benefits of interferon-beta and temozolomide combination therapy for newly diagnosed primary glioblastoma with the unmethylated MGMT promoter: a multicenter study. Cancer 2010. [Epub ahead of print].

108. Bektas M, Johnson SP, Poe WE, et al. A sphingosine kinase inhibitor induces cell death in temozolomide resistant glioblastoma cells. Cancer Chemother Pharmacol 2009;64(5): 1053–8.

109. Bogdahn U, Hau P, Stockhammer G, et al. Targeted therapy for high-grade glioma with the TGF-beta2 inhibitor trabedersen: results of a randomized and controlled phase IIb study. Neuro Oncol 2011; 13(1):132–42.

110. Beal K, Abrey LE, Gutin PH. Antiangiogenic agents in the treatment of recurrent or newly diagnosed glioblastoma: analysis of single-agent and combined modality approaches. Radiat Oncol 2011;6:2.

111. Sampson JH, Heimberger AB, Archer GE, et al. Immunologic escape after prolonged progression-free survival with epidermal growth factor receptor variant III peptide vaccination in patients with newly diagnosed glioblastoma. J Clin Oncol 2010;28(31): 4722–9.

112. Prasad G, Sottero T, Yang X, et al. Inhibition of PI3K/mTOR pathways in glioblastoma and implications for combination therapy with temozolomide. Neuro Oncol 2011;13(4):384–92.

113. McLendon R, Friedman A, Bigner D, et al. Comprehensive genomic characterization defines human glioblastoma genes and core pathways. Nature 2008;455(7216):1061–8.

114. Cheng CK, Fan QW, Weiss WA. PI3K signaling in glioma–animal models and therapeutic challenges. Brain Pathol 2009;19(1):112–20.

115. Maira SM, Stauffer F, Brueggen J, et al. Identification and characterization of NVP-BEZ235, a new orally available dual phosphatidylinositol 3-kinase/mammalian target of rapamycin inhibitor with potent in vivo antitumor activity. Mol Cancer Ther 2008;7(7):1851–63.

116. Opel D, Westhoff MA, Bender A, et al. Phosphatidylinositol 3-kinase inhibition broadly sensitizes glioblastoma cells to death receptor- and drug-induced apoptosis. Cancer Res 2008;68(15):6271–80.

117. Stupp R, Hegi ME, Neyns B, et al. Phase I/IIa study of cilengitide and temozolomide with concomitant radiotherapy followed by cilengitide and temozolomide maintenance therapy in patients with newly diagnosed glioblastoma. J Clin Oncol 2010; 28(16):2712–8.

118. Cohen KJ, Pollack IF, Zhou T, et al. Temozolomide in the treatment of high-grade gliomas in children: a report from the Children's Oncology Group. Neuro Oncol 2011;13(3):317–23.

119. Pollack IF, Hamilton RL, James CD, et al. Rarity of PTEN deletions and EGFR amplification in malignant gliomas of childhood: results from the Children's Cancer Group 945 cohort. J Neurosurg 2006;105(Suppl 5):418–24.

120. Parsons DW, Jones S, Zhang X, et al. An integrated genomic analysis of human glioblastoma multiforme. Science 2008;321(5897):1807–12.

121. Brem H, Piantadosi S, Burger PC, et al. Placebo-controlled trial of safety and efficacy of intraoperative controlled delivery by biodegradable polymers of chemotherapy for recurrent gliomas. The Polymer-brain Tumor Treatment Group. Lancet 1995;345(8956):1008–12.

122. Bota DA, Desjardins A, Quinn JA, et al. Interstitial chemotherapy with biodegradable BCNU (Gliadel) wafers in the treatment of malignant gliomas. Ther Clin Risk Manag 2007;3(5):707–15.

123. Valtonen S, Timonen U, Toivanen P, et al. Interstitial chemotherapy with carmustine-loaded polymers for high-grade gliomas: a randomized double-blind study. Neurosurgery 1997;41(1):44–8 [discussion: 48–9].

124. Westphal M, Hilt DC, Bortey E, et al. A phase 3 trial of local chemotherapy with biodegradable carmustine (BCNU) wafers (Gliadel wafers) in patients with primary malignant glioma. Neuro Oncol 2003;5(2): 79–88.

125. Vredenburgh JJ, Desjardins A, Herndon JE II, et al. Phase II trial of bevacizumab and irinotecan in recurrent malignant glioma. Clin Cancer Res 2007;13(4):1253–9.

126. Pope WB, Lai A, Nghiemphu P, et al. MRI in patients with high-grade gliomas treated with bevacizumab and chemotherapy. Neurology 2006; 66(8):1258–60.

127. Vredenburgh JJ, Desjardins A, Reardon DA, et al. The addition of bevacizumab to standard radiation therapy and temozolomide followed by bevacizumab, temozolomide, and irinotecan for newly diagnosed glioblastoma. Clin Cancer Res 2011;17(12): 4119–24.

128. Mendelsohn J, Baselga J. The EGF receptor family as targets for cancer therapy. Oncogene 2000; 19(56):6550–65.

129. Wong ET, Gautam S, Malchow C, et al. Bevacizumab for recurrent glioblastoma multiforme: a meta-analysis. J Natl Compr Canc Netw 2011;9(4):403–7.

130. de Groot JF, Yung WK. Bevacizumab and irinotecan in the treatment of recurrent malignant gliomas. Cancer J 2008;14(5):279–85.

131. Norden AD, Young GS, Setayesh K, et al. Bevacizumab for recurrent malignant gliomas: efficacy, toxicity, and patterns of recurrence. Neurology 2008;70(10):779–87.

132. Friedman HS, Prados MD, Wen PY, et al. Bevacizumab alone and in combination with irinotecan in recurrent glioblastoma. J Clin Oncol 2009;27(28): 4733–40.

133. Salmaggi A, Gaviani P, Botturi A, et al. Bevacizumab at recurrence in high-grade glioma. Neurol Sci 2011;2(Suppl 2):S251–3.

134. Addeo R, Caraglia M, De Santi MS, et al. A new schedule of fotemustine in temozolomide-pretreated patients with relapsing glioblastoma. J Neurooncol 2011;102(3):417–24.

135. Scoccianti S, Detti B, Sardaro A, et al. Second-line chemotherapy with fotemustine in temozolomide-pretreated patients with relapsing glioblastoma: a single institution experience. Anticancer Drugs 2008;19(6):613–20.

136. Kreisl TN, Kim L, Moore K, et al. Phase II trial of single-agent bevacizumab followed by bevacizumab plus irinotecan at tumor progression in recurrent glioblastoma. J Clin Oncol 2009;27(5):740–5.

137. Hofer S, Elandt K, Greil R, et al. Clinical outcome with bevacizumab in patients with recurrent

high-grade glioma treated outside clinical trials. Acta Oncol 2011;50(5):630–5.

138. Reardon DA, Desjardins A, Peters KB, et al. Phase II study of carboplatin, irinotecan, and bevacizumab for bevacizumab naive, recurrent glioblastoma. J Neurooncol 2011. [Epub ahead of print].

139. Vredenburgh JJ, Desjardins A, Herndon JEII, et al. Bevacizumab plus irinotecan in recurrent glioblastoma multiforme. J Clin Oncol 2007;25(30):4722–9.

140. Reardon DA, Desjardins A, Vredenburgh JJ, et al. Metronomic chemotherapy with daily, oral etoposide plus bevacizumab for recurrent malignant glioma: a phase II study. Br J Cancer 2009; 101(12):1986–94.

141. Hasselbalch B, Lassen U, Hansen S, et al. Cetuximab, bevacizumab, and irinotecan for patients with primary glioblastoma and progression after radiation therapy and temozolomide: a phase II trial. Neuro Oncol 2010;12(5):508–16.

142. Pu JK, Chan RT, Ng GK, et al. Using bevacizumab in the fight against malignant glioma: first results in Asian patients. Hong Kong Med J 2011;17(4):274–9.

143. Lamborn KR, Chang SM, Prados MD. Prognostic factors for survival of patients with glioblastoma: recursive partitioning analysis. Neuro Oncol 2004; 6(3):227–35.

144. Ballman KV, Buckner JC, Brown PD, et al. The relationship between six-month progression-free survival and 12-month overall survival end points for phase II trials in patients with glioblastoma multiforme. Neuro Oncol 2007;9(1):29–38.

145. Franceschi E, Brandes AA. Clinical end points in recurrent glioblastoma: are antiangiogenic agents friend or foe? Expert Rev Anticancer Ther 2011; 11(5):657–60.

146. Thompson EM, Frenkel EP, Neuwelt EA. The paradoxical effect of bevacizumab in the therapy of malignant gliomas. Neurology 2011;76(1):87–93.

147. Kirson ED, Dbaly V, Tovarys F, et al. Alternating electric fields arrest cell proliferation in animal tumor models and human brain tumors. Proc Natl Acad Sci U S A 2007;104(24):10152–7.

148. Stupp R, Kanner A, Engelhard H, et al. A prospective, randomized, open-label, phase III clinical trial of NovoTTF-100A versus best standard of care chemotherapy in patients with recurrent glioblastoma. J Clin Oncol 2010;28(Suppl 18): [abstract: LBA2007].

149. Bronzino J. The biomedical engineering handbook. Boca Raton (FL): CRC, IEEE Press; 1995. p. 1–1656.

150. Burnette RR, Ongpipattanakul B. Characterization of the pore transport properties and tissue alteration of excised human skin during iontophoresis. J Pharm Sci 1988;77(2):132–7.

151. Cho MR, Thatte HS, Silvia MT, et al. Transmembrane calcium influx induced by ac electric fields. FASEB J 1999;13(6):677–83.

152. Orrenius S, McCabe MJ Jr, Nicotera P. Ca(2+)-dependent mechanisms of cytotoxicity and programmed cell death. Toxicol Lett 1992;64–65(Spec No): 357–64.

153. Bock HC, Puchner MJ, Lohmann F, et al. First-line treatment of malignant glioma with carmustine implants followed by concomitant radiochemotherapy: a multicenter experience. Neurosurg Rev 2010;33(4):441–9.

Superselective Intra-Arterial Cerebral Infusion of Novel Agents After Blood–Brain Disruption for the Treatment of Recurrent Glioblastoma Multiforme: A Technical Case Series

Benjamin J. Shin, BS[a], Jan-Karl Burkhardt, MD[a],
Howard A. Riina, MD[a], John A. Boockvar, MD[a,b],*

KEYWORDS

- Glioblastoma multiforme • Intra-arterial chemotherapy
- Bevacizumab • Cetuximab • Temozolomide

Every year approximately 12,000 cases of glioblastoma multiforme (GBM) are newly diagnosed in the United States,[1] constituting the most common primary brain tumor. GBM carries a grim prognosis with a 2-year survival rate after diagnosis of approximately 26.5%,[2,3] even with a multidisciplinary treatment including surgical resection followed by radiation therapy and concomitant temozolomide.[4] Once the tumor recurs, patients are treated with several chemotherapeutic agents, such as bevacizumab and irinotecan, which have been shown to improve progression-free survival and overall survival.[5] Because treatment effects are modest and nothing to date has been shown to extend life satisfactorily, there is a great need for novel therapeutics. Several novel therapeutic modalities are under study and development, including immunotherapies involving tumor vaccines[6] and selective intra-arterial (IA) delivery of chemotherapeutics.[7]

Application of IA delivery of chemotherapeutics to treat malignant gliomas was introduced into clinical practice decades ago with the IA infusion of carmustine by an intracarotid approach.[8] These early studies showed no survival difference between IA and intravenous administration and even revealed a high complication rate, such as white matter necrosis or blindness in patients treated with the IA approach, which most likely occurred as a result of unselective catheter use and direct infusion of toxic agents.[9–11] Recently, however, modern specialized microcatheters are better able to selectively deliver drugs to distal tumor vessels to enhance local drug delivery.[12,13] At our institution, we use specialized microcatheters for superselective infusion of bevacizumab, cetuximab, and temozolomide. Our phase I trial revealed that the use of IA bevacizumab after blood–brain barrier disruption (BBBD) for recurrent GBM is safe and well tolerated.[7]

[a] Department of Neurological Surgery, New York–Presbyterian Hospital, Weill Cornell Medical College, 525 East 68th Street, Box 99, New York, NY 10021, USA
[b] Department of Neurological Surgery, Weill Cornell Brain Tumor Center, Weill Cornell Medical College, New York–Presbyterian Hospital, 525 East 68th Street, Box 99, New York, NY 10021, USA
* Corresponding author. Department of Neurological Surgery, Weill Cornell Brain Tumor Center, Weill Cornell Medical College, New York–Presbyterian Hospital, 525 East 68th Street, Box 99, New York, NY 10021.
E-mail address: jab2029@nyp.org

Neurosurg Clin N Am 23 (2012) 323–329
doi:10.1016/j.nec.2012.01.008
1042-3680/12/ ... ee front matter © 2012 Elsevier Inc. All rights reserved.

Here, we present a technical case series of patients who received IA delivery of bevacizumab, cetuximab, or temozolamide after BBBD with mannitol. We describe the technical aspects of the procedure and the hospital course and 1-month imaging. All patients were included in an Institutional Review Board–approved phase I clinical trial to determine safety and tolerability. These data support the rationale to export the results to larger studies to evaluate the efficacy of this modality.

ILLUSTRATIVE CASES
Case One: BBBD/IA Bevacizumab

History and examination
The patient is a 52-year-old woman, who presented after subtotal resection of a right temporal lobe GBM in June 2009 at a community hospital followed by 2 months of radiation therapy and temozolamide chemotherapy. Chemotherapy was complicated by a hematologic toxicity including thrombocytopenia and neutropenia. In January 2010, there was evidence of tumor progression on magnetic resonance imaging (MRI). The subinsular enhancing component increased in size, whereas the right temporal lesion remained stable (**Fig. 1**A). Because of her history of neutropenia, additional temozolomide therapy was not recommended, and the patient entered our phase I trial for IA infusion of bevacizumab after BBBD with mannitol in February 2010.

IA treatment: technical description
After obtaining consent, the patient was placed in the supine position in the angiography suite under general anesthesia. The right common femoral artery was found by palpation, and a 19-gauge single-wall needle was inserted into this artery. We replaced the needle with a 6F catheter sheath connected to continuous heparin saline flush. Then, a 5F Torcon catheter was advanced into the right common carotid artery over a 0.035-in angled guidewire. A right common and internal carotid artery angiogram were performed to ensure anterograde flow. Intravenous heparin was then administered after measurement of a baseline activated clotting time (ACT). An Excelsior SL 10 microcatheter angled 45 degrees was then advanced into the right M1 segment over a Synchro 2 soft microwire. After removal of the microwire, 10 mL of 25% mannitol solution was infused for 2 minutes (see **Fig. 1**B). Then, we infused 13 mg/kg of bevacizumab in 36 mL of saline for 36 minutes; postinfusion angiogram excluded arterial vessel damage.

Immediate postoperative course
Postoperative hospital course was unremarkable and immediate follow-up MRI demonstrated a decreased in size in the heterogenous enhancement of the right temporofrontal mass and decreased F-18 fluorodeoxyglucose (FDG) uptake on positron emission tomography scan in the same area (see **Fig. 1**A).

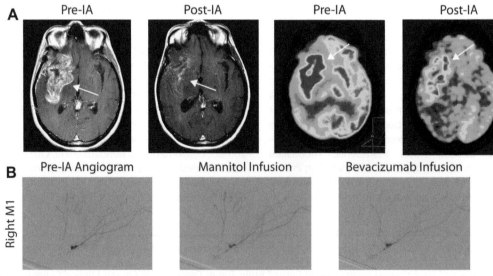

Fig. 1. (*A*) T1 axial magnetic resonance image (MRI) with contrast and fused metabolic positron emission tomography imaging before and 1 month after IA bevacizumab with BBBD treatment. A decrease in the heterogenous enhancement of the right temporofrontal mass on MRI (*arrows*) and a diminished F-18 fluorodeoxyglucose uptake in the same area are present (*arrows*). (*B*) Lateral fluoroscopic imaging of the pre-IA angiogram, after mannitol infusion, and after bevacizumab infusion. The right M1 segment of the right middle cerebral artery was selectively catheterized for infusion of mannitol and bevacizumab to treat the right temporofrontal lesion.

Case Two: BBBD/IA Temozolamide

History and examination

A 40-year-old man who presented in the emergency room with a 2-week history of nausea, vomiting, lethargy, and lower-extremity weakness became bradycardic with loss of consciousness. MRI revealed a heterogenous enhancing mass in the parasagittal left frontal lobe. The patient underwent craniotomy and gross total resection of the left parasagittal frontal lesion and was started on 2 months of chemoradiation with temozolomide. In January 2011, the patient reported clinical progression with some blurry vision in the left eye. MRI revealed recurrent left frontal mass with increased involvement of the corpus callosum (**Fig. 2**A). At this point, the patient was enrolled in our Phase I IA temozolamide trial.

IA temozolamide treatment: technical description

In February 2011, the patient was consented for selective IA infusion of temozolamide after BBBD with mannitol. The right common femoral artery was palpated, and a 19-gauge needle was inserted and then exchanged for a 6F catheter sheath connected to a continuous heparin saline flush. A 6F Envoy catheter was then advanced into the left common carotid artery over a 0.035-in guidewire under fluoroscopic guidance. Diagnostic angiograms were performed for the left common and internal carotid arteries to ensure normal anterograde flow. Afterward, heparin was administered intravenously after measurement of a baseline ACT. Then, using roadmap guidance, an Excelsior SL 10 microcatheter angled to 45 degrees was advanced into the A1-A2 junction over a Synchro 2

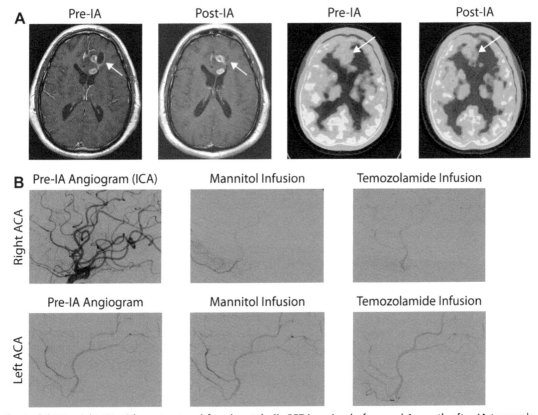

Fig. 2. (*A*) T1 axial MRI with contrast and fused metabolic PET imaging before and 1 month after IA temozolomide with BBBD treatment. There is decreased size in the cystic component of the left frontal mass on MRI (*arrows*) and decreased F-18 FDG uptake in the left frontal parasagittal lesion (*arrows*). (*B*) Lateral fluoroscopic imaging of the pre-IA angiogram, mannitol infusion, and temozolamide infusion. The right A1 segment and left A1-A2 junction of the right and left anterior cerebral artery, respectively, were selectively catheterized for infusion of mannitol and temozolamide to treat the left pericallosal frontal lesion, which may be crossing the midline over the corpus collosum.

soft microwire. After removal of this microwire, 10 mL of 25% mannitol was infused for 2 minutes (see **Fig. 2**B). Then, 83 mL of temozolamide (199 mg) was infused for 60 minutes. Postinfusion angiography was performed to ensure no arterial injury had occurred. The catheter was then advanced into the right common carotid artery under fluoroscopic guidance. An angiogram was performed for the right common and internal carotid arteries to ensure normal anterograde flow followed by intravenous heparin. Just as for the left anterior cerebral artery, 10 mL of 25% mannitol and subsequent 22 mL of temozolamide (53 mg) was infused into the right A1 segment.

Immediate postoperative course

Postoperative hospital course was unremarkable and 1-month follow-up MRI is illustrated in **Fig. 2**A, which demonstrated decrease in size of the cystic component of the left frontal mass and decreased FDG uptake in the left frontal parasagittal lesion.

Case Three: BBBD/IA Cetuximab

History and examination

This 61-year-old male patient presented with ataxia and memory difficulties and subsequently underwent resection of a posterior right parietooccpital GBM in December 2008. Postoperatively, the patient underwent radiation therapy and temozolamide chemotherapy for only 6 weeks because of noncompliance. He was then continued on maintenance temozolamide for 6 months. In August 2009, the patient was started on bevacizumab in addition to temozolamide. While on this treatment regimen, the patient progressed on MRI, showing a 3.5-cm enhancement in the parietal lobe and new heterogeneous enhancement in the right posterior lobe. Irinotecan was added to his treatment. From March 2010 to July 2010, the patient also underwent gamma knife radiation. Bevacizumab was discontinued in August 2010. At that point, the patient reported visual deficit and decreased ambulation. He denied seizures or weakness. However, MRI revealed increased signal enhancement and mass effect within the right parietal, temporal, and occipital lobes (**Fig. 3**A). In September 2010, the patient underwent a right parietal craniotomy and subtotal resection of brain tumor by the senior author (J.B.). Postoperative MRI revealed persistent T2 hyperintensity in the left lateral thalamus and residual tumor. Pathology showed robust (70%) expression of epidermal growth factor receptor on immunohistochemistry.

IA cetuximab treatment: technical description

In October 2010, after obtaining informed consent, the patient was prepped for IA infusion of cetuximab and placed in the angiography suite under general anesthesia. The right common artery was found by palpation, and a 19-gauge needle was inserted. The needle was replaced by a sheath (5F catheter), which was connected to a continuous source of heparin saline flush. A guide catheter (6F catheter) was fluoroscopically advanced to the right common carotid artery over a 0.035-in guidewire. An angiogram was then performed in the posteroanterior and lateral projections to ensure anterograde flow into the right common, external, and internal carotid arteries. An ACT was measured, and heparin was given intravenously. The guide catheter proceeded into the right internal carotid catheter. An Excelsior SL 10 microcatheter angled to 45 degrees was advanced over a Silverspeed 14 microwire and placed into the M1 segment of right middle cerebral artery using the roadmap technique (see **Fig. 3**B). Repeat angiogram was performed to ensure anterograde flow.

After removal of the microwire, 10 mL of 25% mannitol was injected through the microcatheter for 2 minutes. After a postinfusion angiogram, 210 mg of cetuximab (100 mg/m^2) solution mixed in 105 mL of normal saline was infused for 30 minutes (see **Fig. 3**B). To ensure no arterial injury, postinfusion angiography was performed for the right M1 segment. Afterward, a 6F guide catheter was replaced by a smaller 5F catheter, which was advanced into the right vertebral artery over a guidewire. A right vertebral artery angiogram was performed to ensure anterograde flow. The microcatheter was then inserted into the right posterior cerebral artery (P1 segment), and 10 mL of 25% mannitol and 210 mg (100 mg/m^2) cetuximab was infused as previously described for the M1 segment (see **Fig. 3**B). Again, a repeat angiogram of the P1 segment was performed to ensure no arterial injury.

Immediate postoperative course

Postoperative hospital course was unremarkable and immediate follow-up MRI is as illustrated in **Fig. 3**A, which demonstrated decreased in size of the right parietal periventricular lesion.

DISCUSSION
Bevacizumab, Cetuximab, and Temozolomide in GBM

We describe in this case series the technical aspects of selective arterial infusion of cetuximab, bevacizumab, and temozolamide after BBBD.

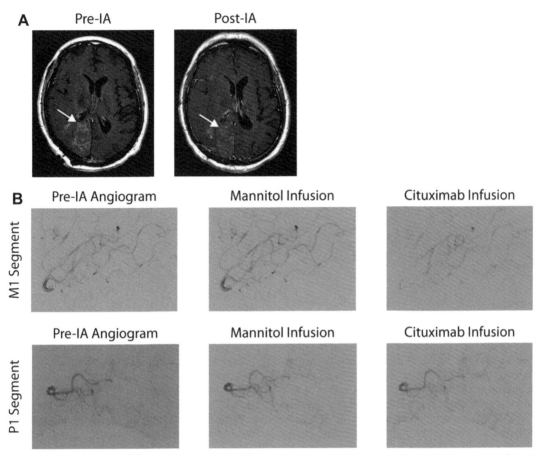

Fig. 3. (*A*) T1 axial MRI with contrast before and 1 month after IA cetuximab with BBBD treatment. There is a decrease in the size and enhancement of the right periventricular parietal lesion (*arrow*) from pre-IA to post-IA treatment. (*B*) Fluoroscopic imaging of the pre-IA angiogram, mannitol infusion, and cetuximab infusion. The right P1 and M1 segments of the right posterior cerebral artery and middle cerebral artery, respectively, were selectively catheterized for infusion of mannitol and cetuximab to treat the right periventricular parietal lesion.

Cetuximab, an epidermal growth factor receptor antibody, has been used intravenously in conjunction with irinotecan for the treatment of metastatic colorectal cancer and is currently in off-label use for recurrent GBM.[14] Likewise, bevacizumab, a vascular endothelial growth factor (VEGF) antibody, has been used intravenously with irinotecan for recurrent GBM.[15] However, survival after the intravenous application of these drugs is still unsatisfying and needs to be optimized. Although temozolamide has been successfully used as first-line chemotherapy in newly diagnosed GBMs,[3] no such success was achieved after the tumor recurred.[16] Up to now, the ideal treatment regimen for recurrent GBM is still missing and novel treatment modalities are needed to improve survival after GBM recurrence. At our institution, we recently completed a phase I trial[7,17] investigating the use of superselective IA infusion of bevacizumab after BBBD for the treatment of recurrent malignant glioma. We found that this

modality is safe and well tolerated. The maximum tolerated dose for IA cetuximab and temozolomide are still under investigation. The three patients in this case series received 13 mg/kg bevacizumab, 4.6 mg/kg cetuximab, and 2 mg/kg temozolomide, respectively. All of the patients in this case series were included in either phase I or II trials, so outcomes and longer-term side effects will be evaluated in a separate study.

Superselective IA Cerebral Infusion and BBBD

Previous studies have shown that superselective IA chemotherapy increases the concentration of Tc-hexamethylpropyleneamine compared with the equivalent intravenous route.[18] In addition to increased parenchyma drug concentrations, localized IA therapy may prevent more systemic effects, as shown by our study.[7] To further increase local drug delivery disruption of the BBB is an established method. Passive transfer

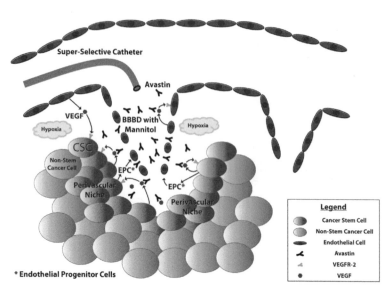

Fig. 4. Example of selective intra-arterial niche disruption and delivery using mannitol and bevacizumab. In addition to intravascular VEGF, VEGF within the perivascular niche needs to be targeted to disrupt mitogenic signaling and the generation of endothelial and tumor progenitor cells. This model can also be applied to cetuximab, temozolamide, or any drug designed to target signaling involving GBM stem-like cells. Cancer stem cell, endothelial progenitor cell.

across any membrane is proportional to both the concentration gradient and the diffusion coefficient of the membrane itself. To increase the diffusion coefficient, the BBB itself can be disrupted. Osmotic disruption of the BBB has been shown to increase uptake of monoclonal antibodies.[19] Although in malignant gliomas it is widely believed that the BBB is disrupted and not intact, Sarin and colleagues[20] showed that the maximal pore size of 12 nm in solid malignant brain tumors allows for only a partial opening of the BBB. Because the BBB is discontinuously open, we believe that agents with a bigger size, such as bevacizumab (size of 15 nm), reach the extravascular space more reliably after BBBD. Therefore, by using IA infusion and disrupting the BBB, we increase the concentration gradient and the transfer coefficient, thereby maximizing transfer of chemotherapy across the BBB.

Selective IA Niche Disruption and Delivery

By disrupting the BBB by IA fusion, we allow for maximal concentration of the infused drugs into the perivascular space known as the "perivascular niche." Calabrese and colleagues[21] have shown that cancer stem cells interact with endothelial cells in this niche and more specifically brain tumor blood vessels maintain the brain cancer stem-like cells and promote the growth of xenografts derived from stem-like cancer cells. Bevacizumab reduces the number of self-renewing tumor cells and especially inhibits the growth of xenografts derived from Daoy-positive cells. In addition, cancer stem-like cells themselves can also become endothelial cells under VEGF signaling, and bevacizumab prevents the maturation of

these tumor endothelial progenitors.[22] As shown in the illustrative sketch (**Fig. 4**), VEGF needs to be targeted within the perivascular niche to disrupt mitogenic signaling and the generation of endothelial and maintenance of tumor progenitor cells. We believe that selective IA niche disruption and delivery is needed to allow monoclonal antibodies, such as bevacziumab, to enter the perivascular niche at a clinically sufficient concentration.

SUMMARY

In this technical case series, we have shown some examples of superselective IA cerebral infusion of chemotherapeutic drugs after BBBD with mannitol. Superselective IA cerebral infusion and selective IA niche disruption and delivery of bevacizumab, cetuximab, and temozolomide are safe methods for the treatment of patients with GBM. Treatment efficacy needs to be further determined in larger ongoing phase II and III trials. It is hoped that this technical case series provides a framework to impact positively the treatment of patients with recurrent GBM.

REFERENCES

1. Hess KR, Broglio KR, Bondy ML. Adult glioma incidence trends in the United States, 1977-2000. Cancer 2004;101:2293.
2. Davis FG, Freels S, Grutsch J, et al. Survival rates in patients with primary malignant brain tumors stratified by patient age and tumor histological type: an analysis based on Surveillance, Epidemiology, and End Results (SEER) data, 1973-1991. J Neurosurg 1998;88:1.

3. Stupp R, Mason WP, van den Bent MJ, et al. Radiotherapy plus concomitant and adjuvant temozolomide for glioblastoma. N Engl J Med 2005;352:987.

4. Khasraw M, Lassman AB. Advances in the treatment of malignant gliomas. Curr Oncol Rep 2010;12:26.

5. Buie LW, Valgus J. Bevacizumab: a treatment option for recurrent glioblastoma multiforme. Ann Pharmacother 2008;42:1486.

6. Sampson JH, Archer GE, Mitchell DA, et al. An epidermal growth factor receptor variant III-targeted vaccine is safe and immunogenic in patients with glioblastoma multiforme. Mol Cancer Ther 2009;8:2773.

7. Boockvar JA, Tsiouris AJ, Hofstetter CP, et al. Safety and maximum tolerated dose of superselective intra-arterial cerebral infusion of bevacizumab after osmotic blood-brain barrier disruption for recurrent malignant glioma. Clinical article. J Neurosurg 2011;114:624.

8. Hochberg FH, Pruitt AA, Beck DO, et al. The rationale and methodology for intra-arterial chemotherapy with BCNU as treatment for glioblastoma. J Neurosurg 1985;63:876.

9. Ashby LS, Shapiro WR. Intra-arterial cisplatin plus oral etoposide for the treatment of recurrent malignant glioma: a phase II study. J Neurooncol 2001; 51:67.

10. Shapiro WR, Green SB, Burger PC, et al. A randomized comparison of intra-arterial versus intravenous BCNU, with or without intravenous 5-fluorouracil, for newly diagnosed patients with malignant glioma. J Neurosurg 1992;76:772.

11. Silvani A, Eoli M, Salmaggi A, et al. Intra-arterial ACNU and carboplatin versus intravenous chemotherapy with cisplatin and BCNU in newly diagnosed patients with glioblastoma. Neurol Sci 2002;23:219.

12. Hasegawa H, Allen JC, Mehta BM, et al. Enhancement of CNS penetration of methotrexate by hyperosmolar intracarotid mannitol or carcinomatous meningitis. Neurology 1979;29:1280.

13. Neuwelt EA, Howieson J, Frenkel EP, et al. Therapeutic efficacy of multiagent chemotherapy with drug delivery enhancement by blood-brain barrier modification in glioblastoma. Neurosurgery 1986; 19:573.

14. Van Cutsem E, Kohne CH, Hitre E, et al. Cetuximab and chemotherapy as initial treatment for metastatic colorectal cancer. N Engl J Med 2009;360:1408.

15. Vredenburgh JJ, Desjardins A, Herndon JE II, et al. Bevacizumab plus irinotecan in recurrent glioblastoma multiforme. J Clin Oncol 2007;25:4722.

16. van den Bent MJ, Brandes AA, Rampling R, et al. Randomized phase II trial of erlotinib versus temozolomide or carmustine in recurrent glioblastoma: EORTC brain tumor group study 26034. J Clin Oncol 2009;27:1268.

17. Riina HA, Fraser JF, Fralin S, et al. Superselective intraarterial cerebral infusion of bevacizumab: a revival of interventional neuro-oncology for malignant glioma. J Exp Ther Oncol 2009;8:145.

18. Namba H, Kobayashi S, Iwadate Y, et al. Assessment of the brain areas perfused by superselective intra-arterial chemotherapy using single photon emission computed tomography with technetium-99m-hexamethyl-propyleneamine oxime: technical note. Neurol Med Chir (Tokyo) 1994;34:832.

19. Neuwelt EA, Specht HD, Barnett PA, et al. Increased delivery of tumor-specific monoclonal antibodies to brain after osmotic blood-brain barrier modification in patients with melanoma metastatic to the central nervous system. Neurosurgery 1987;20:885.

20. Sarin H, Kanevsky AS, Wu H, et al. Physiologic upper limit of pore size in the blood-tumor barrier of malignant solid tumors. J Transl Med 2009;7:51.

21. Calabrese C, Poppleton H, Kocak M, et al. A perivascular niche for brain tumor stem cells. Cancer Cell 2007;11:69.

22. Wang R, Chadalavada K, Wilshire J, et al. Glioblastoma stem-like cells give rise to tumour endothelium. Nature 2010;468:829.

The Role of Avastin in the Management of Recurrent Glioblastoma

Jennifer A. Sweet, MD, Michelle L. Feinberg, MD, Jonathan H. Sherman, MD*

KEYWORDS

- Recurrent glioblastoma • Treatment malignant glioma
- Angiogenesis • Angiogenic switch • VEGF • Antiangiogenic
- Bevacizumab • Avastin • Radiation necrosis

Glioblastoma multiforme (GBM) is a malignant cerebral neoplasm of glial cell origin, accounting for 17% of all primary central nervous system tumors.[1] It has been classified by the World Health Organization as a grade IV malignancy and, thus, associated with rapid disease progression and a universally fatal outcome.[2] The prognosis for patients diagnosed with GBM is dismal, with an estimated 5-year survival rate of only 3.4%.[1] The current standard of treatment of newly diagnosed glioblastomas entails aggressive surgical resection with postoperative radiotherapy and chemotherapy, consisting of temozolamide, an oral alkylating agent.[3,4] Such treatment has improved the overall survival to a median of 12 to 15 months, compared with the previously sited 8 to 10 months.[5,6] However, although patients are living longer with this disease, recurrence proves to be unavoidable, with one study quoting an overall median survival of 6.25 months.[7]

The propensity for glioblastomas to recur can, in part, be explained by their ability to promote endothelial vascular proliferation.[6] The marked increase in vascular density largely accounts for their aggressive and invasive behavior.[8] These neoplasms exhibit an overexpression of vascular endothelial growth factor (VEGF), a promoter of angiogenesis.[9] Increased VEGF expression results in microvascular proliferation and accelerated tumor growth and has been linked to poor prognosis.[8,10]

Novel therapies aimed at arresting angiogenesis and tumor growth have come to play an integral role in the management of recurrent GBM. One such therapy is bevacizumab (Avastin), a recombinant monoclonal immunoglobulin (Ig) G_1 antibody that received Food and Drug Administration (FDA) approval in 2009 for the treatment of recurrent GBM.[11] Avastin acts by inhibiting the binding of VEGF to endothelial cell receptors. It is thought through inhibition of VEGF binding, tumor neovascularization, and, thus, tumor growth can be minimized. The proposed effect of the drug is supported by its radiographic findings of decreased contrast enhancement of tumors on magnetic resonance imaging (MRI).[11] However, the correlation of reduced tumor burden, as seen on imaging, with a progression-free survival (PFS) is uncertain. It is argued that Avastin's ability to neutralize VEGF results in the stabilization of the blood-brain barrier, which can prevent radiographic enhancement and, thus, mask tumor growth.[11] This article reviews the use of Avastin, its clinical applications, and its role in the treatment paradigm of recurrent GBM.

Disclosures: Funding sources, none.
Conflicts of interest: None.
Department of Neurological Surgery, George Washington University Medical Center, 2150 Pennsylvania Avenue, Northwest Suite 7420, Washington, DC 20037, USA
* Corresponding author.
E-mail address: jsherman0620@gmail.com

Neurosurg Clin N Am 23 (2012) 331–341
doi:10.1016/j.nec.2012.02.001
1042-3680/12/$ – see front matter © 2012 Elsevier Inc. All rights reserved

ANGIOGENESIS
The Angiogenic Switch

Angiogenesis is the process by which new blood vessels sprout from existing blood vessels.[12] Although angiogenesis is essential in normal vascular development, it can also be seen in many pathologic processes, including tumorigenesis.[13,14] New blood vessels develop in response to a hypoxic environment and the increased demand for oxygen and nutrients.[12,15] However, in pathologic conditions, this neovascularization is persistent and does not resolve by the reestablishment of adequate vascular perfusion.[12,15] In this setting, there is a transition from a physiologic prevascular environment to a pathologic vascular setting. This model of tumor angiogenesis was first introduced by Dr Judah Folkman in 1971 and is commonly referred to as the angiogenic switch (**Fig. 1**).[13,16,17]

The angiogenic switch provides 2 distinct advantages to tumor cells. The first and perhaps more significant benefit is the direct blood supply afforded to tumors by this neovascularization. In general, tumors that have access to a sufficient blood supply will continue to have exponential growth.[18] As described by Dr Folkman, there is a highly interdependent relationship between tumor cells and endothelial cells within the capillaries of a neoplasm, such that their rates of growth are contingent on each other.[16] The second advantage of neovascularization is the ability for tumor vessels to indirectly support malignant cells in an environment called the vascular niche.[19] This niche consists of small nests of dormant neoplastic cells. Neighboring endothelial cells supports these quiescent cells, yet their dormancy maintains a resistance to treatments, such as radiation and chemotherapeutic agents. Thus, neovascularization, which occurs in response to the angiogenic switch, provides tumors with a distinct growth advantage and proliferative autonomy when compared with normal cells.[14]

The mechanism by which this angiogenic switch occurs is a complex series of events. As tumors enlarge and compress neighboring blood vessels, there is a decrease in blood supply leading to hypoxia.[20] Tumors growing to a size as small as 1 to 2 mm can outgrow the local blood supply, triggering an angiogenic process.[12,15] The decreased partial pressure of oxygen tension in the tissue induces an upregulation of a transcription factor, hypoxia-inducible factor (HIF).[21] During times of normal oxygenation, HIF is kept at low levels by ubiquitin proteasome-dependent protein degradation, mediated by various tumor suppressor genes.[21] In cases of tumorigenesis, however, there is a loss of tumor suppressor function and HIF levels remain elevated.[12,15] This condition results in increased expression of proangiogenic factors, such as VEGF, basic fibroblast growth factor (FGF), and transforming growth factor-β, and a concomitant decrease in antiangiogenic factors, including interferon-α and thrombospondin-1.[13] The result is the stimulus for the angiogenic switch, which allows the growth of new capillaries and consequently the continued growth of a malignant tumor.[13]

Vascular Endothelial Growth Factor

VEGF has been shown to play a key role in the regulation of both normal and abnormal angiogenesis and it is commonly overexpressed in solid

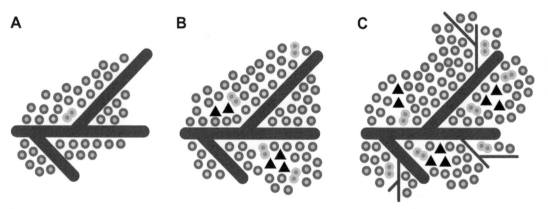

Fig. 1. Angiogenesis in high-grade gliomas. Tumor growth begins with malignant cells inhabiting regions adjacent to normal blood vessels (*A*). As the number of tumor cells increase at a rapid rate, as occurs in high-grade gliomas, the cells outgrow their previous blood supply and become hypoxic and necrotic (*B*). The hypoxic environment stimulates new blood vessel development, which in turn promotes further tumor growth (*C*). The blood vessels are depicted in red, the tumor cells are yellow, normal cells are blue, mitotic cells are green, and necrosis is demonstrated with purple triangles. (*Data from* Bergers G, Benjamin L. Tumorigenesis and the angiogenic switch. Nat Rev Cancer 2003;3(6):401–10.)

tumors.[14] VEGF is a member of the VEGF/platelet-derived growth factor gene family.[13] It binds to 2 tyrosine kinase receptors, VEGF receptor-1 (VEGFR-1 or Flt-1) and VEGF receptor-2 (VEGFR-2 or Flk-1/KDR). Both of these receptors predominantly occupy the surface of vascular endothelial cells.[13] When VEGF binds to the VEGFR-2 receptor, it signals downstream pathways, such as the phosphatidylinositol 3'OH kinase/AKT, to induce angiogenesis, vascular permeability, and mitogenesis.[22] In contrast, the binding to the VEGFR-1 receptor is thought to have negative feedback on VEGFR-2 signaling, monocyte migration, and endothelial cell secretion of proteases and growth factors.[12,15]

In one study, levels of VEGF and other proangiogenic factors were quantified by enzyme-linked immunosorbent assay in patients with primary and recurrent malignant gliomas. Twelve patients with primary GBM, 26 patients with recurrent GBM, and 7 patients with recurrent anaplastic astrocytoma underwent surgery for tumor resection and placement of an Ommaya reservoir into the resection cavity. Intracavitary fluid was drawn from the Ommaya reservoir between 2 to 12 weeks, before receiving chemotherapeutic treatment, and VEGF levels within the fluid were measured. The VEGF levels in the plasma of patients were also evaluated and compared with the plasma levels in 23 healthy controls. The VEGF levels in the plasma of patients were found to be higher than that of the controls ($P = .04$). When comparing the plasma and intracavitary VEGF levels in patients, the intracavitary levels proved to be higher. Finally, the VEGF levels were highest in the intracavitary fluid of patients with recurrent GBM, followed by patients with primary GBM. Intracavitary levels were lowest in patients with recurrent anaplastic astrocytomas. The study also showed a trend toward longer survival with lower intracavitary VEGF levels in the patients with recurrent glioblastomas.[23] As a result, more therapies are aimed at inhibiting the activity of VEGF and, thus, arresting angiogenesis, (**Fig. 2**).

Avastin

One of the more recognized antiangiogenic drugs available is Avastin, a recombinant monoclonal IgG$_1$ antibody derived from the murine VEGF monoclonal antibody.[6,9,14] The protein sequence is composed of 7% murine VEGF-binding residues incorporated into a human IgG framework constituting the other 93% of the protein sequence.[24] Experimental studies with Avastin show neutralization of all isoforms of human VEGF.[13] Treatment with Avastin results in a dose-dependent inhibition of tumor growth and a reduction in tumor density, diameter, and permeability.[13] For instance, patients who received greater than or equal to 0.3 mg/kg of intravenous Avastin demonstrate nondetectable serum levels of VEGF.[25]

In addition to neutralizing VEGF, Avastin has also been found to return tumor vasculature to a more physiologic state.[26] In nonmalignant blood vessels, there is a delicate balance between proangiogenic and antiangiogenic signaling mechanisms. This balance allows for the development of proper support structures, such as pericytes and basement membranes.[10] In tumors, however, the proangiogenic state is favored, resulting in aberrant blood vessels, irregular basement membranes, and discontinuous endothelial lining.[10,13] In effect, there is a leaky and unorganized vascular network with hyperpermeable membranes, which ultimately increases pressure in the interstitial space within tumors.[13,27] As a result, there is impaired delivery of oxygen and cytotoxic agents from the blood to

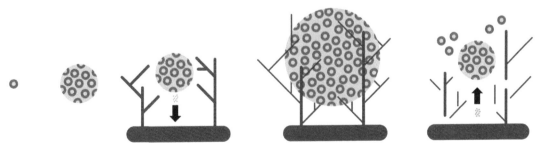

Fig. 2. Angiogenic switch and antiangiogenic theory. Tumor growth begins with a dormant nest of tumor cells, which slowly proliferate. As the tumor grows, it secretes proangiogenic factors and induces neovascularization. Tumor growth will continue as long as there is a sufficient network of blood vessels to support this growth. This process is the angiogenic switch. Antiangiogenic agents aim to inhibit the proangiogenic factors. (*Data from* Bergers G, Benjamin L. Tumorigenesis and the angiogenic switch. Nat Rev Cancer 2003;3(6):401–10.)

the tumor. Moreover, the hypoxic environment may impair the effects of any chemotherapy and radiation that is delivered to tumor cells.[13,28] By restoring the function of abnormal tumor vessels, Avastin indirectly promotes the delivery of cytotoxic agents to tumor cells while reducing leakage into the interstitial space.[13,24,29]

As alluded to earlier, anti-VEGF treatment may also enhance the effects of radiation in addition to chemotherapy. Gorski and colleagues[30] determined a dose-dependent increase in VEGF levels in tumors treated with ionizing radiation both in vitro and in vivo using mouse models. In the in vitro model, VEGF levels were initially 3 times higher in tumors concomitantly irradiated than in those that were not, and levels remained elevated for 14 days ($P = .032$).[30] The in vivo mouse model further demonstrated this synergy, showing no inhibition of tumor growth with anti-VEGF therapy alone, 68.8% inhibition of tumor growth with radiation alone, and 83.4% inhibition of tumor growth with a combined therapy ($P = .046$).[30]

AVASTIN IN CLINICAL TRIALS
Results in Other Malignancies

Angiogenesis is a common pathologic process in several types of malignancies. Similarly, the use of Avastin has been applied to the treatment of other, nonglial neoplastic processes. In 2004, the drug was FDA approved as a first-line agent with 5-florouracil chemotherapy for the treatment of colorectal cancer. In 2006, Avastin was approved as a second-line treatment with 5-fluorouracil/leucovorin/oxaliplatin -4 for colorectal cancer and as a first-line treatment of patients with unresectable or metastatic nonsquamous, non–small cell lung cancer in combination with carboplatin and paclitaxel. The approval for colorectal and lung cancer was based on randomized clinical trials that showed a statistically significant improvement in overall survival. In 2008, the FDA approved Avastin, in conjunction with paclitaxel, as a first-line treatment of metastatic breast cancer because of a single clinical trial in an accelerated approval process.[31] However, in 2010, the FDA began efforts to revoke their approval of the drug for the treatment of breast cancer after data from 5 randomized clinical trials failed to show improvement in overall survival or quality of life.[31]

Glioblastoma

The development of agents targeting VEGF for the treatment of GBM has also been under investigation. Initial trials with Avastin showed promising response rates, and the drug was thought to be a breakthrough in the treatment of glioblastoma.[32,33] In 2009, Avastin was granted accelerated FDA approval as a single-agent therapy for patients with recurrent glioblastoma. A phase II, noncomparative, multicenter trial (AVF3708 g) evaluated the efficacy of Avastin alone and in combination with irinotecan in patients with recurrent glioblastoma. All patients included in this study had histologically confirmed glioblastoma at either their first or second recurrence previously treated with radiotherapy and temozolomide. Patients were stratified by Karnofsky score and by first or second relapse. They received Avastin 10 mg/kg intravenously every other week and were observed for 6 months. Outcomes were compared with historical data with patients with 6-month PFS receiving either salvage therapy or irinotecan.[32]

The 2 primary endpoints in this study were 6-month PFS and objective response rates. The 6-month PFS was defined as the percentage of patients who were alive and progression free at the end of the 24-week period. The objective response rate was defined as either a complete or partial response seen on MRI taken at least 4 weeks apart. This study showed a 6-month PFS of 42.6% in the Avastin alone group and 50.3% in the Avastin and irinotecan group. Additionally, there was no reported investigator-determined clinical progression. These results were significantly superior to the historical controls.[32]

Based on the results of this trial, Genentech applied for accelerated approval of Avastin for monotherapy of recurrent glioblastomas. When the FDA reviewed this study, it reanalyzed the data using an exact 6-month cutoff instead of the 5.52-month cutoff used in the published study, which changed the PFS to 36.0%. The FDA did not include the results of the Avastin and irinotecan arm because that could have confounded the results. Additionally, the FDA excluded the objective response rate data from the trial because they determined that the characteristic histology of pseudopalisading necrosis of glioblastomas gives the tumor an irregular configuration that cannot be accurately measured on MRI. The FDA refused to grant accelerated approval based on these results alone until a confirmatory study with randomized controls rather than historical controls proved Avastin's efficacy.[31]

A single-arm single-site study was performed on patients with histologically confirmed recurrent glioblastoma previously treated with radiotherapy and temozolomide. In the study, patients received Avastin, 10 mg/kg every 14 days on a 28-day cycle. Patients who were noted to have progression of tumor growth during the study were asked to participate in a companion trial with the addition of irinotecan. MRI and positron emission tomography (PET) scans were performed at treatment onset and then again after 4 weeks. The primary end point in this study was PFS at 6 months, which was found to be 29%, with a median PFS of 16 weeks. Based on the Macdonald criteria, the overall response rate was 35%. In assessing the flu-deoxyglucose F 18 uptake measured by PET scan 4 weeks after the start of treatment, this uptake was diminished in 49%, equal to the baseline in 37% and increased compared with the baseline in 14% of patients. In this study, Avastin was generally well tolerated.[33]

Adverse Events

Inhibition of VEGF by Avastin occurs throughout the body and is not specific to tumor angiogenesis.[5] Its effects on normal vascular function and angiogenesis have lead to reports of several serious adverse events.[34] Perhaps the most commonly reported and often the most devastating complication is intracranial hemorrhage. Severe hemorrhage is estimated to occur 5 times more frequently in patients treated with Avastin than those receiving standard chemotherapy.[34] Wound infection and wound healing are additional potential complication because the drug may preclude adequate blood for wound healing.[34] A large cohort study analyzed the incidence of wound complications in patients undergoing abdominal surgery for colon cancer and found it to be directly related to the interval between surgery and the initiation of treatment.[35]

In the initial AVF3708 g trial of Avastin therapy in patients with glioblastomas, 98.8% of the patients experienced adverse events, with 26.2% of patients in the Avastin arm experiencing serious complications.[32] The most common findings were fatigue (45.2%), headache (36.9%), and hypertension (29.8%). A total of 46.4% of the patients in the Avastin-only arm of the study experienced grade 3 or higher adverse events. The most common of these were hypertension (8.3%), convulsion (6%), and fatigue (3.6%).[32] A total of 18 patients discontinued Avastin during this study because of the adverse events, which included cerebral hemorrhage, fatigue, seizure, myocardial infarction, reversible posterior leukoencephalopathy, infection, gastrointestinal perforation, and others.[32] In the National Cancer Institute 06-C-0064E trial, the most frequent adverse events were thromboembolism (12.5%), hypertension (12.5%), hypophosphatemia (6%), and thrombocytopenia (6%).[33]

EVALUATION OF CLINICAL EFFICACY
The Macdonald Criteria

Despite the promising therapeutic benefits of Avastin and other antiangiogenic treatments for the treatment of glioblastoma, several questions remain unanswered. Perhaps the most debated issue is the correlation between radiographic PFS and the clinical outcome of patients. Many studies that examine the efficacy of Avastin use as their end point the radiographic PFS and the objective response rate as determined by the Macdonald criteria.[11,32,36] The Macdonald criteria measure the response rate of glioblastomas to treatment, based on the size of contrast enhancement on T1-weighted MRI.[36] This size is determined by calculating the product of the maximal cross-sectional diameter of the enhancing tumor in 2 dimensions. Tumor progression is defined as a 25% increase in the 2-dimensional size.[36] In this way, 4 categories are analyzed, including a complete response (CR), a partial response (PR), stable disease, and progressive disease.[36] Using the Macdonald criteria, such studies demonstrate an improvement in PFS with Avastin compared with historical controls.[32] In part, it was the ability of Avastin to reduce contrast enhancement as early as 24 hours after the first dose that generated the enthusiasm for the drug and the approval for its use.[11] In fact, the Oncologic Drugs Advisory Committee stated: "objective response could be an adequate surrogate for clinical benefit under the proper parameters."[11]

The Macdonald criteria also factors into its determination of PFS the neurologic condition of patients and their use of steroids.[36] Steroid use is of particular importance because both steroids and Avastin have been shown to reduce vasogenic edema.[37] Reduction in surrounding edema not only improves radiographic findings but it also affects clinical symptoms because GBM-associated edema may contribute to the morbidity and mortality associated with the disease.[38] Decreased cerebral edema, even in the absence of tumor reduction, has been shown to have survival benefits.[37] Consequently, without recognizing the confounding effects of steroids, clinical and radiographic improvement can be erroneously attributed to Avastin. However, Avastin is attributed to the reduction in vasogenic edema independent of steroids by restoring a normal tumor vasculature and decreasing vessel permeability. In fact, multiple studies have shown a decrease in steroid dependence for patients on Avastin.[32,33]

Response Assessment Neuro-Oncology Working Group

Although not part of the Macdonald criteria, evaluation of the fluid attenuated inversion recovery (FLAIR) sequences on MRI may aid in measuring tumor response to antiangiogenic therapy. Some patients, after being treated with anti-VEGF agents, develop tumor progression that is infiltrative but does not enhance on postcontrast T1-weighted images.[39] However, such changes may be evident as increased signal attenuation on the FLAIR sequences on MRI.[39] It is thought that this is caused by the normalization of blood vessels by antiangiogenic therapy, which may mask tumor enhancement without affecting tumor growth and progression.[39] To develop a better method in evaluating neurooncology patients, the Response Assessment Neuro-Oncology (RANO) Working Group was established.

In addition to many other items, the RANO Working Group took into account the nonenhancing portions of tumor.[40] The changes seen on the T2/FLAIR that are suggestive of infiltrative tumor are mass effect, infiltration of the cortical ribbon, and location outside the radiation field.[40] One criticism of the RANO criteria is that it does not specify the degree of T2/FLAIR changes necessary to constitute progression. However, like T1 contrast enhancement, T2/FLAIR signal abnormality is nonspecific and may be a result of the effects of radiation, demyelination, ischemic injury, changes in corticosteroid doses, infection, seizures, and postoperative changes.[39] The Macdonald and RANO criteria and their primary differences are highlighted in **Table 1**.

The Macdonald Criteria Revisited

Much controversy exists regarding the validity of these methods for assessing tumor size and growth. In 2010, Wen and Macdonald and colleagues[36,40] reported the several limitations of the Macdonald criteria that have since been recognized since its original implementation. Primarily, the irregular shape of a glioblastoma makes calculating its 2-dimensional shape very difficult and inaccurate while also causing a strong interobserver variability.[40] In addition, only the primary area of tumor burden and not the infiltrative disease can be visualized with contrast enhancement.[8] As stated previously, the decreased contrast enhancement on MRI is thought to result in decreased permeability of the blood-brain barrier caused by the known effect of Avastin to normalize abnormal tumor vessels.[11,41] As such, this antitumor response may be more appropriately termed a pseudoresponse.[41,42] Furthermore, peripheral tumor cells and tumor cells that have invaded normal brain parenchyma are supplied by nontumoral vessels, which do not enhance with contrast.[8] Contrast enhancement can also be influenced by several factors, such as corticosteroid dose, radiologic technique, treatment-related inflammation, seizure activity, postsurgical changes, ischemia, subacute

radiation effects, and radiation necrosis.[40] Finally, after initial chemoradiation for glioblastoma, a transient increase in size known as pseudoprogression can occur in 20% to 30% of patients without actual tumor progression, which eventually resolves.[40] Consequently, patients with pseudoprogression included in clinical studies for recurrent gliomas could result in a falsely high response rate.[40]

Norden and colleagues[42] compared both the PFS and overall survival of patients treated with cytotoxic chemotherapy protocols with gimatecan and edotecarin as compared with patients treated with Avastin. The investigators' primary aim was to determine if treatment with Avastin results in a true survival benefit. In this study, the chemotherapy group displayed a PFS of 33%, 11%, and 6% at 3, 6, and 9 months respectively, with a median PFS of 8 weeks. In the Avastin group, the median PFS was 22 weeks with 70%, 40%, and 21% at 3, 6, and 9 months. These results showed a significant difference between the 2 treatment modalities with a P value of 0.01. However, the results do not hold for overall survival. In the chemotherapy group, median overall survival is 39 weeks, with 89%, 65%, and 54% at 3, 6, and 9 months, whereas the median overall survival for the Avastin group was only 37 weeks, with 91%, 74%, and 53% at 3, 6, and 9 months. The investigators in this study and several others concluded that Avastin improves PFS but has no significant effect on overall survival.[43]

Treatment After Avastin

Besides radiographic findings, another point of contention regarding patients with recurrent GBM previously treated with Avastin involves re-recurrence and disease progression after therapy. Under these circumstances, decision making becomes increasingly difficult because few treatment options remain.[44] Patients that received standard Avastin therapy had a mean time to disease progression of 4 months.[45] In retrospective analyses, there is no significant difference in the rate of distant recurrences between patients treated with Avastin and those who were not.[46] In fact, repeated studies demonstrate that patients previously treated with Avastin had extremely poor responses to any further treatment.[33] Kriesl and colleagues[33] studied a cohort of 19 patients with tumor progression treated with Avastin as a monotherapy or in combination with irinotecan.[33] None of the patients responded to either monotherapy or combination therapy and their median PFS was 30 days. In a prospective phase II study, Khasraw and colleagues[47] treated patients with recurrent GBM with daily temozolomide. They showed that

Table 1
Macdonld and RANO criteria

	Macdonald Criteria (using Contrast-Enhanced T1-Weighted Images)	RANO Criteria
Complete response	Imaging: complete absence of enhancing disease for a minimum of 4 wk with no new lesion formation Steroid dose: no corticosteroids Clinical assessment: clinical improvement	Imaging: complete absence of enhancing disease for a minimum of 4 wk with no new lesion formation T2/FLAIR images: stable or improved nonenhancing lesions Steroid dose: no corticosteroids Clinical assessment: clinically stable or improved
Partial response	Imaging: a 50% reduction in cross-sectional area from baseline of all measurable enhancing lesions for a minimum of 4 wk with no new lesion formation Steroid dose: stable or reduced corticosteroid dose Clinical assessment: clinically stable or improved	Imaging: A 50% reduction in cross-sectional area from baseline of all measurable enhancing lesions for a minimum of 4 wk with no new lesion formation; stable nonmeasurable lesions T2/FLAIR: stable or improved nonenhancing lesions Steroid dose: stable or reduced corticosteroid dose Clinical assessment: clinically stable or improved
Stable Response	Imaging: Does not meet criteria for CR, PR, or progression Clinical assessment: clinically stable	Imaging: does not meet criteria for CR, PR, or progression T2/FLAIR: stable nonenhancing lesions Steroid dose: stable or reduced corticosteroid dose
Progression	Imaging: an increase in cross-sectional area from baseline of 25% of enhancing lesions or the development of any new lesions Clinical assessment: clinical deterioration	Imaging: an increase in cross-sectional area from baseline of 25% of enhancing lesions or the development of any new lesions T2/FLAIR: increase in nonenhancing lesions Steroid dose: stable or increased corticosteroid dose Clinical assessment: clinical deterioration

Data from Wen P, Macdonald D, Reardon D, et al. Updated response assessment criteria for high-grade gliomas: response assessment in neuro-oncology working group. J Clin Oncol 2010;28(11):1963–72.

patients who previously received Avastin had a 6-month PFS of 14% compared with 36% in patients who did not receive prior treatment.[47]

Despite these reported failed treatments, there is no consensus as to why the use of Avastin yields resistance to future treatments. Some investigators have found that patients with progression after Avastin therapy developed perivascular fibrosis, which limited the amount of subsequent drug delivery to the tumor.[45] It has also been postulated that antiangiogenic therapy alters the phenotype of the tumor, creating a highly infiltrative compartment that is independent of angiogenesis.[44] In a separate hypothesis, treatment with Avastin and other antiangiogenic drugs results in hypoxia and a central region of tumor

necrosis, whereas the remaining neoplastic tissue is preserved. The viable tumor surrounding the central necrotic core is, thus, unaffected by the antiangiogenic affects of the drug, leaving it free to infiltrate adjacent non-neoplastic parenchyma.[45] Because of hypoxia and metabolic deprivation, the still-viable cells in the periphery become increasingly invasive and grow outwards toward already-existing blood vessels. This process of anti-VEGF–treated tumors being able to form invasive satellite tumors is known as their ability to coopt existing vessels.[48] This process may explain why antiangiogenic treatment may even cause an increase in tumor invasion that is not seen radiographically and an accelerated resistance to alternate therapies.[45]

OTHER ANTIANGIOGENIC DRUGS

Although much attention has been directed at Avastin and its role in the treatment of recurrent GBM, numerous antiangiogenic drugs are also under investigation. **Table 2** lists several of these agents and their target of action. Cilengitide is a cyclic arginineglycine-aspartic acid-containing peptide inhibitor of αVβ3 and αVβ5 integrin receptors, which is necessary for tumor invasion and migration through cellular matrix interactions. A phase II trial with 81 patients with recurrent glioblastoma randomized patients to either 500 mg or 2000 mg of cilengitide twice weekly. In this study, the median overall survival was 9.9 months in the cohort receiving the 2000-mg dose compared with 6.5 months in the cohort receiving 500 mg (results not significant). Patients receiving cilengitide tolerated the medication well with no significant toxicities. The most common adverse event from treatment was fatigue (n = 3) and the most common serious adverse event was convulsion (n = 2).[43]

Aflibercept is a recombinant fusion protein of the extracellular domains of VEGF fused to the Fc portion of immunoglobulin G1. The drug binds to both VEGF and placental growth factor (PIGF). PIGF is a key mediator in angiogenesis by enhancing the activity of VEGF signaling by activation of VEGF receptor 1 and contributes to the angiogenic switch in cancer. PIGF levels are markedly increased in patients with recurrent glioblastoma. The North American Brain Tumor Coalition phase II trial was the first clinical trial of aflibercept in recurrent glioblastoma. Despite promising phase I results, the primary end point of this trial was not met because only 7.7% of patients were alive and progression free at the end of 6 months.[45]

Another antiangiogenic therapy, XL184, is a tyrosine kinase inhibitor that affects several receptors, including VEGF receptor 2. A recent phase II cohort study of patients with progressive glioblastoma treated with XL184 showed an overall response rate of 30% (11/37), with a medial PFS of 16 weeks. However, there was no response to XL184 in the patients who had previously been treated with another antiangiogenic compound, although the median PFS was the same in both groups. The most common serious adverse effects associated with XL184 were fatigue (20%), transaminase elevation (12%), and thromboembolic events (10%). The results with XL184 are encouraging and may hold promise in future trials.[44]

Like XL184, cediranib is an oral receptor tyrosine kinase inhibitor but it blocks all VEGF receptors. In a phase II study, 31 patients with recurrent glioblastoma were administered 45 mg/d of cediranib until their tumor progressed or there was unacceptable drug toxicity. At the end of the study, 25.8% of the patients were alive and progression free after 6 months, with 56.7% of patients showing a partial radiographic response. The grade 3/4 toxicities include hypertension (4/31), diarrhea (2/31), and fatigue (6/31).[49]

OTHER APPLICATIONS OF AVASTIN
Intra-arterial Avastin

The role for Avastin and other antiangiogenic agents is not limited to intravenous administration for the treatment of malignancy. In 2009, neurosurgeons at New York-Presbyterian Hospital/Weill Cornell Medical Center were the first to inject intra-arterial (IA) Avastin directly into the tumor bed.[50] In this procedure, known as superselective IA cerebral infusion, an angiogram is performed to identify the abnormal vasculature supplying the tumor. IA mannitol is then injected in an effort to disrupt the blood-brain barrier. Avastin is subsequently injected into the arterial vessels supplying the tumor, with the goal of improving penetration of the drug to the tumor bed without increasing the overall systemic effects of the drug.[50]

The first clinical study to assess the safety and efficacy of superselective IA cerebral infusion was conducted from 2009 to 2010 in patients with recurrent glioblastomas.[51] The study included 20 patients divided into 2 groups according to their prior treatment. Ten patients never received prior treatment with Avastin, whereas 10 patients were previously treated with intravenous Avastin. In the study, all participants were given IA mannitol

Table 2 Antiangiogenic agents and their targets	
Antiangiogenic Agent	**Target**
Avastin	VEGF
Thalidomide	Basic FGF
Vatalanib	VEGF receptor, platelet-derived growth factor receptor
Cilengitide	Integrin receptors
Aflibercept	VEGF, placental growth factor
XL 184	Receptor tyrosine kinase
Cediranib	VEGF receptor, receptor tyrosine kinase
Sunitinib	Receptor tyrosine kinase
CT-322	VEGF receptor-2

Data from Beal K, Abrey L, Gutin P. Antiangiogenic agents in the treatment of recurrent or newly diagnosed glioblastoma: analysis of single-agent and combined modality approaches. Radiat Oncol 2011;6:2.

followed by escalating doses of 2 to 15 mg/kg of IA Avastin. The radiographic effects of the therapy were assessed with MRI before treatment, immediately after therapy, and 28 days later.[51]

Radiographic assessment was based on the RANO working group's study, evaluating the area and volume of T1 contrast enhancement and perituomoral FLAIR signal changes. In the Avastin-naive group, there was a median reduction of area and volume of tumor enhancement by 34.7% and 46.9% respectively. In comparison, the median reduction of area and volume in the comparison group was 15.2% and 8.2% respectively ($P = 0.02$ and 0.06 respectively). There was no significant difference between groups regarding the reduction of tumor perfusion on MRI. The signal attenuation on FLAIR was increased in 2 (10.5%) patients and stable in 8 (42.1%) patients in the Avastin-naive group compared with the previously treated group in which 3 (30%) patients had increased signal and 7 (70%) patients had stable findings on FLAIR.[51]

In this study, IA Avastin was observed to be relatively safe, with no grade 3, 4, or 5 adverse events reported.[51] The grade 2 adverse events were seizures in 2 patients and an acneiform rash in 1 patient. Two patients with a history of pulmonary embolus had new-onset pulmonary emboli during the observation period. One procedure-related stroke with the inflation of the endovascular balloon was reported.[51]

Although this study had a small sample size, it demonstrated the safety and efficacy of IA Avastin for the treatment of recurrent GBM. All of the patients in the group not previously treated with Avastin and two-thirds of the patients who had been previously treated with Avastin showed a meaningful reduction in tumor size according the RANO group's study.[51] These results are also superior to the 50% response rate to intravenous Avastin.[52] Additional investigation into IA Avastin is ongoing.

Treatment of Radiation Necrosis

Avastin may also have applications outside the inhibition of tumor growth. Radiation necrosis is a result of injury to the local tissue, which may occur after radiation therapy. The characteristic appearance of radiation necrosis on MRI is difficult to distinguish from tumor itself, with an area of central necrosis and surrounding vasogenic edema.[53] Radiation necrosis is caused by endothelial cell injury, resulting in a breakdown of the blood-brain barrier with subsequent edema and hypoxia.[54] The hypoxia induces an upregulation of VEGF that causes increased vessel permeability and tissue necrosis.[54] Therefore, it is theorized

that radiation necrosis may respond to treatment with Avastin. A randomized, controlled, double-blinded study comparing Avastin with a placebo control showed that patients treated with Avastin for radiation necrosis had a 59% decrease in the edema as seen on FLAIR on MRI. This result is in stark contrast to the 14% increase in edema on FLAIR sequences in the placebo group.[55] Additionally, there was a 63% decrease in contrast enhancement seen on T1-weighted postcontrast MRI in the Avastin group compared with a 17% increase in enhancement in the placebo group. Although the study sample was small, these results are very promising for the treatment of radiation necrosis.[55]

SUMMARY

The development of antiangiogenic therapy for malignancy is an ever-evolving area of research. With regard to glioblastoma, Avastin is the most studied and is currently approved for recurrent disease. The significant reduction in tumor enhancement on MRI in early studies generated significant excitement concerning the ability of Avastin to improve overall survival in this difficult patient population. However, as Avastin continues to be studied, it is evident that although there is an increase in PFS there is no change in overall survival as compared with historical controls. Currently, several therapies targeting the different mediators of angiogenesis, including endothelial cell growth factor ligands and receptors, placental growth factor, fibroblast growth factor, and angiopoietins, are under investigation. As data from these studies are evaluated, it will become evident which antiangiogenesis inhibitors display efficacy and in what combination chemotherapeutic regimen they should be administered.

REFERENCES

1. CBTRUS, Hinsdale IL. Statistical report: primary brain tumors in the United States, 2004-2007. Central Brain Tumor Registry of the United States; 2011.
2. Louis D, Ohgaki H, Wiestler O, et al. The 2007 WHO classification of tumours of the central nervous system. Acta Neuropathol 2007;114(2): 97–109.
3. Stupp R, Mason W, van den Bent M, et al. Radiotherapy plus concomitant and adjuvant temozolomide for glioblastoma. N Engl J Med 2005;352(10): 987–96.
4. Narayana A, Golfinos J, Fischer I, et al. Feasibility of using bevacizumab with radiation therapy and temozolomide in newly diagnosed high-grade glioma. Int J Radiat Oncol Biol Phys 2008;72(2):383–9.

5. Shirai K, Siedow M, Chakravarti A. Antiangiogenic therapy for patients with recurrent and newly diagnosed malignant glioma. J Oncol 2012;2012: 193436.

6. Daumas-Duport C, Scheithauer B, O'Fallon J, et al. Grading of astrocytomas. A simple and reproducible method. Cancer 1988;62(10):2152–65.

7. Wong E, Hess K, Gleason M, et al. Outcomes and prognostic factors in recurrent glioma patients enrolled onto phase II clinical trials. J Clin Oncol 1999;17(8):2572–8.

8. Onishi M, Ichikawa T, Kurozumi K, et al. Angiogenesis and invasion in glioma. Brain Tumor Pathol 2011;28(1):13–24.

9. Buie L, Valgus J. Bevacizumab: a treatment option for recurrent glioblastoma multiforme. Ann Pharmacother 2008;42(10):1486–90.

10. Jain R, di Tomaso E, Duda D, et al. Angiogenesis in brain tumors. Nat Rev Neurosci 2007;8(8):610–22.

11. Cohen M, Shen Y, Keegan P, et al. FDA approval summary: bevacizumab (Avastin) as treatment of recurrent glioblastoma multiforme. Oncologist 2009;14(11):1131–8.

12. Ferrara N. Pathways mediating VEGF-independent tumor angiogenesis. Cytokine Growth Factor Rev 2010;21(1):21–6.

13. Gerber H, Ferrara N. Pharmacology and pharmacodynamics of bevacizumab as monotherapy or in combination with cytotoxic therapy in preclinical studies. Cancer Res 2005;65(3):671–80.

14. Presta L, Checn H, O'Connor S, et al. Humanization of an anti-vascular endothelial growth factor monoclonal antibody for the therapy of solid tumors and other disorders. Cancer Res 1997; 57(20):4593–9.

15. Chung A, Ferrara N. Developmental and pathological angiogenesis. Annu Rev Cell Dev Biol 2011; 27:563–84.

16. Folkman J. Tumor angiogenesis: therapeutic implications. N Engl J Med 1971;285(21):1182–6.

17. Fine H, Figg W, Jeackle K, et al. Phase II trial of the anti-angiogenic agent thalidomide in patients with recurrent high grade gliomas. J Clin Oncol 2000;18(4):708–15.

18. Folkman J. Tumor angiogenesis. Adv Cancer Res 1974;19(0):331–58.

19. Calabrese C, Poppleton H, Kocak M, et al. A perivascular niche for brain tumor stem cells. Cancer Cell 2007;11(1):69–82.

20. Hanahan D, Folkman J. Patterns and emerging mechanisms of the angiogenic switch during tumorigenesis. Cell 1996;86(3):353–64.

21. Dayan F, Mazure N, Brahimi-Horn M, et al. A dialogue between the hypoxia-inducible factor and the tumor microenvironment. Cancer Microenviron 2008;1(1):53–68.

22. Waltenberger J, Claesson-Welsh L, Siegbahn A, et al. Different signal transduction of KDR and Flt1, to receptors for vascular endothelial growth factor. J Biol Chem 1994;269(43):26988–95.

23. Salmaggi A, Eoli M, Frigerio S, et al. Intracavitary VEGF, bFGF, IL-8, IL-12 levels in primary and recurrent glioma. J Neurooncol 2003;62(3):297–303.

24. Moen M. Bevacizumab: in previously treated glioblastoma. Drugs 2010;70(2):181–9.

25. Gordon M, Margolin K, Talpaz M, et al. Phase I safety and pharmacokinetic study of recombinant human anti-vascular endothelial growth factor in patients with advanced cancer. J Clin Oncol 2001; 19(3):843–50.

26. Jain R. A new target for tumor therapy. N Engl J Med 2009;360(25):2669–71.

27. Kim K, Li B, Houck K, et al. The vascular endothelial growth factor proteins: identification of biologically relevant regions by neutralizing monoclonal antibodies. Growth Factors 1992;7(1):53–64.

28. Dickson P, Hamner J, Sims T, et al. Bevacizumab-induced transient remodeling of the vasculature in neuroblastoma xenografts results in improved delivery and efficacy of systemically administered chemotherapy. Clin Cancer Res 2007;13(13): 3942–50.

29. Jain R. Normalizing tumor vasculature with anti-angiogenic therapy: a new paradigm for combination therapy. Natl Med 2001;7(9):987–9.

30. Gorski D, Beckett M, Jaskowiak N, et al. Blockage of the vascular endothelial growth factor stress response increases the antitumor effects of ionizing radiation. Cancer Res 1999;59(14):3374–8.

31. United States Food, Drug Administration. FDA briefing document oncology drug advisory committee meeting STN 125085/191 and 192 (bevacizumab). Rockville (MD): US Department of Health and Human Services; 2010.

32. Friedman H, Prados M, Wen PY, et al. Bevacizumab alone and in combination with irinotecan in recurrent glioblastoma. J Clin Oncol 2009;27(28):4733–40.

33. Kreisl T, Kim L, Moore K, et al. Phase II trial of single-agent bevacizumab followed by bevacizumab plus irinotecan at tumor progression in recurrent glioblastoma. J Clin Oncol 2009;27(5):740–5.

34. Gressett S, Shah S. Intricacies of bevacizumab-induced toxicities and their management. Ann Pharmacother 2009;43(3):490–501.

35. Sugrue M, Purdie D, Feng P, et al. Serious wound healing complications (WHCs) in patients (pts) with metastatic colorectal cancer (mCRC) receiving bevacizumab (BV) as part of a first-line regiment: results from the BRITE Observational Cohort Study (OCS). J Clin Oncol 2008;26(Suppl 15):[abstract: 4105].

36. Macdonald D, Cascino T, Schold S, et al. Response criteria for phase II studies of supratentorial malignant glioma. J Clin Oncol 1990;8(7):1277–80.

37. Kamoun W, Ley C, Farrar C, et al. Edema control by cediranib, a vascular endothelial growth factor

receptor-targeted kinase inhibitor, prolongs survival despite persistent brain tumor growth in mice. J Clin Oncol 2009;27(15):2542–52.

38. Silbergeld D, Rostomily R, Alvord E. The cause of death in patients with glioblastoma is multifactorial: clinical factors and autopsy findings in 117 cases of supratentorial glioblastoma in adults. J Neurooncol 1991;10(2):179–85.

39. Quant E, Wen P. Response assessment in neuro-oncology. Curr Oncol Rep 2011;13(1):50–6.

40. Wen P, Macdonald D, Reardon D, et al. Updated response assessment criteria for high-grade gliomas: response assessment in neuro-oncology working group. J Clin Oncol 2010;28(11):1963–72.

41. Thompson E, Dosa E, Kraemer D, et al. Correlation of MRI sequences to assess glioblastoma multiforme treated with bevacizumab. J Neurooncol 2011;103(2):353–60.

42. Norden A, Drappatz J, Muzikansky A, et al. An exploratory survival analysis of anti-angiogenic therapy for recurrent malignant glioma. J Neurooncol 2009;92(2): 149–55.

43. Reardon D, Fink K, Mikkelsen T, et al. Randomized phase II study of cilengitide, an integrin-targeting arginine-glycine-aspartic acid peptide, in recurrent glioblastoma multiforme. J Clin Oncol 2008;26(34):5610–7.

44. Beal K, Abrey L, Gutin P. Antiangiogenic agents in the treatment of recurrent or newly diagnosed glioblastoma: analysis of single-agent and combined modality approaches. Radiat Oncol 2011;6:2.

45. de Groot J, Lamborn K, Chang S, et al. Phase II study of aflibercept in recurrent malignant glioma: a North American Brain Tumor Consortium study. J Clin Oncol 2011;29(19):2689–95.

46. Platten M, Dorner N, Hofer S, et al. Evaluation of distant spread in bevacizumab-treated versus control-treated patients with malignant gliomas: a matched-pair study. J Clin Oncol 2010;28(Suppl 15): [abstract: 2064].

47. Khasraw M, Abrey L, Lassman A, et al. Phase II trial of continuous low dose temozolomide (TMZ) for recurrent malignant glioma (MG) with and without prior exposure to bevacizumab (BEV). J Clin Oncol 2010;28(Suppl 15):[abstract: 2065].

48. Rubenstein J, Kim J, Ozawa T, et al. Anti-VEGF antibody treatment of glioblastoma prolongs survival but results in increased vascular cooption. Neoplasia 2000;2(4):306–14.

49. Batchelor T, Duda D, di Tomaso E. Phase II study of cediranib, an oral pan-vascular endothelial growth factor receptor tyrosine kinase inhibitor, in patients with recurrent glioblastoma. J Clin Oncol 2010; 28(17):2817–23.

50. Riina H, Fraser J, Fralin S, et al. Superselective intra-arterial cerebral infusion of bevacizumab: a revival of interventional neuro-oncology for malignant glioma. J Exp Ther Oncol 2009;8(2):145–50.

51. Boockvar J, Tsiouris A, Hofstetter C, et al. Safety and maximum tolerated dose of superselective intra-arterial cerebral infusion of bevacizumab after osmotic blood-brain barrier disruption for recurrent malignant glioma. Clinical trial. J Neurosurg 2011; 114(3):624–32.

52. Vredenburgh J, Desjardins A, Reardon D, et al. Experience with irinotecan for the treatment of malignant glioma. Neuro Oncol 2009;11(1):80–91.

53. Brandsma D, Stalpers L, Taal W, et al. Clinical features, mechanisms, and management of pseudoprogression in malignant gliomas. Lancet Oncol 2008;9(5):453–61.

54. Rahman M, Hoh B. Avastin in the treatment for radiation necrosis: exciting results from a recent randomized trial. World Neurosurg 2011;75(1):4–5.

55. Levin V, Bidaut L, Hou P, et al. Randomized double-blind placebo-controlled trial of bevacizumab therapy for radiation necrosis of the central nervous system. Int J Radiat Oncol Biol Phys 2011;79(5): 1487–95.

Management of Multifocal and Multicentric Gliomas

Chirag G. Patil, MD, MS*, Paula Eboli, MD, Jethro Hu, MD

KEYWORDS

- Multifocal • Multicentric • Glioma • Glioblastoma
- Treatment

The diffuse nature of gliomas has long confounded attempts at achieving a definitive cure. Superradical hemispherectomies were performed in the early years of neurosurgery; yet even these desperate efforts could not prevent tumor from recurring on the contralateral side. With the advent of computed tomography and magnetic resonance imaging (MRI), it became increasingly apparent that gliomas could have a multifocal or multicentric appearance. Treating these tumors is the summit of an already daunting challenge, because the obstacles that must be surmounted to treat gliomas in general, namely, their heterogeneity, diffuse nature, and ability to insidiously invade normal brain, are more conspicuous in this subset of tumors.

EPIDEMIOLOGY

Malignant gliomas represent the most common primary brain tumor in adults. Median survival of patients with glioblastoma after optimal treatment continues to be less than 15 months.[1] Although most gliomas have been described as solitary lesions, multifocal/multicentric lesions have been described with an incidence ranging from 0.5% to 20%.[2–8] Most of the data available specifically regarding multifocal tumors are in the form of case reports or small series. Chamberlain and colleagues[9] described the radiographic patterns of relapse in 80 patients with glioblastoma multiforme (GBM). At diagnosis, 10% of patients had multifocal or multicentric disease, whereas at first recurrence this proportion increased to 14%. Salvati and colleagues[7] published a series on

25 patients with multicentric tumors and reported that these multicentric tumors represented 2% of all malignant tumors in their series. Silbergeld and colleagues[10] reported that 17% of 117 adult patients with supratentorial GBM examined post mortem by autopsy had multifocal disease.

Multicentric/focal gliomas can either be multiple at the time of diagnosis or develop later in the disease process. Kyritsis and colleagues[11] described 51 patients with multifocal/multicentric gliomas; 26 of the patients had simultaneous lesions at the time of diagnosis, whereas the other 25 developed multifocality later. In 14 of the 51 patients, no apparent dissemination route was identified, and the tumors were classified as multicentric gliomas. The rest of the patients showed different patterns of spread from the primary site, and the tumors were classified as multifocal. The investigators described the meningeal-subarachnoid space as the most frequent dissemination route, followed by the subependymal route, intraventricular route, and direct brain penetration.[11]

DEFINITION: MULTIFOCAL VERSUS MULTICENTRIC TUMORS

Multicentric gliomas were first described by Bradley[12] in 1880. Based on the points brought up by Russell and Rubinstein, Batzdorf and Malamud[2] described the criteria to differentiate multifocal from multicentric tumors in 1963. The investigators described multifocal tumors as those that can be explained as the result of growth or dissemination via established routes: (1) commissural or other

Department of Neurological Surgery, Cedars-Sinai Medical Center, Los Angeles, CA, USA
* Corresponding author. Center for Neurosurgical Outcomes Research, Maxine Dunitz Neurosurgical Institute, Department of Neurosurgery, Cedars-Sinai Medical Center, 8631 West Third Street, Suite 800E, Los Angeles, CA 90048.
E-mail address: chiragpatil@gmail.com

Neurosurg Clin N Am 23 (2012) 343–350
doi:10.1016/j.nec.2012.01.012
1042-3680/12/$ – see front matter © 2012 Elsevier Inc. All rights reserved.

pathways, such as the corpus callosum; (2) cerebrospinal fluid channels, either through subarachnoid spaces or the ventricular system; and (3) local metastasis through satellite formation in the immediate vicinity of the main tumor. Multicentric tumors were defined as those that represent widely separated lesions, for example, those in different hemispheres and whose origin cannot be explained following the pathways mentioned earlier. Multicentric tumors also include those tumors separated in time.[2] Although these definitions can be used to separate patients with multifocal gliomas from those that harbor multicentric tumors, the clinical or prognostic significance between these 2 clinical entities remains unclear.

PATHOGENESIS

The pathogenesis of multicentric tumors is unknown. In 1960, Willis[13] introduced the theory of initiation and promotion that allows unlinked proliferation of neoplastic cells at different topographic locations[4] and suggested that multicentric lesions could result from a 2-step process. In the first stage called initiation, a large area or perhaps the entire brain undergoes neoplastic transformation and becomes more susceptible to neoplastic growth. In the second stage called promotion, the neoplastic proliferation occurs in multiple sites through different sources of stimulation, such as hormonal, biochemical, or even viral.[14,15] The increased prevalence of multicentric tumors in patients with germline p53 mutations and neurofibromatosis type I (with germline mutation of the NF1 tumor suppressor gene) is likely explained by the mechanism by which the germline mutation serves as the initiating hit.[16,17] The idea of initiation and promotion also makes sense in the context of the cancer stem cell hypothesis, as elaborated later.

Despite this theory, most cases of multicentric tumors and all cases of multifocal tumors are more likely to develop because of the unique propensity of glioma cells to invade normal brain and migrate long distances. (Claes and colleagues[15] aptly compared glioma cells to guerilla warriors capable of invading individually or in small groups and abusing preexisting supply lines.) In 1940, the neuropathologist Hans-Joachim Scherer[18] described secondary structures of glioma growth along existing cytoarchitectural elements, such as neurons, white matter tracts, and blood vessels. In 1997, Geer and Grossman[19] suggested that interstitial fluid flow along white matter tracts could be a potentially important mechanism for the dissemination of glioma cells, explaining that glioma cells are inherently capable

of migration along white matter tracts to distant areas of the brain. Hefti and colleagues[4] found most multicentric glioma lesions to be located along known migrational pathways of glioma cells and, therefore, suggested that active migratory processes are involved in the development of these lesions. The investigators also described a time-related dependency for multicentricity and concluded that with the advent of radical tumor resection, adjuvant therapies, better local control, and longer life expectancy, the incidence of multicentric/multifocal gliomas is likely to increase.

PATHOLOGY

Pathologically, most multicentric/multifocal gliomas can be classified as GBM.[2,7] However, anaplastic astrocytoma, anaplastic oligoastrocytoma, gliosarcoma, oligodendroglioma, and ependymoma with multicentric and multifocal features have been described.[2,7,20] These tumors do not exhibit any specific histologic features that could differentiate them from similar unifocal gliomas.[2] In most cases, the histology of separate lesions is similar, with variations comparable to those visualized in different areas of the same tumor.[2] However, less commonly, multicentricity can also occur as a combination of different histologic tumors, for example, anaplastic astrocytoma and glioblastoma, low-grade astrocytoma and anaplastic astrocytoma, and low-grade astrocytoma and glioblastoma.[5,7,21] Most multicentric gliomas occur supratentorially, but combined lesions in both supratentorial and posterior fossa have also been described.[2,7,8,22,23]

DIAGNOSIS

MRI with contrast is the modality of choice for evaluating brain tumors. Glioblastomas, brain metastases, and central nervous system (CNS) lymphomas share similar enhancement patterns on MRI, and no definitive characteristics can differentiate multifocal/multicentric GBM from metastatic disease or CNS lymphoma.[3,22,24] Very recently, Wang and colleagues[25] reported the use of a combination of MRI diffusion tensor imaging (DTI) and dynamic susceptibility contrast-enhanced (DSC) MRI to differentiate glioblastomas from metastases and lymphoma. Using DTI and DSC parameters, the investigators were able to differentiate GBM from metastases and lymphoma with a sensitivity of 89% and specificity of 93%.

Although important strides are being made to radiographically differentiate between these pathologic conditions, tissue diagnosis with surgical biopsy remains the standard of care for all gliomas including multifocal/multicentric tumors.

TREATMENT
Surgical Management

There are no clearly defined guidelines in the literature on the surgical management of multifocal or multicentric gliomas. Some investigators favor a conservative surgical approach with the use of stereotactic biopsy for accurate diagnosis while avoiding risk of neurologic deficit or hemorrhage.[22,26] Other investigators have suggested that aggressive resection of the contrast-enhancing portions of multifocal/multicentric tumors yields better overall survival compared with patients with solitary malignant gliomas. These investigators have recommended craniotomy or even multiple craniotomies with maximal safe resection.[3,7]

Hassaneen and colleagues[3] recently described the use of multiple craniotomies in the management of multifocal and multicentric glioblastomas in 20 patients and used a matched cohort of patients with solitary GBM for comparison. The investigators, however, were not able to compare their results with those of a group of patients with multicentric/multifocal glioblastomas who were treated only with biopsy. An overall survival of 9.7 months was reported in the multifocal/multicentric group after aggressive surgical resection with multiple craniotomies. This result was similar to that of the matched control group with single tumors who had a median survival of 10.5 months ($P = .34$). The investigators concluded that multiple craniotomies resulted in a survival period comparable with that of patients undergoing surgery for a single lesion, with no increase in complication rate or postoperative morbidity.[3] Therefore, these investigators recommended maximal safe resection of the enhancing tumors to maximize survival in select patients with multifocal/multicentric tumors.

Salvati and colleagues[7] described the largest series of 25 patients with multicentric high-grade gliomas according to the criteria defined by Batzdorf and Malamud.[2] In their series, similar to Hassaneen and colleagues,[3] the average survival of patients who underwent surgical resection was 9.5 months. Patients with tumors in inaccessible or eloquent locations underwent biopsy and had an average survival of 2.8 months. Based on their data and experience, the investigators concluded that patients with accessible tumors should undergo surgical resection of all tumors and the rest should undergo stereotactic biopsy to obtain histologic diagnosis.[7]

Radiation Therapy

The standard treatment of malignant glioma, specifically GBM, involves conformal radiotherapy (RT) of 60 Gy encompassing the tumor volume and margin. However, historically, whole brain radiotherapy (WBRT) has been used for the treatment of multifocal/multicentric tumors with or without a boost to the tumor. The inclusion of whole brain fields has been recently questioned, given that most failures occur within the original tumor volume and that limited doses can be delivered to the entire brain.[27]

Showalter and colleagues[27] reported outcomes of 50 patients with multifocal or multicentric GBMs who were treated with WBRT (n = 16) or conformal RT (n = 34). The median survival was 8.1 months. The investigators found no difference in the time to progression or overall survival in patients treated with WBRT versus those treated with conformal RT. All patients had local recurrence, and no recurrences were seen distant from the original foci in the absence of significant local progression. Therefore, the investigators concluded that conformal RT is as efficacious as WBRT and that radiation of whole brain fields may not be necessary.[27] A limited field radiation may better optimize cognitive outcomes and functional status, given the evidence of decline in neurocognitive outcomes in patients undergoing WBRT for brain metastases.[28]

The efficacy of stereotactic radiosurgery (SRS) in the treatment of malignant gliomas is not clearly established. Several retrospective reviews suggest a survival benefit when SRS is used after conventional RT for focal residual or recurrent disease. For example, Pouratian and colleagues[29] reported a median survival of 16.2 months in 48 patients with GBM who underwent Gamma Knife radiosurgery and concluded that this suggests an improved survival compared with the median survival of 14.6 months reported by the pivotal randomized controlled trial by Stupp and colleagues.[1] However, the only randomized controlled trial assessing the efficacy of SRS before RT failed to show any benefit.[30] Many investigators, however, continue to believe that SRS has a role in the management of patients after RT for small, residual, inaccessible, or recurrent foci.[29,31]

Chemotherapy

There is currently no clinically proven chemotherapy that specifically targets multifocal or multicentric glioblastoma. In general, the standard treatment of a newly diagnosed glioblastoma consists of fractionated involved-field radiation therapy combined with the oral alkylating agent temozolomide, followed by cycles of adjuvant temozolomide. An international phase III trial demonstrated a median survival of 14.6 months with this regimen.[1] Many patients with glioblastoma are also treated at some point with the anti-angiogenic agent bevacizumab. Bevacizumab, an intravenously administered monoclonal antibody, inhibits the vascular endothelial growth factor (VEGF) and was approved by the Food and Drug Administration, in 2009, for the treatment of recurrent glioblastoma. Although the survival benefit is modest, treatment with bevacizumab is well tolerated and often improves quality of life.

Great effort has gone into identifying subpopulations of patients who may respond better (or worse) to a particular treatment. It is now well established that patients with tumors that possess a methylated O6-methylguanine-DNA methyltransferase (MGMT) promoter are more likely to respond well to chemotherapy with temozolomide than those with tumors that possess an unmethylated MGMT promoter.[32,33] Yet temozolomide is the current first-line chemotherapeutic agent for patients with tumors that possess an unmethylated MGMT promoter. Our therapeutic armamentarium is not currently robust or sophisticated enough to further tailor treatments, and the same holds true for the subset of patients with multifocal/multicentric glioblastoma; they may not do as well as the others, but clearly no better treatment option exists. In addition, with the ability to hit a near-limitless number of targets, chemotherapy holds great promise. Furthermore, we can use our knowledge of pathophysiology to design rational treatment strategies for patients with multifocal/multicentric glioblastoma. Promising areas of research include targeting invasion, targeting glioma stem-like cells, and using immunotherapy.

Targeting invasion

Tumor invasion confounds traditional modes of treatment in multiple ways. Locally directed therapies, such as surgical resection and intracavitary therapies, may not reach the leading invasive edge of the tumor. This inaccessibility is obviously the case with multifocal/multicentric tumors. In addition, the blood-brain barrier is much more likely to be intact along the leading edge of the tumor, which poses a significant challenge for systemically delivered therapies. Only 2% of low–molecular weight drugs (and no high–molecular weight drugs) are able to penetrate an intact blood-brain barrier.[34] Lastly, several lines of evidence suggest that invasiveness and proliferation are inversely correlated. Tumor growth factor β, for example, stimulates invasion but suppresses proliferation.[35] Furthermore, glioma cells selected for their migratory capacity in vitro demonstrate a slower growth rate than their unselected counterparts, and analysis of glioma biopsies has shown decreased proliferation rates in the white

matter and infiltrated cortex compared with solid tumor.[36,37] Most traditional chemotherapy drugs are selectively toxic to cells that divide rapidly. Therefore, in addition to being exposed to less chemotherapy, tumor cells along the invasive edge are also less susceptible to the effects of chemotherapy.

There has also been concern that treatment with antiangiogenic agents may promote tumor invasiveness. In 2001, Kunkel and colleagues[38] showed that when mice implanted with human G55 glioma cells were treated with DC101 (a monoclonal antibody against VEGF receptor 2), the number of satellite tumors increased significantly, even though the overall tumor volumes were reduced. On histopathologic examination, tumor cells were seen migrating long distances along host vessels and in the subarachnoid space. Several retrospective reviews of imaging patterns at recurrence after antiangiogenic therapy seemed to further justify this concern. In a review of 26 patients treated with bevacizumab, Norden and colleagues[39] reported that 4 patients (15%) presented with distant disease at relapse. Similarly, Iwamoto and colleagues[40] found that 6 of 37 patients (16%) treated with bevacizumab had multifocal disease at relapse. Only 46% of the patients in this bevacizumab-treated group developed enhancing local disease at relapse, much lower than the 90% to 95% rate of local recurrence reported in studies performed in the preantiangiogenic era. These studies suggest that multifocal/multicentric disease may become more commonplace now that antiangiogenic therapy is well established. However, subsequent studies have not found an increased risk of remote or multifocal relapse after treatment with bevacizumab.[9,41] Regardless of whether antiangiogenic therapy itself increases the risk of multifocal/multicentric disease, it seems likely that as median survival continues to improve and more patients survive beyond first, second, and third relapses, the incidence of multifocal/multicentric disease will increase.

Invasion requires the coordination of several distinct cellular processes, each of which can potentially be targeted. First, glioma cells must dissociate from the tumor mass and form contacts with the extracellular matrix (ECM). CD44, tenascin-C, neural cell adhesion molecule, cadherins, and integrins play critical roles in this process. In a rat gliosarcoma model, intratumoral injection of an anti-CD44 monoclonal antibody resulted in decreased brain invasion.[42] Tenascin-C is an ECM glycoprotein that is ubiquitously expressed by glioma cells. A radiolabeled monoclonal antibody against tenascin-C has been developed, but the intracavitary injection used to deliver this treatment may fail to reach the leading invasive edge it was designed to target. The cyclic pentapeptide cilengitide is an inhibitor of the integrins $\alpha_v\beta_3$ and $\alpha_v\beta_5$. These integrins are expressed on both endothelial and glioma cells, suggesting that cilengitide may target both angiogenesis and invasion. Having demonstrated activity and safety in several phase I and II trials, cilengitide is currently being evaluated in phase III trials for the treatment of patients with glioblastoma.

After detachment from the tumor mass, the ECM must be degraded and remodeled to allow for cell movement. This process involves matrix metalloproteinases (MMPs), urokinase plasminogen activator and its receptor, cathepsin, and the family of multidomain membrane-associated proteins known as a disintegrin and metalloproteinase. A randomized placebo-controlled phase II trial of the MMP inhibitor marimastat showed negative results, perhaps because of compensatory activity by other enzymes.[43]

Finally, the cellular machinery responsible for cell migration must be activated. For movement to occur, lamellipodia and filopodia interact with the ECM at adhesion complexes. These complexes consist of an integrin core in association with numerous other proteins, including focal adhesion kinase (FAK), which has been shown to be overexpressed in glioma, particularly at the infiltrating edge. In vitro studies demonstrate that inhibiting FAK decreases invasiveness.[44]

The initiation and coordination of cellular processes that lead to invasion result from activation of specific signal transduction pathways. In particular, the receptor tyrosine kinases, epidermal growth factor receptor (EGFR) and c-Met, as well as the nonreceptor tyrosine kinase Src drive glioma invasiveness, although all these pathways have pleiotropic effects beyond triggering invasion. The small molecule EGFR inhibitors erlotinib and gefitinib have been evaluated in multiple clinical trials for glioblastoma, with only modest results. An earlier study suggested that EGFR inhibitors may be more effective for tumors that possess the EGFRvIII mutation and wild-type PTEN, but subsequent studies have not validated this finding.[45] In a small retrospective review, the multikinase inhibitor dasatinib (which inhibits Src, BCR-ABL, c-KIT, ephrin type-A receptor 2, and platelet-derived growth factor β) demonstrated little activity after bevacizumab failure in patients with heavily pretreated GBM.[46] Results of multicenter clinical trials on dasatinib are currently pending. Rilotumumab, a monoclonal antibody against hepatocyte growth factor/scatter factor, the ligand for c-Met, was recently evaluated in a phase II clinical trial for patients with recurrent glioblastoma. Again, little activity was seen.[47] The overall lack of efficacy seen in clinical trials to date may be because of coactivation of multiple signaling pathways. Combination therapy may, therefore, be required.

Targeting glioma stem-like cells

In 2003, Singh and colleagues[48] demonstrated that cancer cells with stem-like properties are present within brain tumors. Unlike the more differentiated cells that comprise the bulk of a tumor, cancer stem cells are capable of continual proliferation and self-renewal. Because these cells are relatively quiescent, they are resistant to radiation therapy and traditional cytotoxic chemotherapy. It has long been thought that these glioma stem-like cells may preferentially reside in specific niches such as the subventricular zone (SVZ) in which nonneoplastic neural stem cells are known to exist. Glantz and colleagues[49] theorize that the inability of locally directed therapies to permanently eradicate tumor may be because of the continued presence of glioma stem-like cells in the SVZ. These cells may possess the ability to migrate out of the SVZ into the surrounding brain tissue far away from the primary tumor using the same scaffolding used in neural development. Lim and colleagues[50] showed that glioblastomas contacting the SVZ and infiltrating cortex are much more likely to have multifocal disease (56%) at diagnosis than tumors found in other locations. Multifocal/multicentric tumors may, therefore, be more enriched with glioma stem-like cells than their solitary counterparts, thus adding to the treatment challenge.

Even as the cancer stem cell hypothesis is being debated and refined, targeting glioma stem-like cells has become an area of active research. Normal stem cells are regulated by signaling pathways that play an important role in development, such as the SHH, Wnt, and Notch signaling pathways. Dysregulation of these pathways can lead to the development of cancer stem cells, and inhibitors of these pathways are currently being evaluated for clinical use. Nitric oxide signaling has recently been shown to play an important role in glioma stem cell proliferation.[51] A multicenter phase II dendritic cell vaccine trial in which the autologous dendritic cells used in the vaccine are primed against antigens that are highly expressed by cancer stem cells is currently underway. Glantz and colleagues[49] suggest that because glioma stem-like cells may reside in the SVZ, cerebrospinal fluid (CSF)-directed therapies may have better efficacy than systemically delivered therapies. Chemotherapeutic agents instilled directly into the CSF only penetrate a few millimeters into the brain parenchyma, so the efficacy of this strategy is unclear. To date, no clinically proven method of eradicating glioma stem-like cells exists.

Immunotherapy

One of the most promising areas of oncology research is immunotherapy, and the immunotherapeutic approach may prove to be a particularly effective strategy against multifocal/multicentric glioblastoma. After all, few, if any, pharmaceutical compounds are able to seek out and destroy foreign pathogens as robustly and specifically as the immune system. Several clinical trials using immune-priming adjuvant therapies (such as polylysine and carboxymethylcellulose, a toll-like receptor 3 ligand) or dendritic cell vaccines have been performed or are underway. To date, no trial results that specifically address efficacy for multicentric/multifocal gliomas have been reported. However, using a rat multifocal glioblastoma model (in which rats were injected with glioma cells in each hemisphere), King and colleagues[52] demonstrated that treatment with adenoviral vectors expressing thymidine kinase and human Flt3L resulted in long-term survival in 50% of the animals. By recruiting macrophages and CD4 cells, the presence of Flt3L helps initiate an immune response that is able to eradicate distant targets. A clinical trial of this therapy is about to commence.

PROGNOSIS

Multifocal and multicentric gliomas have traditionally been thought to have a worse prognosis than solitary tumors. The median survival for these patients has ranged from 2 to 10 months.[3,7,14,27] Salvati and colleagues[7] reported a median survival of 2.8 months for patients who underwent biopsy of their multicentric tumors. These patients had tumors located in inaccessible or eloquent regions. Patients with surgically accessible tumors who underwent surgical resection had a median survival of 9.5 months.[7] Similarly, Hassaneen and colleagues[3] reported a median survival of 9.7 months after aggressive surgical management and concluded that if the enhancing portions of the multifocal/multicentric tumors can be safely resected, outcomes in these patients may be similar to those in patients with solitary disease. Finally, Showalter and colleagues[27] studied 50 patients who underwent RT and multiple therapies for their multifocal malignant gliomas and described a median survival of 8.1 months.

SUMMARY

Multifocal and multicentric tumors magnify many of the challenges one faces when treating patients with malignant gliomas. Issues such as biopsy versus maximal safe resection and optimal choice of anticancer treatments beyond the standard of care are currently under debate and investigation. The subset of patients with multifocal or multicentric gliomas may indeed be more susceptible or resistant to a given therapy compared with those with localized disease. As the knowledge of the disease process increases, the ability to better tailor treatments will also improve.

REFERENCES

1. Stupp R, Mason WP, van den Bent MJ, et al. Radiotherapy plus concomitant and adjuvant temozolomide for glioblastoma. N Engl J Med 2005;352: 987–96.
2. Batzdorf U, Malamud N. The problem of multicentric gliomas. J Neurosurg 1963;20:122–36.
3. Hassaneen W, Levine NB, Suki D, et al. Multiple craniotomies in the management of multifocal and multicentric glioblastoma. Clinical article. J Neurosurg 2011;114:576–84.
4. Hefti M, von Campe G, Schneider C, et al. Multicentric tumor manifestations of high grade gliomas: independent proliferation or hallmark of extensive disease? Cen Eur Neurosurg 2010;71:20–5.
5. Jaskolski D, Zawirski M, Wisniewska G, et al. A case of multicentric glioma of cerebellum and brain. Zentralbl Neurochir 1988;49:124–7.
6. Kato T, Aida T, Abe H, et al. Clinicopathological study of multiple gliomas—report of three cases. Neurol Med Chir (Tokyo) 1990;30:604–9.
7. Salvati M, Caroli E, Orlando ER, et al. Multicentric glioma: our experience in 25 patients and critical review of the literature. Neurosurg Rev 2003;26:275–9.
8. Solomon A, Perret GE, McCormick WF. Multicentric gliomas of the cerebral and cerebellar hemispheres. Case report. J Neurosurg 1969;31:87–93.
9. Chamberlain MC. Radiographic patterns of relapse in glioblastoma. J Neurooncol 2011;101:319–23.
10. Silbergeld DL, Rostomily RC, Alvord EC Jr. The cause of death in patients with glioblastoma is multifactorial: clinical factors and autopsy findings in 117 cases of supratentorial glioblastoma in adults. J Neurooncol 1991;10:179–85.
11. Kyritsis AP, Levin VA, Yung WK, et al. Imaging patterns of multifocal gliomas. Eur J Radiol 1993; 16:163–70.
12. Bradley WL. Case of gliosarcomatous tumors of the brain. Proc Conn Med Soc 1880;2:39–41.
13. Willis RA. Pathology of tumors. London: Butterworths; 1960. p. 811.
14. Ampil F, Burton GV, Gonzalez-Toledo E, et al. Do we need whole brain irradiation in multifocal or multicentric high-grade cerebral gliomas? Review of

cases and the literature. J Neurooncol 2007;85: 353–5.

15. Claes A, Idema AJ, Wesseling P. Diffuse glioma growth: a guerilla war. Acta Neuropathol 2007;114: 443–58.

16. Kyritsis AP, Bondy ML, Xiao M, et al. Germline p53 gene mutations in subsets of glioma patients. J Natl Cancer Inst 1994;86:344–9.

17. Kyritsis AP, Yung WK, Leeds NE, et al. Multifocal cerebral gliomas associated with secondary malignancies. Lancet 1992;339:1229–30.

18. Scherer H. Structural development in gliomas. Am J Cancer 1938;34:333–51.

19. Geer CP, Grossman SA. Interstitial fluid flow along white matter tracts: a potentially important mechanism for the dissemination of primary brain tumors. J Neurooncol 1997;32:193–201.

20. Bassoe P. Multiple ependymal glioma—one tumor of the fourth ventricle, the other of the frontal lobes. Arch Intern Med 1908;2:194–200.

21. Salunke P, Badhe P, Sharma A. Cerebellar glioblastoma multiforme with non-contiguous grade 2 astrocytoma of the temporal lobe in the same individual. Neurol India 2010;58:651–3.

22. Chadduck WM, Roycroft D, Brown MW. Multicentric glioma as a cause of multiple cerebral lesions. Neurosurgery 1983;13:170–5.

23. Mishra HB, Haran RP, Singh JP, et al. Multicentric gliomas: two case reports and a review of the literature. Br J Neurosurg 1990;4:535–9.

24. Wang S, Kim S, Chawla S, et al. Differentiation between glioblastomas and solitary brain metastases using diffusion tensor imaging. Neuroimage 2009;44:653–60.

25. Wang S, Kim S, Chawla S, et al. Differentiation between glioblastomas, solitary brain metastases, and primary cerebral lymphomas using diffusion tensor and dynamic susceptibility contrast-enhanced MR imaging. AJNR Am J Neuroradiol 2011;32:507–14.

26. Marshall LF, Jennett B, Langfitt TW. Needle biopsy for the diagnosis of malignant glioma. JAMA 1974; 228:1417–8.

27. Showalter TN, Andrel J, Andrews DW, et al. Multifocal glioblastoma multiforme: prognostic factors and patterns of progression. Int J Radiat Oncol Biol Phys 2007;69:820–4.

28. Chang EL, Wefel JS, Hess KR, et al. Neurocognition in patients with brain metastases treated with radiosurgery or radiosurgery plus whole-brain irradiation: a randomised controlled trial. Lancet Oncol 2009;10: 1037–44.

29. Pouratian N, Crowley RW, Sherman JH, et al. Gamma Knife radiosurgery after radiation therapy as an adjunctive treatment for glioblastoma. J Neurooncol 2009;94:409–18.

30. Souhami L, Seiferheld W, Brachman D, et al. Randomized comparison of stereotactic radiosurgery followed by conventional radiotherapy with carmustine to conventional radiotherapy with carmustine for patients with glioblastoma multiforme: report of Radiation Therapy Oncology Group 93-05 protocol. Int J Radiat Oncol Biol Phys 2004;60:853–60.

31. Elliott RE, Parker EC, Rush SC, et al. Efficacy of gamma knife radiosurgery for small-volume recurrent malignant gliomas after initial radical resection. World Neurosurg 2011;76:128–40 [discussion: 161–2].

32. Hegi ME, Diserens AC, Gorlia T, et al. MGMT gene silencing and benefit from temozolomide in glioblastoma. N Engl J Med 2005;352:997–1003.

33. Hegi ME, Liu L, Herman JG, et al. Correlation of O6-methylguanine methyltransferase (MGMT) promoter methylation with clinical outcomes in glioblastoma and clinical strategies to modulate MGMT activity. J Clin Oncol 2008;26:4189–99.

34. Pardridge WM. Blood-brain barrier drug targeting: the future of brain drug development. Mol Interv 2003;3:90–105, 151.

35. Merzak A, McCrea S, Koocheckpour S, et al. Control of human glioma cell growth, migration and invasion in vitro by transforming growth factor beta 1. Br J Cancer 1994;70:199–203.

36. McDonough W, Tran N, Giese A, et al. Altered gene expression in human astrocytoma cells selected for migration: I. Thromboxane synthase. J Neuropathol Exp Neurol 1998;57:449–55.

37. Schiffer D, Cavalla P, Dutto A, et al. Cell proliferation and invasion in malignant gliomas. Anticancer Res 1997;17:61–9.

38. Kunkel P, Ulbricht U, Bohlen P, et al. Inhibition of glioma angiogenesis and growth in vivo by systemic treatment with a monoclonal antibody against vascular endothelial growth factor receptor-2. Cancer Res 2001;61:6624–8.

39. Norden AD, Young GS, Setayesh K, et al. Bevacizumab for recurrent malignant gliomas: efficacy, toxicity, and patterns of recurrence. Neurology 2008;70:779–87.

40. Iwamoto FM, Abrey LE, Beal K, et al. Patterns of relapse and prognosis after bevacizumab failure in recurrent glioblastoma. Neurology 2009;73:1200–6.

41. Wick A, Dörner N, Schäfer N, et al. Bevacizumab does not increase the risk of remote relapse in malignant glioma. Ann Neurol 2011;69:586–92.

42. Gunia S, Hussein S, Radu DL, et al. CD44s-targeted treatment with monoclonal antibody blocks intracerebral invasion and growth of 9L gliosarcoma. Clin Exp Metastasis 1999;17:221–30.

43. Levin VA, Phuphanich S, Yung WK, et al. Randomized, double-blind, placebo-controlled trial of marimastat in glioblastoma multiforme patients following surgery and irradiation. J Neurooncol 2006;78:295–302.

44. Liu TJ, LaFortune T, Honda T, et al. Inhibition of both focal adhesion kinase and insulin-like growth factor-I receptor kinase suppresses glioma proliferation in vitro and in vivo. Mol Cancer Ther 2007;6:357–1367.

45. Mellinghoff IK, Wang MY, Vivanco I, et al. Molecular determinants of the response of glioblastomas to EGFR kinase inhibitors. N Engl J Med 2005;353: 2012–24.

46. Lu-Emerson C, Norden AD, Drappatz J, et al. Retrospective study of dasatinib for recurrent glioblastoma after bevacizumab failure. J Neurooncol 2011;104:287–91.

47. Wen PY, Schiff D, Cloughesy TF, et al. A phase II study evaluating the efficacy and safety of AMG 102 (rilotumumab) in patients with recurrent glioblastoma. Neuro Oncol 2011;13:437–46.

48. Singh SK, Clarke ID, Terasaki M, et al. Identification of a cancer stem cell in human brain tumors. Cancer Res 2003;63:5821–8.

49. Glantz M, Kesari S, Recht L, et al. Understanding the origins of gliomas and developing novel therapies: cerebrospinal fluid and subventricular zone interplay. Semin Oncol 2009;36:S17–24.

50. Lim DA, Cha S, Mayo MC, et al. Relationship of glioblastoma multiforme to neural stem cell regions predicts invasive and multifocal tumor phenotype. Neuro Oncol 2007;9:424–9.

51. Eyler CE, Wu Q, Yan K, et al. Glioma stem cell proliferation and tumor growth are promoted by nitric oxide synthase-2. Cell 2011;146:53–66.

52. King GD, Muhammad AK, Curtin JF, et al. Flt3L and TK gene therapy eradicate multifocal glioma in a syngeneic glioblastoma model. Neuro Oncol 2008;10:19–31.

Index

Note: Page numbers of article titles are in **boldface** type.

Printed and bound by CPI Group (UK) Ltd, Croydon, CR0 4YY

03/10/2024

01040356-0006